T0201013

PERSONALITY-DISORDERED PATIENTS

Treatable and Untreatable

PERSONALITY-DISORDERED PATIENTS

Treatable and Untreatable

By

Michael H. Stone, M.D.

Professor of Clinical Psychiatry, Columbia College of
Physicians and Surgeons, New York, New York

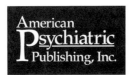

American Psychiatric Publishing, Inc.

Washington, DC
London, England

Note: The author has worked to ensure that all information in this book is accurate at the time of publication and consistent with general psychiatric and medical standards. As medical research and practice continue to advance, however, therapeutic standards may change. Moreover, specific situations may require a specific therapeutic response not included in this book. For these reasons and because human and mechanical errors sometimes occur, we recommend that readers follow the advice of physicians directly involved in their care or the care of a member of their family.

Books published by American Psychiatric Publishing, Inc., represent the views and opinions of the individual authors and do not necessarily represent the policies and opinions of APPI or the American Psychiatric Association.

Copyright © 2006 American Psychiatric Publishing, Inc.
ALL RIGHTS RESERVED

Manufactured in the United States of America on acid-free paper
09   08   07   06   05   5   4   3   2   1
First Edition

Typeset in Adobe's Janson Text and VAGRounded.

American Psychiatric Publishing, Inc.
1000 Wilson Boulevard
Arlington, VA 22209-3901
www.appi.org

Library of Congress Cataloging-in-Publication Data
Stone, Michael H., 1933-

  Personality-disordered patients : treatable and untreatable / by Michael H. Stone.
-- 1st ed.
    p. ; cm.
  Includes bibliographical references and index.
  ISBN 1-58562-172-2 (pbk. : alk. paper)
  1. Personality disorders--Patients--Treatment. 2. Psychotherapy. I. Title.
  [DNLM: 1. Personality Disorders--therapy. 2. Psychotherapy.
 WM 190 S879p 2005]
 RC554.S765 2005
 616.85'81--dc22

                                                            2005022750

British Library Cataloguing in Publication Data
A CIP record is available from the British Library.

CONTENTS

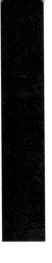

PREFACE

Of the many tasks Dr. Otto Kernberg has addressed throughout his career, one of the most important has been the application of the scientific method to psychoanalysis and to the psychoanalytically oriented therapy of patients with borderline personality disorder. All forms of psychotherapy are mixtures of art and science, but for too long psychoanalytic therapy and the way in which it worked were subjects surrounded with mystery and haze. In recent years, the precision Dr. Kernberg has brought to the analysis of videotaped sessions of transference-focused psychotherapy with borderline patients has lifted much of the haze and removed much of the mystery. He and his colleagues at the Personality Disorder Institute have developed a manual for carrying out this form of therapy, and this accomplishment has contributed to the refinement of technique in treating patients with borderline and other severe disorders of personality. Dr. Kernberg's influence, when we first met, spurred my own interest in personality disorders, and borderline personality most especially, to which I have now devoted half my life.

This book deals with the whole range of personality disorders, from the mildest and most successfully treated to those of the greatest malignancy, where successful treatment is only a wish, not a realizable venture. The emphasis in this book is not on the "how-to" aspects of treatment but on the amenability of the various disorders to amelioration by any method of therapy whatsoever. With which kinds of patients is therapy likely to succeed? With which is failure almost a certainty?

Success with the treatment of personality disorders is at best a long and painstaking process that effects only modest changes. Symptoms can often be alleviated dramatically; personality is, as it should be, highly resistant to change. Personality is the skin that separates us from the outside world.

Psychotherapists do not aim to make radical changes in a patient's personality, but rather to smooth down the rough edges with fine sandpaper—to make the abrasive person more polite, the impulsive person more restrained, and so on.

In my clinical work I have come to realize that a large number of factors help determine, within the broad domain of personality disorders, which patients are likely to respond well to psychotherapeutic interventions and which will prove most resistive. These factors, and relevant clinical examples, are discussed in the early chapters. Because the main instrument therapists use in this work is their own personality, inevitably there is much subjectivity in how therapists go about their work and in the range of patients with whom they have the best results. This is the "art" with which the science of psychotherapy is necessarily mixed. Illustrations of this phenomenon are offered in the middle sections of the book. The final chapters are taken up with the most severe aberrations of personality and with the limitations these conditions impose on therapists' efficacy. Some may take this discussion as a counsel of despair, but realism and honesty should compel us to acknowledge these limitations. To this end, I offer in the last chapter some rather extreme examples that I hope make this point clear.

My gratitude goes also to Dr. Glen O. Gabbard, who reviewed the manuscript as it was unfolding and gave me many helpful recommendations and suggestions for improving its substance. No less important, the serenity and calmness of my wife Beth's personality created an optimal atmosphere for carrying out the lengthy task of authorship.

AMENABILITY TO TREATMENT IN THE REALM OF PERSONALITY DISORDER

For the past quarter century, the *Diagnostic and Statistical Manual of Mental Disorders* (of which the latest version is the text revision of the fourth edition, DSM-IV-TR [American Psychiatric Association 2000]), has apportioned the various entities into two broad divisions: one devoted to symptom disorders (Axis I) and the other to disorders of personality (Axis II). Some voices have been raised in criticism of this division as too arbitrary and inelastic. Persons with the symptom of agoraphobia, for example, often manifest avoidant personality. Provided they confine themselves to the safety of home, only the latter is apparent. If they are forced to venture outside, the related symptom disorder quickly reaches the level at which it is clinically recognizable. Still, the bipartite division has one special virtue, especially for our purposes. Symptoms are defined as uncomfortable conditions for which the term *ego-dystonic* is customarily used. It is unpleasant and disadvantageous to be depressed, schizophrenic, bulimic; to be unable to touch a doorknob for fear of germs; or to be "phobic" about entering an elevator. Personality disorders, in contrast, are constellations of personality traits. Unlike symptoms, personality traits are almost invariably *ego-syntonic*, which implies that the person who possesses the traits is comfortable about them. Epidemiological study suggests that perhaps one-sixth of the population has a symptom disorder (Regier and Robbins 1991). Perhaps as many also meet the criteria for one of the personality disorders described in the categories of Axis II. But *everyone* has a personality of some sort, and the dividing line between pathology and averageness or normality is not always easy to draw.

Personality is fundamentally an aggregate of the ways in which we habitually, predictably, and enduringly relate to other people. These "ways," taken one by one, are the individual *traits* of personality. If one thinks of the Kantian division of *mind* into three main partitions—*thought, feeling,* and *behavior*—traits can generally be assigned to one of these divisions. Traits such as solicitousness, pedantry, open-mindedness, and bigotry, for example, belong to the sphere of thought. In the sphere of feeling we can place traits such as calmness, moodiness, mercuriality, and irascibility. In the sphere of behavioral traits are generosity, miserliness, impulsivity, abrasiveness, tactfulness, and contemptuousness. Our vocabulary is richer in negative than in positive traits (Stone 1993), probably because of the high survival value (in evolutionary terms) of noticing qualities in other people that may threaten us physically or psychologically. Thus, there are more than a dozen shades and gradations of *dishonesty*, whereas honesty needs few qualifiers.

People show different arrays of traits on different occasions, depending on the persons with whom they are momentarily interacting, the task at hand, or the social setting, but once we know a person well, we are usually able to describe how that person is "in general" with a few apt trait adjectives. If, for example, we are describing someone whose demeanor differs markedly depending on the social status of the others he or she is interacting with, we have little trouble finding pairs of trait words for such "bifurcated" personalities. A co-worker, for example, may be "ingratiating toward the higher-ups but abrupt and mean-spirited with his subordinates." An attorney may be loyal to her staff, charming to her clients, but a "tigress" in the courtroom. Variations of this sort tend to be more marked in those with definable personality disorders.

Because of this tendency, therapists cannot always rely on the impressions their patients make on them, because they see only "one side" of a patient's personality. The "disorder" of the personality disorder may indeed manifest itself primarily with the patient's spouse, parents, children, boss, or neighbors, and without access to the key outside parties—the so-called *collaterals*—the therapist may remain blind to where the trouble is and to how intense it is. Alcohol and other psychoactive substances can radically alter the outward expression of personality (usually in most unfavorable ways), and the personality of some persons may be genuinely calm, pleasant, and well controlled *except* when they are abusing a substance. A personality disorder is present, but it is apparent only to those who see or interact with the person when he or she is under the influence of the drug. The extreme example of this phenomenon is encountered in certain serial killers whose personalities have a Jekyll-and-Hyde quality, with the negative aspects emerging under the influence of alcohol (Stone 1998).

The distinction between trait and behavior is not absolute. Certain behaviorally oriented traits, such as impulsivity, exist along a spectrum. At some point on the spectrum the trait passes over into abnormal, pathological behavior and becomes a *symptom*. The trait adjective ceases to be a descriptor of everyday personality and morphs into the language of Axis I. Some persons, for example, are characteristically vehement or hostile, perhaps even mildly combative, but if they become repetitively assaultive, such violence is better regarded as symptomatic behavior—with profound legal implications. If asked to describe the personality of such a person, we do not ordinarily say, "Oh, he's assaultive." We might say, "He's very hostile and aggressive...always has been" (i.e., in personality). "And lately, he's been arrested four times for assault" (i.e., there have been eruptions of highly pathological behavior). Some trait words wear a double cloak—sometimes pertaining to personality, at other times to symptomatic behavior. But unless otherwise specified, I use the word *trait* here to signify a perdurable characteristic of an individual—a *personality* feature.

With about 600 trait adjectives in the English language, we can give a full characterization of almost all persons. Five hundred of these terms describe negative or maladaptive traits; the remainder, positive traits (Stone 1993, pp. 104–108). We encounter very few people who show not even one trait that is mildly irritating, socially disadvantageous, alienating, or obnoxious, even though their "negative" traits may be so few and so mild as to fall far short of constituting an Axis II disorder. Cultural factors enter into the equation. Some persons may be experienced as quite acceptable and ordinary within their own culture, only to be found timid or aggressive or overly fussy when transplanted into a different culture whose norms do not mesh with those of the original culture. Examples will be given later in this chapter in the "Cultural Factors" section.

With respect to the ego-syntonic nature of most personality traits, there are two special points to be made, both relevant to the issue of amenability to treatment. *First*, there are a small number of traits that people are generally willing both to acknowledge and to complain about. Traits, in other words, can sometimes be ego-dystonic. Mostly, these traits center on shyness and unassertiveness. Occasionally one also hears a person complain of being a "neatnik"—that is, overly meticulous about where each dish, desk object, article of clothing, and so on must be placed. Others admit that they can't seem to throw anything away. The neatnik exemplifies one of Freud's "triad" of traits characteristic of the obsessive person: orderliness, obstinacy, and parsimony (Freud 1908/1953). Hoarding may cease being a *trait* and may shade into one of the *symptoms* of obsessive-compulsive disorder, as in the case of a patient who slept on the floor because his bed and sofa were filled many feet high with newspaper clippings and magazine articles going back decades. He knew there was something wrong with that pattern, and he wished to conquer this habit. In therapeutic work with personality-disordered patients, it is reasonable to assume that a treatment alliance can be formed more easily with patients who already wish to give up certain traits than with patients who persistently disclaim having any traits that need modification.

Second, not all the descriptors of the personality disorders listed in DSM are *traits* in the dictionary sense of that term. This is especially true of borderline personality disorder (BPD). Among the descriptors (or "items") of BPD are symptomatic behaviors, such as self-destructive acts; peculiarities of mind, such as identity disturbance; and maladaptive interpersonal patterns, such as stormy interpersonal relationships. Antisocial personality disorder is also defined by means of a mixture of traits and behaviors. The presence of symptoms among the descriptive features of a personality disorder affects amenability to treatment of that disorder, rendering some aspects of the disorder easier to resolve and other aspects more difficult. True personality traits, such as stinginess, haughtiness, or clinginess, are seldom modifiable by medication. But in some patients the mood lability of BPD may stem from bipolar II disorder and may be correctable through the use of mood stabilizers. As for the combativeness of an antisocial person, what matters is not so much the tendency for aggressive behavior but rather the true personality traits that lurk behind the scenes. Where there is self-centeredness and dismissiveness, treatability will be adversely affected. If remorse is present, amenability to treatment may be much better.

With these remarks as prelude, we can begin to examine in greater detail the qualities that conduce to, or enhance, amenability to treatment. Here "treatment" refers specifically to *verbal psychotherapy* in whatever forms may be appropriate. Psychotherapy, as opposed to pharmacotherapy, is the cornerstone of treatment for personality disorders—to the extent that we focus on the traits peculiar to each disorder. Medications have their role in treatment when symptoms accompany the disorder in question. This is true primarily in the case of BPD, inasmuch as borderline patients almost without exception exhibit symptoms of one sort or another. It is for this reason that the practice guideline for the treatment of BPD published by the American Psychiatric Association (2001) contains a section devoted to the suggested pharmacotherapeutic agents for the symptoms routinely noted in BPD, including anxiety, mood fluctuations, and cognitive disturbances. The indications for the use of medications (anxiolytics, mood stabilizers, antidepressants, neuroleptics) relate to whichever symptom(s) are present in each particular patient. Amenability to psychotherapy relates to personality characteristics embedded deeply within the psyche of the patient.

For didactic purposes it is useful to discuss the various amenability factors separately, although several of these factors are interrelated and conceptually overlapping.

ABILITY TO THINK ABOUT ONESELF AND OTHERS AND TO IDENTIFY FEELINGS

Several terms in psychiatry relate to people's ability to think about themselves and others on the psychological plane. Another set of terms refers to the benefits of having this ability if it has developed optimally and to the adverse consequences of an impaired ability for this kind of abstraction.

Some of the terms concern largely conscious processes. *Introspection*, for example, is the ability to stand apart from the immediacy of one's emotional state, even while one is experiencing a strong emotion. Introspection implies the ability to think about what one is feeling and to give the appropriate names for the emotions, then to speculate about the factors to which the emotion of the moment was a response. In the psychotherapeutic setting, introspection ideally involves identifying the circumstances from the recent past that contributed to a new emotional state and at the same time making good guesses, based on awareness of one's early history, to identify the influences from one's past that might have been brought to bear on the current emotional reaction.

The Latinate term *introspection* translates quite simply as *looking into oneself*. The most well-integrated patients, including those with personality disorders, are capable of simultaneously experiencing an emotion and thinking about it, pondering the probable reasons for its emergence. These individuals can be subjective and objective at the same time. In contrast, patients with poorly integrated mental functioning—such as those with BPD—do not easily show this kind of simultaneity. They tend to be either engulfed in a strong emotion—so much so that they are unable to think about how the emotion came about—or detached from emotion. In the latter situation, they may talk during their sessions in an expressionless manner about events or experiences that ordinarily would have elicited a strong emotion. As Judd and McGlashan (2003) explained, "When not emotionally involved in a situation, most BPD patients can employ empathy.... Once they are threatened or in an intense state of need, their analytic abilities disappear and they become highly self-centered, concrete, and context-bound" (p. 186). Besides introspection, there is also *introspectiveness*, a character trait corresponding to the habit of actively thinking about the possible connections between feeling states—one's own or those of other key persons in one's life—and the factors that may underlie these states.

In contrast to the conscious process of introspection, *empathy* refers to an essentially unconscious process by which one grasps intuitively—that is, with an immediacy that does not require conscious thought and deliberation—the emotional state of another person. Empathy is an outward-directed capacity, and in contemporary parlance it also includes the quality of compassion. To grasp the feeling state of another, yet without the accompanying compassion, is called simply "mind-reading" (Baron-Cohen 2003). It is possible, for example, to mind-read another's feelings accurately without necessarily caring much about the welfare of that person. Empathy, in the fuller sense, allows us to figure out that a child crying in a crowded place has probably been separated from its mother; the compassionate component directs us to soothe the child and to help it find its mother.

Peter Fonagy, who with colleagues developed an elegant schema for understanding the development of borderline states (Fonagy 2001; Fonagy and Higgitt 1989), employed the term *mentalization*, referring to a "specific symbolic function"—the reflective function—that "enables children to conceive of others' beliefs, feelings, attitudes, desires, hopes, knowledge, imagination, pretense, plans, and so on" (Fonagy 2001, p. 165). In a normal nurturing environment, mentalization can be discerned in children beginning around age 4 years, but it "is gradually acquired over the first few years of life" (Bateman and Fonagy 2004, p. 36). A burgeoning sense of self and other is noticeable in children of that age. They are beginning to attach names to their feeling states and to realize that their parents and siblings and other people think and feel in ways similar to the way they as children think and feel. Whereas empathy is unidirectional—referring to one's understanding of another's mental states—mentalization is bidirectional, because it embraces one's understanding of the mental states of self and other.

As Bateman and Fonagy emphasized, mentalization develops optimally in the context of a secure child-parent (or child-caregiver) relationship that permits the child to make sense of the subjective states of self and other.

This faculty fails to develop properly or is seriously deranged where child-parent relationships have been from the beginning habitually strained, hindering the development of secure attachment. Instead, pathological forms of attachment occur, and such forms are characteristic of persons who later develop borderline personality. Probably it would be more accurate to say that persons who show serious flaws in their capacity to mentalize are labeled as "borderline" rather than to say that borderline persons show faulty mentalization. Clinicians, for example, notice the faulty mentalization during an interview with a prospective patient and then decide that "borderline" is the proper name for the condition. In addition, there may be a subgroup of persons who initially receive a diagnosis of "borderline" (once they are brought to the attention of clinicians) because they speak of repeated acts of self-mutilation and suicidal behaviors. Subsequently, the clinician notices the impairment in their mentalizing capacity.

Psychological mindedness and mentalizing, identified by whatever terms one prefers, taken together, become the oil for the engine of psychotherapy. This is not to say that psychotherapy cannot "run" in their absence; rather, it will run more smoothly, more efficiently, and with a better chance that its goals will be realized if patients have a reasonable degree of these qualities. In the case of BPD, as Fonagy pointed out, early insecurity, childhood traumata, and a high innate tendency to emotional arousal can impede the development of mentalization. Yet this capacity can be enhanced during the course of a sensitively conducted psychotherapy, such that the borderline patient may emerge later on with a more secure form of attachment and a better ability to mentalize (Bateman and Fonagy 2004). This enhancement will include an improved ability to recall and to reflect on traumatic experiences that may have been inaccessible to consciousness for many years. In the chapters that follow I discuss the typical levels of psychological mindedness and capacity for mentalizing found in each major category of personality disorder, as well as how these levels affect both the patient's amenability to major psychotherapeutic approaches and the patient's prognosis.

Another mental faculty that deserves consideration is *intelligence*. High intelligence is certainly not a prerequisite to the development of adequate psychological mindedness. Many persons and, by extension, many patients whose general intelligence is no less than brilliant have a meager capacity for self-reflection. Sometimes this situation comes about chiefly through an innate predisposition to a kind of *affect-blindness*. (I prefer this term to the clumsy half-Latin/half-Greek *alexithymia*, whose meaning is by no means clear on the surface). Persons with a predisposition to affect-blindness seem to be strangers to the world of emotion, are scarcely able to identify their own feeling states (apart, perhaps, from profound rage), and are similarly at a loss, through their lack of empathy, in picking up the nuances of feeling in even the people within their intimate circle. In other instances, this state comes about as a result of repetitive traumatic experiences early in life that cripple the machinery of mentalization, as Fonagy has described.

Apart from these otherwise normally intelligent but emotionally handicapped persons, there are others whose psychological mindedness is compromised because their general intelligence falls well below average. Persons with very low intelligence often have difficulty making the kinds of rapid connections and assessments necessary to the identification of emotional states in themselves and in others. They often show impaired access to memories of past events that may be related to their current problems in relating to others, and they are less quick to grasp the impact of their behavior on the feelings and reactions of others. Because one of the aims of psychotherapy is expansion of awareness of what affects one's reactions and of how one's attitudes and behavior affect the reactions of others, low intelligence hinders amenability to therapy.

Another important factor that may contribute to affect-blindness is head injury that results in damage to the frontal lobe centers that mediate emotional comprehension and social decision-making. Such injury may occur as a result of trauma, disease, or extreme fever. Clinicians in private practice and those who work in the ordinary psychiatric settings of clinic or hospital may never encounter personality-disordered patients in whom head injury has played a major role. But as many as one-half or more of the patients in forensic hospitals have experienced severe head injury—through accidents or severe maltreatment by caretakers—of the sort that ushers in a marked alteration of personality. The famous story of the nineteenth-century railroad worker Phineas Gage, as recounted by Damasio (1994), is illustrative of this phenomenon. Gage was an earnest, honorable, and well-regarded worker before a blasting accident in which an iron bar passed through his head. Although he survived, he underwent a drastic change in personality, becoming rude, irritable, and self-centered. Damasio determined that the iron bar had severely damaged the ventromedial (orbital) prefrontal region of the frontal lobe (the region that appears to subserve social decision-making), impairing Gage's ability to relate empathically and compassionately to others. Presumably, his capacity for introspection was grossly impaired as well.

CHARACTER

It is customary to divide the broad topic of personality into two components: *temperament* and *character* (Cloninger et al. 1999). Temperament refers to innate factors, either genetic or constitutional (i.e., influenced by variables of fetal development), that influence the emerging personality. Character refers to the facets of personality that are shaped primarily by postnatal influences, which consist chiefly of the interactional patterns between caretakers and the child but which also include other environmental (including cultural) factors. These distinctions are of course not so neat in life as they are on paper. Certain peculiarities of temperament may exert strong effects on the development of character, such that the two streams of influence merge and blend. Imagine someone born with what Kraepelin (1921) called the irritable temperament, one of the four temperaments associated with manic-depression. A child with this innate predisposition may be quite difficult for the parents to handle, becoming angry or tending to have a tantrum in reaction to minor stresses that most children take in stride. The child may end up being reprimanded, at times harshly, much more than the other siblings. He may then experience the world as a hostile place, develop sharply polarized views of people, and become self-centered, alienated, and vengeful—all in relation to the negative interactions he has provoked because of his irritability. For this child, an abnormal temperament prejudices or skews the environmental influences, creating an abnormality of character that would not have come about had the child's temperament been calmer, the child more tractable, and the parents more easygoing.

The family of the murderer Gary Gilmore, the subject of a lengthy biography by Norman Mailer (1979), provides a telling example. Gary was one of four brothers born in a family where the father was a brutally punitive, irascible alcoholic. All the sons, as recounted in the moving essay by one of the brothers, Mikal Gilmore (1991), were beaten repeatedly by their father for the most minor offenses or for no offense at all. Gary was the rebellious one, the one with the irritable temperament from the day he was born. Whereas for most children, punishment fosters obedience in reaction to the anxiety engendered by the fear of further punishment, Gary proved immune to this socializing mechanism. The harder his father beat him, the more hostile and defiant Gary became. The three brothers with calmer temperaments grew up as law-abiding, sociable citizens. Gary grew up to be abusive, assaultive, violent, tyrannical, morbidly jealous, and criminal.

In everyday parlance the word *character* denotes the set of values and standards by which a person lives and that become embodied in the person's actions toward others habitually and predictably throughout the entire life course. Thus, someone may speak of another by saying, "She has a sterling character," or of some other person (such as the ill-fated Gary Gilmore) by saying, "He has a rotten character." In this nontechnical usage of *character* we are no longer making fine distinctions between genetic and environmental influences; we are referring to the final amalgam of these influences as they give form to the individual's moral structure (or lack of it). This nuance of the word *character* is the one that Freud had in mind when he wrote his comments about amenability to psychoanalytic treatment 100 years ago: "One should look beyond the patient's illness and form an estimate of his whole personality; those patients who do not possess a reasonable degree of education and a fairly reliable character should be refused" (Freud 1904/1953, p. 263).

Good character is an important factor—one may say a *vital* factor—in amenability to psychotherapy of any sort, not just psychoanalytic psychotherapy. The assessment of character becomes an indispensable exercise in the initial encounter with a patient seeking psychotherapeutic help. Where, along the spectrum of character, does the patient fit? At one extreme are persons of incorruptible character, such as that of the "whistle-blowers" who are willing to sacrifice job and status in order to uphold a social virtue or to stand up for what is morally right, albeit socially inconvenient. This kind of character led Roger Boisjoly, an aerospace engineer working in the company that made parts for the Challenger space shuttle, to put his complaint in writing—at the cost of his job—that the O-rings, when chilled, would not provide sufficient safeguard for the astronauts. This kind of character was also reflected in the actions of Cynthia Cooper, Coleen Rowley, and Sherron Watkins, who were named *TIME* magazine's "Persons of the Year" in 2002 for their fearless confrontation of financial misdeeds and other serious oversights in the large organizations where they were employed.

A personality trait applicable to persons of this sort is *integrity*. Integrity in this context signifies a special combination of honesty and courage—specifically, the courage to stand up for one's convictions, regardless of the consequences. Because of the element of courage, this quality goes well beyond the honesty—commendable as it is—involved in returning someone's wallet found in the street or in a taxi. Integrity writ large was reflected in the actions of Count Claus von Stauffenberg, who led the plot to assassinate Hitler in July 1944 and was later executed (Petrova and Watson 1995). Similarly, Niklas Frank, the younger son of Hans Frank, Hitler's appointed governor general of occupied Poland, wrote a stinging denunciation of his father (who was hanged after the Nuremberg trials in 1946), emerging as the only child of a high-ranking Nazi to transcend family loyalty to adhere to a higher morality (Frank 1991; Posner 1991). We are fortunate that many people in ordinary life show admirable levels of integrity—for example, parents who do not automatically come to the defense of a child who has gotten into trouble at school (for cheating on homework or hurting another child) but who take the time to listen to the teacher or the family of an injured party and take corrective measures if their own child was truly at fault.

Persons with the kind of good character that facilitates psychotherapy need not display the courage of a whistle-blower or a von Stauffenberg. It suffices if the person is honest, reliable, and thoughtful of others. In the setting of psychotherapy, good character may be displayed in such acts as coming on time to the sessions, notifying the therapist in advance of an appointment that will be missed or of a late arrival, discussing vacation plans well in advance, taking care of the bill in a responsible manner, and so forth.

At the other extreme, *bad* character asserts itself through an opposite set of attributes, including dishonesty, unreliability, and contemptuousness. These traits are included in the criteria for both *antisocial* and *narcissistic* personality disorders as outlined in DSM-IV-TR. These disorders overlap conceptually, insofar as both are characterized by an overarching quality of self-centeredness. Both disorders happen also to have been placed in the dramatic cluster—Cluster B—in DSM Axis II, along with BPD and histrionic personality disorder. The criteria for narcissistic personality disorder, however, may be met by some persons who, although they are remarkably self-centered, are quietly so and are not in the least "dramatic" in their behavior. By the same token, many narcissistic patients are haughty, scornful, and egotistical, but in no way novelty-seeking, extraverted, or dramatic in their self-presentation. Some successful businessmen who occupy high-level corporate positions are of this type. If they seek therapy, they prove to be challenging patients, not because of any antisocial traits but because of their dismissiveness, which creates a roadblock in the development of a therapeutic alliance.

Before discussing some other aspects of character that affect amenability to treatment, an explanation of a third usage of the term *character* is needed. Freud and the pioneering generation of psychoanalysts spoke of various kinds of character—for example, depressive, phobic, compulsive, narcissistic, and hysteric character—that are now considered varieties of personality. Wilhelm Reich (1949) used the phrase *"aristocratic character"* (p. 180), instead of the current *narcissistic personality*, and *"passive-feminine character"* for the current *dependent personality*. The word *personality* was rarely used by Freud or by the first generation of psychoanalysts, and it has come into common use only in the past 50 years.

Still other ingredients of character besides integrity and honesty affect amenability to treatment. Another is the *ability to take criticism*, which in turn implies a measure of humility. In dealing with patients with personality disorders, therapists frequently find themselves at pains to point out something negative about the patient's habitual way of thinking, feeling, or behaving in various key situations. Psychotherapy in the realm of personality disorders is all about overturning old habits and gradually replacing them with better ones. Some of the old habits may be maladaptive, self-defeating, hurtful to others, or rude, and it falls to the therapist eventually to mention these habits. This discussion is often experienced by the patient as an attack (however gently mounted) against an aspect of his or her personality that is ego-syntonic and therefore off-limits to criticism.

Fortunately, not all personality-disordered patients are equally touchy about the therapist's entry into these sensitive areas. Patients with anxious cluster (Cluster C) disorders are generally better at taking criticism than are those with Cluster A and Cluster B disorders, but even that generalization is too broad. Some patients with obsessive-compulsive personality disorder are rigid and easily offended, whereas many with histrionic personality disorder or with *hysteric character* (the original and milder form of that disorder that is described in the psychoanalytic literature) (Kernberg 1984, p. 80) respond with less defensiveness to a therapist's confrontations about troublesome habits.

Patients with pronounced narcissistic traits, as well as those with antisocial traits, however, often take umbrage at the mildest of suggestions or confrontations about the negative facets of their personalities. This tendency is doubled for those with paranoid personality disorder. Even here, one must distinguish between patients whose predominant traits belong to other disorders (especially of the anxious cluster) but who manifest a few paranoid traits and those whose personalities are predominantly and grossly paranoid, who have minimal ability to take criticism.

A few clinical examples may make these distinctions clearer:

> **A man in his 40s** had worked for a number of years in the research section of a large corporation in New Jersey. He had emigrated to the United States from an Eastern Bloc country where his family had endured considerable persecution for their religious and political views. His culture and life experiences were much different from those of his co-workers and the company executives, leaving him with the feeling that he didn't fit in and was not well liked. He saw himself as the victim of prejudice—an impression that seemed all the more convincing to him when a less qualified man was given a promotion that he felt he deserved. Yet in other areas of his life, paranoid traits were not apparent. He and his wife had a circle of friends and relatives with whom relations were harmonious. Therapy went smoothly, and there was no paranoid tinge in the transference relationship. It is always difficult to get a good grasp of a patient's workplace complaints, because patients sel-

dom permit a therapist to contact a boss or co-workers, lest the inquiry compromise the patient's employment. I was never able to assess the validity of my patient's complaint related to his workplace. Eventually the troublesome situation was circumvented when he decided to go into business on his own. He was now his own boss, and he was in control of his own fate. The new venture became quite successful. The stimuli that had set in motion his paranoid reactions at the old company were no longer in the picture, and the paranoid trend was no longer active.

A 26-year-old man sought help because of depression and panic attacks. These symptoms had been sparked by an incident while he was in graduate school. A male professor had invited him home and had then proceeded to make a sexual pass at him. The patient's sexual orientation was homosexual, but he experienced great shame over his orientation, due in great part to his having been molested in adolescence by two male relatives. Initially he was suspicious toward me, albeit for a different set of reasons. He was convinced I was "stronger" than he was and was simply biding my time until I decided to "beat him up." He was also convinced that I was contemptuous of his having come from a "poor" background and that I would rather "treat a Rockefeller for nothing" than treat him for my usual fee.

The first of these distortions was the more glaring, as he was athletically built and I was twice his age. In reality, he was the only patient in my 40 years of private practice who made me fearful for my physical safety. It was only when I told him of my apprehension that he grew calmer and more comfortable with me. The second distortion took longer to resolve. Unbeknownst to my patient, I had great admiration for him because of his immersion in the study of foreign languages, a pursuit that corresponded to my lifelong avocation. He eventually began to see me as an ally—his only ally in a dangerous and menacing world.

An example of his continued paranoid thinking about strangers came some months later, in connection with a subway ride. It chanced that a young woman was sitting next to him while he was reading the newspaper, studiously avoiding any contact with others. The woman asked him, "Sir, could I possibly borrow that section of the paper when you've finished with it?" He glared at her, so he told me, and then continued to immerse himself in the paper. She got off the train at the next stop, muttering some unkind remark at him under her breath. He heard it as "faggot." Because a day barely went by without his imagining someone calling him by that name, my view was that what he thought he heard was more a projection of his own self-condemnation than an accurate perception. I tried to deal with his paranoid reaction in this manner: "Don't you think it possible that if you were not so uncomfortable with even harmless-seeming strangers like that girl, you might have said something to her that would have preserved your distance, yet not offended her? Suppose you'd said something diplomatic just to put her down gently, like 'Excuse me, ma'am, but I really need both parts of the paper for a meeting I'm going to, so I'm afraid I can't share it with you; I hope you'll understand.'" To which he replied: "The bitch didn't deserve it!" I couldn't get him to understand that he had "converted" her into a bitch by his needlessly hostile response to her. This pattern was characteristic of his reactions during the 3 years I worked with him. In that period he made significant improvements in his work life. From being unemployed, he returned to graduate school and received promotions in his job at a library. But he remained a loner, and his paranoid personality was unresponsive to anything I could suggest to him about the innocuousness of ordinary people. His ability to take criticism remained as feeble as it had been at the outset.

Still another quality relating to character is *likeability*. Likeability differs from the other qualities because it is not a character trait, per se, but rather is a derivative of several traits—a *conglomerate* trait. It also differs from other qualities in that it reflects directly the attitude of other persons. Unlike impulsivity, greediness, moodiness, calmness, or curiosity (all of which register on a neutral observer), likeability implies subjectivity—the reaction of the observer to the person in question. In the context of psychotherapy, the observer is the therapist.

There is probably a close correlation between likeability and the concept of affability or friendliness and thus between likeability and one of the main elements in the *Five-Factor Model* of personality—*agreeableness* (Trull and McCrae 2002; Wiggins and Pincus 2002). And yet likeability and agreeableness are not the same. Therapists do better work and have better success with patients they like than with those they dislike or cannot bring themselves to like during the initial phases of treatment. Thus likeability is a highly important factor in amenability to treatment. But likeability in the therapist-patient setting is not the same as in the person-to-person settings of everyday life, because a therapist may like and like working with patients who have many facets of personality that the therapist does not admire or that rub the therapist the wrong way. Certain qualities related to character traits—for example, perseverance and motivation—and even external qualities such as attractiveness, social class, and cultural factors weigh in the balance. Similarity of interests between patient and therapist, as in the case of the language student discussed earlier, may contribute to the therapist's liking a patient who in other respects is, at the outset at least, hostile, dismissive, unappreciative, or otherwise difficult to connect with. Therapists may like patients whom they find intriguing or whose courage or colorful way of speaking they admire, but whom they would never warm up to at all, were they to meet socially. Paradoxically, a therapist may find some patients immensely likeable because of their charm but rather quickly may come to regard them as scarcely amenable to treatment of any kind. These patients are the "con artists" and psychopaths whose particularities are discussed later (Chapter 9, "Untreatable Personality Disorders").

Suffice it to say at this point that amenability to treatment does not rest on likeability alone, as much as on a combination of likeability, good character, psychological mindedness, and another Five-Factor Model superordinate trait, *openness*. Openness refers to a constellation of traits having to do with the willingness to consider alternative ideas (that is, openness to other persons) and the willingness to expose aspects of one's own life history, including embarrassing aspects, to another person (that is, openness about oneself). Openness facilitates the dialogue between therapist and patient, wherein the "noble rhetoric" (a term suggested by Spillane [1987]) of the therapist ultimately effects salutary changes in the patient's personality. The therapist's rhetoric includes a number of techniques, including the *mutative interpretations* of which psychoanalysts Strachey (1937) and Valenstein (1962) wrote, but also the various skeins of supportive therapy—exhortations, suggestions, validating remarks, and sympathetic comments—whose interweaving fosters the desired shifts in and maturation of the patient's personality.

Another highly subjective feature of likeability becomes noticeable in therapists who work in institutional settings. When patients are assigned on rotation to the members of a treatment team, it often turns out that each therapist thinks his or her own patients are the nicest to work with, are the ones with the best prognosis, and so forth, and is glad not to have been "stuck" with some of the patients assigned to colleagues. This phenomenon is akin to the reaction of parents to their newborn babies, who are regularly experienced as "beautiful" by the parents yet (exceptions aside) as ordinary-looking by outsiders. In the therapeutic setting, this phenomenon obviously works to the benefit of the patients, because their therapists feel inspired to do their best work on behalf of their own patients. In working with personality-disordered patients, this irrational parental love becomes the fuel that keeps therapists going during phases of the work when the patient seems recalcitrant, unreachable, or hopeless.

The following example concerns a patient who seemed not likeable at first, but whom I found myself liking anyway:

> **The patient was a young surgeon** about to finish his residency training. His treatment consisted of twice-weekly psychoanalytically oriented psychotherapy. He showed prominent narcissistic traits, including a sense of specialness, a preoccupation with fame and power, and a tendency to criticize and humiliate others. This tendency showed itself in the transference early on, when he would draw attention with considerable scorn to all manner of things about my person: my suit jacket had only three buttons instead of four, which to him meant it was cheap goods; my ears stuck out too far; I wore the same tie day in and day out; and so forth.

The only child of divorced parents, he had endured endless and withering criticism from his mother. His father rarely saw him and made it plain he could not wait for their visits to be over. Underneath the patient's scorn was envy of me spurred by the fact that I wrote books and had become a professor, something he aspired to do. He had drive and ambition and was already a champion tennis player. I respected him for these qualities and felt he could realize his ambitions, so long as he didn't assume, as he tended to do, that a top job would somehow fall into his lap from the heavens, just because he "deserved it" and had had a hard life. I told him after some months of treatment that we could keep the analysis going forever, but his envy would remain untouched unless he channeled his ambition into perfecting some surgical procedure or developing a new procedure and got onto the lecture circuit to tell of his results. If he did so, he would become a "top surgeon" and there would be little left for him to envy. He did exactly that: he developed a complicated procedure for surgery of the head and neck to deal with laryngeal cancer, wrote 10 papers about the procedure, and lectured about it throughout the United States. By the time our treatment was finished, he had become the "number two" man in a surgical department. His envy and bitterness had melted away, and he was able to express gratitude for the help I had offered him. I had felt all along that there was a person of fine character hiding underneath his unpleasant traits. The analysis served as a kind of surgical debridement—as he would have spoken of it—of his bitter exterior. This man started out not very likeable in the ordinary sense of the word but ended up likeable. He was likeable to me in the beginning, but mostly in the abstract sense of his being an unfinished product—a person with potential for emotional health and occupational success, if that potential could be mobilized through treatment. At first, I liked *who-he-could-become*, and this feeling carried me past the initial difficulties. I think therapists often have this experience with their personality-disordered patients.

The kinds of patients in whom likeability and amenability to therapy are most sharply separated are seen mostly in forensic settings. Here are two examples from my experience at a forensic hospital:

A 30-year-old woman had been admitted to a forensic hospital shortly after she stabbed her 7-year-old daughter to death. She was severely depressed at the time and had made a suicide gesture the same day as the murder. For this reason, she was considered not guilty by reason of insanity and was remanded to a forensic facility. The patient and her husband had emigrated to the United States 8 years earlier from an Asian country. Her husband was a domineering and ill-tempered man who was resentful of her having come from a better family and of her being better educated. His anger was greatly intensified after he was fired from his job, at which point he told her that he was taking their daughter back to their home country "to get away from America where women were corrupted" and that she would never see her daughter again. This threat was the precipitant of the murder and suicide gesture.

By the time I got to know the patient she had been in the hospital almost a year. She was no longer clinically depressed. She had in fact a sunny disposition. I hoped to help her develop some insight into the forces that motivated her acts of violence. In line with the impressions of Lewis and Bunce (2003), I couldn't assign one simple motive to the filicidal act. Instead, there seemed to be two major motifs: she wanted to exact revenge against her husband (reminiscent of Medea's behavior) but at the same time she had an "altruistic" impulse—to spare her daughter a life of misery with a cruel father in a poor country. But all my efforts to have her even think about these possibilities fell on deaf ears. Her reactions were similar to those of other women who have killed their children. Because of the shame associated with the act, the topic remains taboo, and these patients' amenability to therapy is generally quite low.

One of the patients assigned to me when I began my clinical work at the forensic hospital was a man in his early 40s who had made a plea of not guilty by reason of insanity when he was arrested some years before for serial sexual homicide. The patient was the picture of joviality and charm. When he had committed his last murder—the one for which he had been arrested—he was under the influence of alcohol and hallucinogens, and hence he had received the diagnosis—incorrect as it turned out to be—of schizophrenia. However, this impression led to his being sent to a forensic hospital rather than to a prison.

Throughout his adolescent years he had been repeatedly tortured (for the facts merited this strong word) by his mother, who would tie him up and whip him for minor infractions, such as coming home late for dinner. In his 20s he began to turn the tables, luring women to isolated places and then subjecting them to torture before killing them.

On the hospital ward, his behavior had always been exemplary. Because of his infectious good humor and his ability to referee disputes among the other patients, the patients voted him their leader and spokesman, and he presented their requests at the regular staff-patient meetings. He was well liked by everyone. In my sessions with him, he showed some superficial insight and was aware that his victimization of women was born of his having been victimized by his mother. But this awareness did not soften his attitude toward women. Despite his claims of being a "different person" now, he would periodically engage in secretive behaviors that gave his truer feelings away. He once manipulated a pen pal into purchasing for him several books on torture, which she was then to send to his "home" (actually, the hospital). Her discovery of his actual address and status dampened her enthusiasm to comply with his request.

For therapists in private practice, where a greater opportunity for choice of patients exists, *amenability to treatment* is affected to a considerable degree by the preferences of each individual therapist; that is, by the personality of the therapist, not just by the personality of the prospective patient. In a community of any size, where each therapist knows many colleagues on a social as well as on a professional basis, referrals are often made according to assumptions that certain colleagues will work especially well with certain kinds of patients. This matching goes beyond the matter of gender preference, where certain patients insist on working with a female or with a male therapist. A female incest victim, for example, may feel too uncomfortable, in the beginning at least, with a male therapist, although amenability to treatment may be excellent with a female therapist. Some male adolescents feel ill at ease baring their secrets to a female therapist but feel more comfortable with a male therapist. Numerous similar examples could be cited. But here I highlight the particularities and early life experiences that make certain therapists especially competent, for example, in their work with schizophrenic patients; others, with depressed patients; and still others, with borderline patients. In other words, one therapist may find a whole class of patients particularly likeable and enjoyable to work with, while other therapists may fail in their work with these same patients, finding them unlikeable and enervating. The phenomenon here could be akin to that captured by the adage about beauty being in the eye of the beholder. Extremes of beauty, of course, are not dependent on the beholder; they are universals such as, for example, the *Mona Lisa* of the 1490s and actress Hedy Lamarr of the 1940s. Perhaps there are some patients who are so delightful, agreeable, and cooperative that they seem likeable to all therapists. Certainly there are other patients for whom the field is much more limited.

An example of the latter group of patients was a young schizophrenic man I saw in consultation who had recently been discharged from the hospital. His delusions had dissipated, and his speech was now coherent and rational. He was looking for work, although his scruffy dress and poor hygiene inspired a measure of pessimism about his chance for success. I did not find him very likeable, besides which I scarcely knew where to begin to deal with his poor social skills. Instead, I referred him to a colleague, Dr. Harry Albert, who had the reputation of "wearing the hair shirt"—that is, he was known to take on and to do well with psychotic patients whose illnesses most therapists considered too formidable. He felt freer to break the mold of his psychoanalytic training when circumstances called for other modalities, including behavioral techniques. Dr. Albert found diplomatic ways of encouraging this patient to bathe with greater regularity, so as not to mar his chances in the workplace. He once took a morning off to accompany the man to a fashionable men's clothing shop, to help him select an outfit that would be impressive in a job interview. In this way he was able to help this patient to become reintegrated into the community, to find work, and to become self-supporting. Dr. Albert succeeded where others would have failed, in part because he found something likeable in this seemingly unpromising patient.

SPIRITUALITY

Character traits in the overall category of spirituality are found in abundance in persons we feel demonstrate "good character," and the opposites of these traits define a particular type of "bad character." Taken together, the terms and their antonyms make up a spectrum that is useful in assessing amenability to psychotherapy. Elsewhere I published a Scale of Spirituality that contains 20 descriptors at either end of the spectrum (Stone 2000). What I indicate by the term *spirituality* in this context is not religious feeling per se, but rather a combination of *self-transcendence* and *altruism* (putting the feelings and needs of others ahead of one's own). The French word *oblativité* captures the latter concept better than our word altruism. The following word pairs or term pairs are included in the Scale of Spirituality:

- Hopefulness, as opposed to despair
- Forbearance, as opposed to impatience
- Humility, as opposed to false pride
- Orientation toward others, as opposed to self-centeredness
- Faith in self and others, as opposed to disillusion
- Self-acceptance and being at peace with the past, as opposed to self-pity
- Resignation, as opposed to bitterness
- Serenity, as opposed to tormentedness
- Forgiveness, as opposed to grudge-holding
- Compassion, as opposed to hard-heartedness
- Uncomplainingness, as opposed to querulousness
- Self-transcendence, as opposed to giving up easily
- Common decency, as opposed to mean-spiritedness
- Dignity, as opposed to being undignified
- Uprightness, as opposed to moral shabbiness

In addition, the scale includes several phrases whose tone is similar to the values espoused by Alcoholics Anonymous (AA): feeling of a source of power beyond the self (in contrast to cynicism) and respectfulness of others (in contrast to the belief that "everyone is out for himself").

The negative terms belong mostly to the overall concepts of *depression* or perhaps to a kind of irritable depression (despair, disillusion, bitterness, and querulousness) and *narcissism*. Some of the negative terms represent the extremes of narcissism that one confronts in the psychopath (hard-heartedness, moral shabbiness).

One might argue that envy belongs in the list, as another antonym for self-acceptance. When envy is a dominant feature of a patient's personality, amenability to therapy is hampered. In the ancient catalog of the Seven Deadly Sins (pride, envy, gluttony, lust, anger, greed, and sloth), envy is sometimes contrasted with kindness, sometimes (as in the epic poem of the fifth-century writer Prudentius [http://deadlysins.com/virtues.html]) with love. In any case, envy is one of the most corrosive of the negative character traits and one of the most resistant to dynamic therapy. Psychoanalysis may uncover the main roots of a patient's envy, without the resultant insight making much of a dent in the trait.

In work with depressed patients certain positive traits augur for recovery, even in the face of initially strong suicidal feelings, whereas certain negative traits seem to heighten risk. Patients who are oriented toward others, even while in the throes of a deep depression, and who show resignation are able to surmount their depressed feelings and to avoid total despair. Those who are particularly self-centered and bitter tend to linger in their depressed state longer and to remain more deeply depressed. Amenability to therapy is thus a function of the balance between these opposing attributes and of the intensity (or rigidity) of any negative traits.

Some characteristics grouped under the heading of spirituality are character traits in the everyday sense of the term. They are adjectives (or phrases) we might use to describe someone to a third party—for example, she is "dignified," or he is "compassionate." But self-transcendence, correctly designated by Cloninger et al. (1999, p. 39) as a "second-order" character dimension, is a composite. We would not answer the request "Tell me what he's like" with the comment "Oh, he's very self-transcendent." Cloninger et al. listed five first-order traits encompassed in self-transcendence: self-forgetful, acquiescent, spiritual, enlightened, and idealistic. The component of self-forgetfulness, similar to the previously mentioned *oblativité*, involves not so much forgetting one's needs as putting the needs of others ahead of one's own. Self-transcendence as it relates to treatability, however, is not the quality of enlightenment, such as the state of *satori* that a Zen master strives for. The essence of this elusive quality is instead well captured in the German phrase (for which I am indebted to Otto Kernberg) *die Fähigkeit über den eigenen Schatten zu springen*—the ability to "jump over one's own shadow"—that is, the ability to surmount (transcend) one's own personal difficulties, sorrows, and losses, retaining all the while a sense of purposefulness about one's life and goals, as well as an inextinguishable capacity to care about and to involve oneself in the lives of others and in the tasks relevant to the improvement of the community or of the world at large.

Self-transcendence often makes the difference between despair and serious suicidality in patients coping with depression, providing the will to continue on despite the intense sadness and lethargy. The *essence* of self-transcendence may be gleaned in the following example from my days in hematology, before I began my psychiatric training. While working in a chemotherapy unit of a cancer hospital, I had under my care a woman in her mid-20s who was dying of myeloid leukemia and was in the last weeks of her life. Hers was a rare form of the disease in which the cell type was the eosinophil. Patients with eosinophilic leukemia tend to develop restriction of lung movement because the pleura becomes thickened with the invading cells, leading to painful air hunger and breathlessness. Yet this woman remained cheerful, stoical, and candid in talking with the doctors and her family members about her condition and about how little time she had left. More remarkable was that she thought and worried about the fate of the other patients on the unit, all of whom also had terminal cancer of one sort or another. In the minutes before she died, her last words to her husband were that he must promise her he would grant permission for an autopsy, because a girl being treated on the unit was also dying of the same rare condition and the doctors might learn something that could help her.

The following examples concern two depressed patients with contrasting levels of self-transcendence:

A 62-year-old married woman had been chronically depressed since her early 40s. Her mother was a kindly woman, but her father was harsh and punitive toward everyone in the family. After high school, where she had been the beauty queen of her class, she became a stewardess. She later married a well-to-do executive, with whom she had two daughters. During the years of her depression she received courses of electroconvulsive therapy, many different trials of antidepressants, and various courses of psychotherapy. By the time I began treating her, she was showing the vegetative signs of depression, particularly fatigability. This symptom was so marked that it made the simplest tasks seem Herculean. She enjoyed visits with her grandchildren but felt drained of all energy afterward. Church meant a great deal to her, and she and her husband gave generously to its support. But she was usually too tired to attend services. Her husband was a fast-paced, energetic man, but they were sometimes at cross-purposes because she could not keep up with the demands of his active social calendar. This inability was her only complaint, and it was resolved after I met with her and her husband and helped her husband to accept her limitations. In the several years I worked with her, she never spoke of suicidal thoughts, and she accepted her lot with resignation. Although semi-invalided with her depression, she helped to babysit for her grandchildren so that her daughters could have some time to themselves. She involved herself as best she could in various charitable activities, and she expressed gratitude for my not very successful efforts to alleviate her depression. She achieved a measure of *serenity*—another important element of spirituality. Her amenability to therapy was of a high order. She was insightful about the ways in which her harsh upbringing had aggravated her constitutional tendency to depression, a predisposition that she shared with many relatives on her mother's side.

A 62-year-old woman sought treatment for chronic depression. Her symptoms developed after her divorce some 30 years earlier. She had a doctorate in English and had taught at a college until her depression interfered with her ability to work. She had returned home to live with her elderly mother, where she had remained ever since, becoming totally dependent on her mother. Convinced she could not survive if her mother died, she thought she would have to commit suicide after her mother's funeral. In the meantime she fretted constantly about her mother's aches and pains, concerned that they were harbingers of a fatal illness. Most of her days were spent in her bedroom staring out the window or watching television. She had alienated all her former friends through her constant complaining. Her remarks to others alternated between expressions of self-pity and paranoid fears that others were taking advantage of her. She bombarded her daughter—her only child—with demands and complaints, until the daughter obtained an unlisted phone number and broke off relations with her, forbidding her to see her grandchildren. Her response to antidepressants and anxiolytics was minimal, and she had become agoraphobic, seldom venturing outside her house except for her sessions or to buy a newspaper. Even that task grew onerous, as she suspected the newspaper vendor of giving her the wrong change, which spurred arguments with him. In our sessions she dwelled on how attractive she used to be, on how many suitors she once had, and on how much the faculty at the college had admired her writing skills. Now, however, she had given up on life and was merely marking time until her mother died. My efforts to encourage her to resume some of her former activities—to reinsert some meaning in her life—were without success. When she turned 65 years old, her family placed her in an assisted-living facility, although she was still in good health physically and had no signs of dementia. This patient demonstrated the opposite set of characteristics relating to spirituality: bitterness, self-pity, querulousness, and an inability to rise above her difficulties. One consequence of this state of demoralization was her unresponsiveness to supportive therapy.

CANDOR

The root meaning of candor, from the Latin *candidus*, is the quality of being white, bright, glistening (as in in*cand*escent). To be candid is to be frank, open, straightforward. As a character trait, candor is one of the essential ingredients of amenability to psychotherapy. The trait implies honesty in what one reveals to a therapist. A patient's innermost secrets remain hidden for a long time, and trust and comfort must be built up in the therapeutic relationship before it is safe to bring these buried aspects of the self to the surface. But the road to this exposure must be paved with candor.

Candor, in the fullest sense, is an ideal state that one approaches only asymptotically. Even after several years of psychoanalysis, a patient does not reveal *everything* to the analyst. But usually patients with moderate degrees of candor at the outset become more open as time goes on. Embarrassment diminishes, self-acceptance improves, and candor is enhanced. This pattern occurs across the personality disorders, except in antisocial personality disorder. Antisocial persons, especially the subset who meet the criteria for psychopathy, regularly show little candor. Some antisocial persons with moderate degrees of psychopathic traits become more open eventually, in response either to therapy (especially group therapy) or to the passage of time.

For example, a psychiatric resident was treating a man who had shot a policeman who had been trying to arrest him during an armed robbery. The policeman died of his wounds a month after the man's trial. The patient first went to a forensic hospital and later to a civil psychiatric hospital where the resident was in training. Whereas the man had been furious at his trial, complaining that all the sympathy went to the wounded policeman and his wife, he was able, after many months of therapy, to acknowledge that the crime had been his fault. He began to feel sympathy for the widow and her children. In his therapy he was urged to give talks at local high schools about the dangers of drugs, which he had tried to obtain money for in the armed robbery. At this point he demonstrated both candor and self-transcendence, surmounting his criminal past through the confessional lectures. Fortunately, he showed fewer of the narcissistic traits of psychopathy than of the impulsive traits (Harpur et al. 1989), which are often more amenable to treatment (as will be discussed in Chapter 9, "Untreatable Personality Disorders").

Many patients with personality disorders show deficiencies in candor, albeit milder than those seen in psychopaths. Patients with marked obsessive-compulsive traits often show the "isolation of affect" typical of this personality. They avoid revealing negative thoughts and embarrassing memories and avoid expressions of anger. Their discourse is often dry and boring. Yet they may be quite motivated for treatment and reliable about keeping appointments. In that sense their amenability to therapy is good—better, in fact, than that of many hysteric or histrionic patients (here I am using *histrionic* to represent the more extreme form of *hysteric*), who may "emote" in exaggerated ways during sessions but may be so irregular in keeping appointments and so scattered in discourse as to derive little benefit from the therapy. With the obsessive patient, the rigid defense against self-revelation can ultimately be minimized, and this task becomes the first order of business in the treatment. With the resistance lowered, the patient's candor increases, and deeper layers of emotion become more reachable.

Candor is usually more difficult to achieve through therapy in patients with marked paranoid traits than in obsessive-compulsive patients. Paranoid patients customarily externalize the source of their problems, as though the responsibility always lies with others, not with themselves. This tendency works against the enhancement of candor in therapy.

Trauma can exert striking effects on memory and thus on candor. In a lecture on physical trauma, Arthur Green (1996) presented the case of a young man who had been convicted of murder. A videotape that accompanied the lecture showed an interview with the murderer, who painted a rosy picture of his childhood and denied having been beaten by his mother. A second tape showed an interview with his mother, who was able to acknowledge having whipped her son with an electrical cord on many occasions during his early years. Dr. Green's point was that the senseless beatings had set the stage for the outbreak of violence after the young man left home. Ironically, the mother had more candor (and remorse) than her son, who had no access to memories of the beatings or even to the rage that they apparently mobilized and that was taken out on strangers later in his life.

Particularly in cases of sexual trauma or situations that evoke fears of sexual misuse, revelation of the traumatic experiences may be avoided for long periods of time, even in persons who talk candidly about most other matters. An example of this phenomenon—a kind of *candor interrupted*—occurred when I was finishing a "control case" in the course of psychoanalytic training:

> **The patient was married** and had a 5-year-old son. The marriage was very troubled, but she found it difficult to share with me what the main trouble was. Only after a number of months did she trust me enough to tell me that she had caught sight, the year before, of her husband molesting their son sexually when he had inadvertently left the bathroom door open. What had held her back was the realization that once she had spoken the words, she could no longer pretend nothing had happened, and she would have to disrupt her life and divorce her husband. This she did. But there was another worry she could not candidly talk about—until the very last session of her 4-year-long psychoanalysis. In that 800th session, she finally told me that she had feared all along that I was going to ask her to lie undressed on the couch. The therapist she had been in treatment with before she began her analysis with me was a Reichian. Taking a page from the writings of Wilhelm Reich, he believed in "freeing up her character armoring" by massaging her supposedly tightened muscles as she lay naked on the couch. This memory disturbed her so greatly, as well it might, that even after 799 sessions in which I made no such request, she did not quite trust that I *never*

would—until it was crystal clear on the last day, when I still hadn't, that she was safe.

A still more dramatic example of how trauma put candor on hold for a long time in someone otherwise quite eager to expose what had happened is contained in the following vignette:

> **A 19-year-old woman** was admitted to a psychiatric hospital for reasons not immediately clear, although she appeared depressed. Her most striking feature was that she was completely mute and remained so month after month. Various experts interviewed her in consultation ("saw her" would be more accurate, since she herself said nothing), and each came up with a different diagnosis, including severe depression, "elective" mutism (in a presumably willful, negativistic person), and catatonic schizophrenia. She met with her therapist three times a week in what must have been supremely frustrating sessions, because she was no more vocal with the therapist than with the consultants. The therapist happened to be doing research on incest, so the topic was less foreign to her than it was to many other mental health professionals at that time (30 years ago). The therapist began to suspect that incest might have been an antecedent in the patient's history, so she tactfully inquired about this possibility. Then, in the thirteenth month of her hospital stay, the patient revealed, amidst a violent abreaction, that her father, a prominent executive, had carried on an incestuous relationship with her since she was 8 years old. Shortly before her hospitalization, she had become pregnant by him. He had driven her to an abortion clinic far from her home and then abandoned her, leaving her to find her way back by hitchhiking. He warned her that if she ever told anyone the truth about these events, he would kill her. It was at this point she became mute. It took great courage for her to reveal these secrets, although once she did so, her candor rose to a high level.

Occasionally therapists encounter what appears to be a superabundance of candor. Patients with antisocial personality (especially those who exhibit psychopathy) may speak with unusual openness in the very earliest sessions about embarrassing material that is ordinarily kept hidden for a long time. But the revelations are accompanied by a shallowness of affect that makes one suspect the patient's sincerity. Or, such patients may quickly reveal something that is true and shocking, yet not nearly so shocking as what is withheld. A patient might, for example, admit to breaking and entering a house while high on cocaine but omit having murdered an occupant of the house. Another patient might readily speak even about murder, truly telling everything, but with such callousness and lack of concern as to give the lie to the "candor" with which he acknowledges these acts. Such patients show only a kind of pseudo-candor.

MOTIVATION

Motivation for treatment may be understood as a complex of attitudes, composed of such elements as 1) the wish to get help, 2) the wish to continue treatment, and 3) the wish to change (Appelbaum 1972). Wallerstein (1986) emphasized the importance of motivation as a factor influencing amenability to psychotherapy: "Motivation for treatment is universally regarded as one of the central determinants of treatment prospect, almost regardless of the theoretical persuasion of the therapist" (p. 167). Typically, patients seeking therapy are animated by anxiety or some other form of mental discomfort that becomes the *vis a tergo*—the push from behind—propelling them into a treatment that they hope will alleviate their distress. Motivation is a necessary, albeit not sufficient, factor in amenability to treatment, in the personality disorders and in other forms of mental illness. In general, the greater the overall motivation, the greater is the eagerness not only to get help but to pursue therapy to its logical conclusion and to make as many adaptive changes as possible.

Among the personality disorders, including not only the DSM-IV-TR categories but also the varieties not included in DSM-IV-TR (depressive, masochistic, hysteric, hypomanic, passive-aggressive, sadistic, psychopathic), some are associated with high degrees of motivation, and others, with low or negligible motivation. Motivation tends to be adequate or high in patients with Cluster C disorders and in those with hysteric, depressive, or masochistic character structure. The opposite is true in those with antisocial or psychopathic personalities and (to a lesser extent) in narcissistic and schizoid patients.

Therapists seldom see the most hermit-like of schizoid persons, who, if they come for treatment at all, usually come at the urging of relatives (Stone 1996). Gabbard (1994) suggested that schizoid persons adopt a facade of aloofness, underneath which is a yearning for closeness—similar to the situation of the avoidant person, only more severe. In my experience, patients whose personality configuration meets the DSM-IV-TR criteria for schizoid personality disorder and who come voluntarily for therapy do represent the pattern Gabbard described. But other, more prototypically schizoid persons have no motivation for change and no desire for treatment. If coerced into therapy, they tend to quit prematurely. Motivation for help and for change in schizotypal patients is, in contrast, often keen, and amenability to treatment is correspondingly good.

Depending on their degree of immersion in paranoid ideation, paranoid persons vary widely in motivation. Those who come for treatment only at the behest of relatives—and who feel "railroaded" by these concerned and often frantic persons—believe that the trouble is with "the others" and have minimal motivation for treatment. But less severely paranoid persons who experience at the same time significant depression may show excellent motivation. Some accounts by the first generation of psychoanalysts describe work with paranoid patients of this sort, and these patients showed motivation to continue in treatment and to change, not merely to get help (Bjerre 1912; Maeder 1910). Borderline patients generally show high motivation for help, because psychic pain and the quest for attachment are strong. Their impulsivity and the chaotic quality that characterizes the lives of many patients with BPD serve to limit their motivation for continuing therapy. The dropout rate of BPD patients as a group is quite high, approaching 40% (Waldinger and Gunderson 1984).

Motivation is lowest in psychopathic persons and in many antisocial persons, because these persons have a tendency to deny that anything is wrong with their personalities. Commenting on psychopaths, Hare (1993) mentioned, "Unlike other individuals, psychopaths do not seek help on their own. Instead, they are pushed into therapy by a desperate family, or they enter treatment because of a court order" (p. 196). Further, he added that psychopaths resent authority, including that of any therapist, and regard therapy with mockery; therapists are seen by them as persons to be conned.

Antisocial personality disorder is a broader domain than psychopathy and includes some persons with underlying decency of character who felt forced into antisocial ways because of parental rejection, poverty, incestuous misuse, and other adverse environmental factors. Several of the BPD patients with comorbid antisocial personality in the P.I.-500 study, a long-term follow-up of patients hospitalized in 1963–1976 at New York State Psychiatric Institute, were of this sort (Stone 1990). One young man had run away from home after being rejected by his stepmother. He became a heroin addict and stole to support his habit. But after a near-death experience resulting from an overdose, he had an "enlightenment." He realized he was throwing his life away and stopped his heroin use then and there. He now had the motivation to get help and to change. He entered a recovery program and eventually became an employee of Narcotics Anonymous (NA), lecturing to audiences about the dangers of drugs.

The motivation for change is negligible in persons with sadistic personality, apart perhaps for certain persons who batter their sexual partners but who are troubled enough about their cruel behavior to try to overcome it. The outlook for violent criminals with marked sadistic personalities (such as men who commit serial sexual homicide) is, in contrast, utterly bleak (Stone 1998).

Many patients who are motivated to seek help for symptom conditions have in addition one or two annoying personality traits that fall short of meeting the criteria for a DSM-IV-TR disorder. These traits may however exert a destructive influence on important relationships and, to that extent, may be the patient's main problem, even though they may lie outside the patient's awareness. Examples of such traits are *stinginess, contemptuousness*, and *stubbornness. Jealousy* is another highly destructive trait that may exist without enough other paranoid traits to warrant a diagnosis of paranoid personality disorder. Some patients actually acknowledge their jealousy as a serious problem for which they were motivated to seek help.

Such traits highlight the tenacity of habits (habits of mind and the corresponding habits of behavior)—and the persistent efforts therapists must make to overturn these habits. Because motivation to change is central to amenability to treatment in the realm of personality, in many cases the proper motivation must be instilled through the art and persuasiveness of the therapist, often with the cooperation of others in the patient's life who bear the brunt of the undesirable traits.

PERSEVERANCE

In their analysis of the *temperament component* of personality, Cloninger et al. (1994) assigned four qualities to the domain of temperament (i.e., the moderately heritable, stable set of automatic responses to emotional stimuli). The four qualities are 1) harm avoidance, 2) novelty-seeking, 3) reward dependence, and 4) persistence. Persons who scored high in persistence were noted to be *industrious, diligent, hardworking, ambitious, perseverant*, and *perfectionistic* (p. 19). Those who scored low on the persistence scale developed by these authors had traits of *being inactive, being indolent, giving up easily*, and *quitting*. Patients with any of the personality disorders in Axis II tended to show low perseverance. For the *character component* of personality, which relates to family environment and individual life experiences, the main qualities assigned by Cloninger et al. were 1) self-directedness, 2) cooperativeness, and 3) self-transcendence. Among the terms they used to describe the attributes of self-directedness were *mature, reliable, purposeful, resourceful, effective*, and *self-accepting*. Terms describing the attributes of cooperativeness included *empathic, helpful, compassionate, constructive*, and *principled*. Cloninger's group found that persons who scored low in self-directedness and in cooperativeness tended to exhibit a DSM personality disorder; this association was strong enough to merit the conclusion that low self-directedness and low cooperativeness are core features of all personality disorders (Svrakic et al. 1993). One way these features manifested was in the general lack of direction noted in many persons with an Axis II disorder. Those who were young when initially evaluated tended to be uncertain of their occupational goals and tended not to pursue their preparatory education to completion.

Lack of perseverance and low self-directedness are common in personality-disordered patients but nevertheless show bell curve–like variation. In patients in whom these qualities are strikingly low, amenability to treatment is correspondingly low, because lack of perseverance is associated with quitting therapy before any reasonable goals have been realized.

Certain personality-disordered patients show considerable motivation and perseverance to continue therapy but seem unable to persevere in any occupational pursuit or even in the handling of their personal affairs. One of my patients, a humanities professor with marked obsessive-compulsive personality, strove to create a complete catalog of famous writers and composers. He would pursue and then drop the project by turns, such that it was always "80% done." As the years went on, new writers and composers rose to prominence, such that his oeuvre remained, when death overtook him in his 70s, still "80% done."

More common is the patient with good motivation for help and perseverance in the work situation, but little perseverance to see therapy through to its completion. The following vignette is illustrative:

> **A 30-year-old woman** was referred to me for psychotherapy after she had been briefly in treatment with two colleagues. She spoke of not having been comfortable with either of them. The only child of a well-to-do French father who was now nearly 90 years old and a much younger mother, she had been raised in what she called a "golden prison"—a home with elegant furnishings where she was continuously berated by her father as "useless" and "ugly." The men she chose to date humiliated her in ways similar to her father's treatment of her. Yet she remained attached to them. After the first few sessions of history taking, she began to come late to her appointments. In the next-to-the-last meeting of a "therapy" that lasted only 2 months, she told me that she had found it increasingly uncomfortable to come to her sessions. She said that although she found me kindly and avuncular, unlike her father, my appearance and the timbre of my voice were very similar to his, and she could not overcome her fear of me. Given the urgency of the situation—that she was about to break off her treatment—I made what I felt were the appropriate transference interpretations, mentioning that she herself had acknowledged that in my person, as opposed to my outward appearances and voice, I was not the scary father image from which she needed to flee. She gave it one more try but then quit treatment with me and sought the names of some female therapists, in the hope that they would not make her feel that she was in the presence of her father, as had the (now three) male therapists. I think for most patients, even borderline patients, stum-

bling blocks of this sort would not prove insuperable. But this woman, whose level of perseverance was quite low, was unable to work through her fear and remain in treatment.

LIFE CIRCUMSTANCES

The qualities affecting amenability to therapy discussed thus far relate to various characterological and temperamental aspects of personality. A few other factors worthy of consideration are not immediately related to personality. One of them is the life circumstances of a prospective patient. Some of these circumstances are obvious, and others are paradoxical. Obvious life circumstances include youth and dependency on the family (where the key family members are obstructionistic, destructive, or intrusive), poverty, absence of any work history, dependence on disability payments, lack of either education or marketable skills, and old age. The paradoxical circumstances include celebrity and great wealth. All of these factors potentially interfere with optimal amenability to psychotherapy.

Occasionally therapists may encounter adolescent patients who feign a psychiatric disorder in order to extricate themselves from an intolerable life situation. For example, a 15-year-old girl had witnessed her uncle being shot to death and her father wounded in a dispute between Mafia higher-ups. She had also been molested sexually by her father. She realized that she could never get treatment as long as she remained at home, and, because her father was a violent man, she felt she could not register a complaint with a child protective service agency. So she cut her wrists lightly as a suicide gesture, which earned her a "free pass" to the psychiatric hospital, where, under the guise of having "borderline personality," she was safe to tell her story.

In some homes, marital discord, including screaming and physical violence between the spouses, creates an environment inimical to the therapy of any children from the household, regardless of whether they are otherwise amenable to treatment. Poverty imposes great constraints on the availability of therapeutic resources. Personality-disordered patients from poor economic circumstances are usually at the mercy of whatever staff and treatment measures are available at low-cost or free clinics. The treatment staff members often have heavy caseloads, making it difficult to see an individual patient more than once every week or once every other week. Borderline patients, especially those who are seriously depressed or suicidal, would be better served if they were seen twice a week, but such a schedule is rarely possible. Patients may not be able to afford the cost of transportation to and from the clinic, or they may cancel appointments at the last minute because of the frequent crises that punctuate their lives.

The absence or near absence of any work history is another serious impediment to the success of treatment for personality-disordered patients. The disorder may itself be an important contributing factor to the poor work history. Some narcissistic patients, for example, especially as they move into their late 20s or early 30s, avoid jobs that are available to them as being "beneath them," yet they do not have the qualifications or experience to command the higher positions to which they feel unrealistically entitled.

Certain patients with passive-aggressive traits are earmarked (seldom consciously) by a parent to be the parent's companion in old age. By means of humiliating and guilt-provoking remarks, a parent may so undermine the self-confidence of a child as to hinder any step toward emotional and economic independence. Although there is no lack of clinical examples, sometimes a great dramatist captures the essence of this phenomenon with especial poignancy. In *The Beauty Queen of Leenane* by Martin McDonagh (1996), for example, the 40-year-old heroine's last chance at marriage and happiness is quashed by her lonely but also selfish and manipulative mother.

Lack of marketable skills and deficient education are related problems that interfere with treatability, partly because they predispose patients to dependency on the welfare system, including the sectors involved with awarding disability payments. Patients who receive disability payments but who are nevertheless capable of at least part-time work pose a problem in therapy. Disability status, with its secondary gain, creates a cushion that may be useful for a time but may eventually hinder further progress. Some patients who receive disability payments remain unmotivated to return to work unless the prospective job offers at a minimum one-and-a-half times the amount obtained from disability; at this level of compensation, these patients seem to feel it is worthwhile to risk leaving the security of disability insurance.

Of personality-disordered patients, those with borderline, schizotypal, and antisocial personalities are most likely to show poor work histories. To address this factor, Linehan (1993) emphasized skills training in her overall approach to the behavioral therapy of patients with BPD (pp. 329–344). Age also makes a difference, and the longer a patient has put off acquiring the appropriate training and skills, the higher the emotional hurdle to overcome. A 30-year-old person contemplating an entry-level job may feel embarrassed and may give up in advance. How well such embarrassment can be overcome is a measure of the patient's courage.

Amenability to psychotherapy may seem to be high in certain personality-disordered patients, if one looks only at the list of *favorable* characteristics. But when working with BPD patients, therapists are in a much more precarious situation where *suicidality* is a serious issue *and* the patient is living alone. The risk may be reduced if the patient changes his or her living arrangements so as to have a roommate, but one can seldom count on an acquaintance to show the same level of concern in a time of crisis as would a close friend, a lover, or a relative. If therapy is to succeed, the patient may be urged to agree to live in a halfway house or sheltered apartment managed by a psychiatric hospital until he or she is more stable.

It may seem paradoxical that celebrity, political power, or great wealth may adversely affect amenability to therapy. Persons who enjoy these advantages certainly have no trouble affording the cost of therapy, but beyond this one advantage, the disadvantages are numerous. It is not easy to safeguard the privacy of an easily recognized celebrity or a person in a prominent political position. In addition, the famous, the powerful, and the wealthy often pose serious problems in scheduling, because they can, and often must, travel widely and for long periods, thus interrupting the regularity of therapy sessions. When personality disorders are present in such persons, narcissistic traits are apt to be at the forefront, along with dismissiveness and a sense of entitlement and specialness (not so discordant with reality here, but an impediment all the same), all of which tend to create barriers to the formation of a cooperative alliance with the therapist (Stone 1972, 1979). Persons with the level of social success implied in celebrity and political power may have difficulty acknowledging negative personality traits. If they do enter therapy, they may be slow to recognize the authority of the therapist. From the countertransference side, therapists who treat such patients must guard against being so awestruck that they lose their objectivity.

OBJECT RELATIONS

The quality of object relations is an important determinant of amenability to psychotherapy in particular and to psychiatric treatment in general. The *theory of object relations*, as formulated by Kernberg (1976a), refers to the mental constructs (or "structures") each person develops that govern the emerging views of self and other as they form in response to the myriad interactions with people in the external world, especially during the formative years of childhood. In the early years, the people in the external world are primarily parents or other important caretakers, along with siblings and other close relatives. Depending on whether the early relationships are mainly harmonious or mainly chaotic, painful, or destructive, the internalized views of the self and of other persons will be either well integrated or poorly integrated. The interactions with the mother (usually the primary caretaker) and important others are not *all* of the influences that shape the attachment process and object relations. In addition, inborn abnormalities of temperament can predispose certain children to distort their perceptions and reactions to the caretakers. This distortion can lead to abnormalities of object relations even in the presence of parents who are nurturing and adequate in their concern for and understanding of their child. Similarly, abnormal temperament can lead to exaggerated reactions to a rejecting or neglectful parent, over and above what would be noted in siblings in the same family whose temperaments were calmer.

A parent tends to be loved no matter what, thanks to innate tendencies akin to what ethologists have called "imprinting" (Eibl-Eibesfeldt 1989; Lorenz 1965). But if a parent is highly abusive or neglectful, the child may find it quite difficult to entertain an *integrated* image of the other. Instead, *splitting* may occur. In splitting, polar opposite views of self and other are held, as it were, in separate compartments of the mind. Persons who exhibit splitting have difficulty in summoning both the positive and the negative aspects of self and other simultaneously. Instead, they oscillate abruptly between extreme positions, thinking of an offending parent, for example, now as saint, then as monster, and viewing themselves now as a virtuous victim, then as an undeserving wretch. In persons given to this kind of splitting, similar polarization will be discernible in their relationships with lovers, spouses, bosses, and close friends, as well as with the caretakers who may have predisposed them to form these split images originally. Splitting may be seen as a primitive defense mechanism; it is noticeable most prominently in BPD, but it is also found in other severe personality disorders.

Kernberg (1967, 1976b) drew attention to the frequency of splitting mechanisms in personality-disordered patients who show borderline personality organization, a broader concept than BPD. The main criteria for borderline personality organization are an enfeebled sense of identity, coupled with an intact capacity for reality testing in interpersonal relations. Many patients with severe personality disorders, including schizotypal, paranoid, antisocial, and histrionic personality, among others, exhibit borderline personality organization. Thus, splitting and other primitive defenses such as denial, projective identification, and devaluation are encountered over a wide spectrum of personality disorders, not just in BPD. These defenses and the impairments in object relations that are usually found in conjunction with them combine to create obstacles in the course of therapy.

Another relevant concept in this realm is *attachment*. Common attachment styles encountered in personality-disordered patients include the *entangled* (a subset of the preoccupied type) and the *dismissive* types (Fonagy et al. 1995; Main 1996). Each presents particular challenges to the therapist, but it appears that patients who exhibit the *dismissive* attachment style—found frequently among narcissistic, antisocial, and paranoid patients—become the most difficult, if for no other reason than that they are the most prone to trivialize the efforts of the therapist, to deny having any significant personality problems, and to quit treatment prematurely. The high dropout rate noted in work with borderline patients is attributable in good part to the subgroup of BPD patients who show the dismissive attachment style. Fonagy (2001) made a similar point in his discussion of borderline patients.

The attachment style is not, however, the sole aspect of attachment that affects amenability to therapy. Patients with avoidant personality disorder, for example, who usually show an insecure type of attachment, are seldom dismissive. Instead, they hunger for attachment and become overly dependent and clingy toward the therapist, even though in the outside world, they avoid social contact and have few friends and no intimates. The tragedy of this situation is the built-in vicious circle: these patients have no way to test or overturn the pessimistic convictions they start out with—that people won't like them, will think them ugly or uninteresting, and so on—because they have too few interactions with others to allow them to realize that the negative assumptions are quite likely wrong. They deny themselves, in effect, the sort of feedback with the external world that ordinary people rely on to improve the accuracy of their perceptions of themselves and of other people. Hence, for avoidant patients, the negative assumptions harden and become like "absolute facts." Body dysmorphic disorder is common in this group (Phillips et al. 1995), and these patients' drastically negative views about certain parts of their bodies tend to remain untested because they limit close contact with others so severely that they never develop a more realistic self-image. Therapists who treat avoidant patients, especially those functioning at the borderline level (i.e., who meet the criteria for borderline personality organization), have great difficulty in persuading them to reach out to others in various social encounters so that they might in time begin to question their negative assumptions about their personal and physical attractiveness. These patients are highly motivated to seek help and to continue in therapy, but change is frightening for them, so much so that their overall amenability to therapy is impaired.

Well-functioning persons who show, characterologically, great reserve and a certain choosiness about whom they associate with may show the "dismissive" style in *mild* form, without being haughty, snobbish, contemptuous, or otherwise dismissive at a *pathological* level. Only the pathological levels of the attachment styles, if manifested in a patient seeking therapy, lower amenability to treatment and present serious obstacles to that therapy.

The topics of object relations and attachment theory take on special importance in discussions of borderline patients (those with borderline personality organization or the narrower entity, BPD). With borderline patients, it is common, although no less bewildering, for the therapist to encounter paradoxical situations. The patient may hold incompatible views of self and others that oscillate wildly and unpredictably, sometimes even within a single psychotherapy session. Borderline patients typically hunger for love and attachment, yet they often spurn the very attention that a lover may offer and that the patient consciously craves. Writing from the perspective of evolutionary psychiatry, McGuire and Troisi (1998) touched on this paradox: "When [BPD] is viewed in an evolutionary context, the majority of the DSM-IV diagnostic criteria can be interpreted as indices of failed efforts to achieve goals that require others' participation" (p. 197). The BPD item "frantic efforts to avoid real or imagined abandonment," in DSM-IV-TR, relates to this phenomenon. Side by side with the striving for affection is often an equally strong need to repudiate offers of affection or caring when they are made. This puzzling reaction is generally born of a masochistic personality configuration in which there are unconscious guilt feelings that, as Kernberg (1980) pointed out, "bring about an intensification of the patient's resistances and of negative therapeutic reactions— because the patient would then be faced with coming to terms with his libidinal attachment to bad, ambivalently loved objects" (p. 74). In the negative therapeutic reaction, one confronts the paradox wherein the more helpful, kindly, caring, and positive an attitude the therapist displays, the more the patient seems to cringe, reject the help, and threaten to quit the treatment. This tendency of course has a negative impact on amenability to psychotherapy, unless the situation can be salvaged by interpretations (that the patient is able to accept and process) about how unworthy the patient feels at receiving anything warmly positive from the therapist. The more cruel, abusive, and neglectful the primary caretakers actually were, the more likely is this reaction to occur.

For example, a borderline woman in her 20s was the only child of warring parents. When she was 9 years old, her father shot her mother to death with a rifle, but he insisted to his daughter that her mother "committed suicide." He warned her of dire consequences were she ever to reveal the truth. She ended up affiliating herself during her 20s with abusive men, recapitulating her original home life in which she suffered undeservedly at the hands of a tyrannical man. Later, while working with a therapist who was warm and accepting, she became irritated, depressed, and suicidal. When the therapist was able to interpret this paradoxical reaction—and show the patient that she was unnerved by the kindness she nevertheless hungered for—she grew able, slowly, to overcome her self-hatred, her loyalty to the murderous father, and her masochistic need for suffering.

CULTURAL FACTORS

In assessing the influence of cultural factors on the amenability to psychotherapy, we need to look not only at the patients and their varied backgrounds but also at the therapists and their varying levels of familiarity with different cultures. The cultural diversity in the United States is staggering in its complexity, and the strength of the country derives to a great extent from the skills and talents of persons from every nation, every ethnic group, and every religion on earth. People from these groups handle psychological problems in ways that reflect their cultural origins. A form of therapy that may be appropriate for one group may not be ideal for another. Freedom to discuss sensitive personal issues may be seriously constricted in some cultural groups and hardly limited in others. Although the DSM personality disorders can be found across cultures, their distribution differs, such that a personality type encountered frequently in one group may be uncommon in another. The literature includes several articles examining the distribution of personality types across groups—for example, in Swiss versus non-Swiss patients (Baleydier et al. 2003), Vietnamese versus Cambodian immigrants to the United States (Boehnlein et al. 1995), Irish American versus Jewish American families with psychotic relatives (Wylan and Mintz 1976), and Chinese persons with personality disorder (Zheng et al. 2002).

No matter how self-reflective or amenable to therapy in other respects they may be, personality-disordered patients who come from a fundamentalist religious background of any faith often keep certain sectors of their lives off limits with respect to acknowledgment or, if that bridge is crossed, to exploration. Some brief case examples follow:

> **A 40-year-old Muslim woman,** a high school teacher married to an engineer, was referred for therapy because of depression. She had emigrated to the United States at age 19 years, having been accepted at an American college. The next year, she married a man from her country who was also studying in the United States. Their married life had been ungratifying, mostly because she still pined for the young man with whom she had had a brief clandestine affair before moving to the United States. Premarital sex in her culture and especially in her fundamentalist family was more than *harām* (forbidden); it was punished with the utmost severity. Twenty years' exposure to American culture and to people of many religious and ethnic origins had not alleviated her feelings of guilt and sinfulness. I was the first person to whom she told the story of the old affair. Because her amenability to therapy was of a high order in other respects, she persevered in therapy.

For a long time my comments about the harshness of her conscience, especially in view of how blameless her life had been in every other respect, gave her no relief. In her view, I could not comprehend the depth of her feeling about her sin (as she referred to it), because I came from a different culture; therefore, my reassuring remarks rolled too easily off my tongue. Over 2 years of therapy, however, her guilt lessened, and she became more self-accepting. One thing she found helpful was my insistence that she create a hierarchical catalog of sins, assigning her experience of long ago to a place she felt was appropriate within it. She could grasp, looking at her catalog, that her "sin," which had hurt no one, was far down on the list, compared with murder, rape, child beating, verbal abuse, and torture.

A married man in his late 30s had been raised in an ultra-strict Baptist home. Biblical injunctions were taken seriously, and eternal damnation was believed to await those who transgressed. A successful electrician, he had begun to work two jobs to put his wife through law school. While there, she became enamored of a fellow student and made plans to divorce. Her husband, a man of marked compulsive and paranoid traits, regarded divorce as unthinkable. To him, the marriage vows were indissoluble, and to violate them was an unforgivable sin. One day, as she was preparing her exit, he shot her in the leg. At first he fled to a different city. After hiding out in a motel for 2 weeks, he suddenly had a religious experience in which he heard God's voice telling him that he had done wrong and should give himself up to the authorities. He did so and was arrested, but he was found mentally ill and remanded to a forensic hospital, where I became his therapist. At first he was reluctant to talk with me at all. In the eyes of the law he was a man accused of attempted murder. In my eyes, as I made him aware, he was an unusually honorable and earnest man who was at the same time rigidly moralistic and who had allowed himself so little "wiggle room" that he snapped under the impact of his wife's betrayal. By now he was no longer unapproachable regarding therapy. He began to understand that, ironically, his morality was in all likelihood harsher than God's morality. I said that it seemed inconceivable that God would prefer that two people spend the rest of their days scowling at each other in thinly veiled hatred, rather than let the marriage end, permitting one, and probably both, of them ultimately to make a more satisfactory life. He eventually felt this philosophy was acceptable.

A woman from a Chinese family in Hong Kong came to the United States when she was 10 years old. She was now, at age 32 years, a professor at a university who lived alone. In personality, she showed predominantly depressive-masochistic and obsessional traits. Currently she was struggling with the decision of whether to marry a man with whom she had been in a romantic relationship. This issue was the motivating force that led her to seek treatment. The problem was that her boyfriend was an "Anglo" (i.e., Caucasian), which rendered him unacceptable to her very traditional and conservative parents. She in turn was loath to marry someone her parents could not welcome into the family. In the first few sessions with me it became clear that she felt herself in an analogous bind with me. I was supposed

to help her resolve her dilemma, but I too was an "Anglo." I was not someone intimately familiar with her culture, and it was a part of Chinese culture
that one does not reveal personal problems to outsiders. She felt that I could
not be objective and would favor that side of her that wished to remain with
her boyfriend (which was basically what she wanted), and thus I would be
"unfair" to her parents. I was unable to allay her anxieties about these issues,
and after a month she left treatment.

These examples point up some of the resistances that may arise in the
therapy of personality-disordered patients as a result of cultural and religious factors. On the other side of the equation, of course, difficulties may
arise because the therapist is so unfamiliar with the patient's culture as to
hinder the chances of a successful treatment. This situation can occur even
when the patient might be very amenable to psychotherapy, if only the right
therapist were conducting it. The last of the three case examples just presented concerned a Chinese patient. Michael Bond (1991), a Canadian psychologist now living in Hong Kong, and his Chinese colleagues Patrick
Leung and Peter Lee (Leung and Lee 1996) wrote that native-born Chinese tend to regard the acknowledgment of mental problems as shameful
and tend to avoid talking about them even to professionals. Instead, they
often "somatize," that is, ascribe their emotional difficulties to various
bodily complaints.

Patients who are leaders or professional persons in their respective
faiths, including ministers, priests, nuns, and rabbis, may not be comfortable with therapists who are not of their faith, or even who are of their faith
but are not observant. These patients often prefer to work with therapists
who are deeply involved in religion themselves—for example, former
priests or ministers. One cannot measure their amenability to psychotherapy without taking these sensibilities into consideration; that is, they may
be very amenable, but only to treatment with a therapist who has a background similar to their own.

Because amenability to therapy depends rather heavily on the therapist's
openness to the patient's culture, some portion of the opening phase of psychotherapy should be devoted to becoming more familiar with these facets
of the patient's background. The therapist's knowledge of these details may
determine whether the patient feels understood and accepted and thus
whether the treatment is likely to succeed.

IMPACT OF SYMPTOM DISORDERS

Depending on the personality disorder, one or a combination of Axis I
symptom disorders may be present as well and may interfere to varying de-

grees with amenability to psychotherapy. Patients with personality disorders of the dramatic cluster are prone to abuse alcohol or other substances, which can interfere grossly with amenability to psychotherapy. Alcoholism may be found in conjunction with other personality disorders as well. Borderline patients often self-medicate with several different substances at once, using one drug to help them overcome insomnia, another to minimize depression, and still another to keep them alert during the day. One-to-one sessions in psychotherapy have little if any efficacy in curbing substance abuse. Patients exhibiting problems in this area need to enroll in the relevant 12-step program (AA or NA). Refusal to do so augurs poorly for the outcome of psychotherapy, regardless of the therapeutic approach.

Several other symptom disorders are often found in association with personality disorders. Patients with BPD almost invariably have one or more of the following conditions: anxiety disorders and eating disorders (Oldham et al. 1995), attention-deficit/hyperactivity disorder (Fossati et al. 2002), depressive symptoms (Klein and Schwartz 2002), and dissociative disorders or posttraumatic stress disorder (Sar et al. 1999; van den Bosch et al. 2003). Patients with avoidant personality disorder often have anxiety disorders, such as agoraphobia or social anxiety disorder. Patients with obsessive-compulsive disorder often have an accompanying personality disorder; the latter need not be obsessive-compulsive personality disorder, but it usually is one of the anxious cluster disorders (Baer and Jenike 1990). The presence of a personality disorder has been regarded as a negative prognostic factor within the realm of the symptom disorders. For example, Halmi and Kleifield (1996) reported that patients with bulimia nervosa often have a personality disorder that manifests in interpersonal difficulties, impulsivity, lying about their eating habits, and low self-esteem. The personality disorder (BPD is the most common) then gets in the way of overall treatment "by compromising the patient's motivation, participation, and follow-through with treatment" (p. 927).

Severe agoraphobia can interfere with the treatment of a patient with an underlying personality disorder, usually avoidant personality disorder. The agoraphobic patient may find it next to impossible to leave the house to go to the therapist's office; thus, the patient cannot receive the help the therapist might have been able to offer to ameliorate the personality disorder. To get around this "catch-22" situation, a family member or friend may accompany the patient to sessions until psychotherapy and appropriate medications have lessened the intensity of the agoraphobia. At that point, other factors bearing on amenability to therapy—the patient's character, self-reflective capacity, and other qualities (which are often quite favorable in agoraphobic patients)—can finally be mobilized.

TREATABILITY

The treatability factors enumerated and explained in this chapter are summarized in Table 1–1. The table is organized so that therapists may also use it as a guideline for evaluating a prospective patient or a patient who has begun treatment. Most of the factors can be rated along a continuum from high (or "optimal") to low. For the last four factors (G to J), different adjectives are more appropriate. The completed form shows at a glance the patient's strengths and weaknesses concerning amenability to psychotherapy.

REFERENCES

American Psychiatric Association: Diagnostic and Statistical Manual of Mental Disorders, 4th Edition, Text Revision. Washington, DC, American Psychiatric Association, 2000

American Psychiatric Association: Practice Guideline for the Treatment of Patients With Borderline Personality Disorder. Am J Psychiatry 158 (Oct suppl):1–52, 2001

Appelbaum A: A critical re-examination of the concept "motivation for change" in psychoanalytic treatment. Int J Psychoanal 53:51–59, 1972

Baer L, Jenike MA: Personality disorders in obsessive-compulsive disorder, in Obsessive-Compulsive Disorders: Theory and Management. Edited by Jenike MA, Baer L, Minichiello WE. Chicago, IL, Yearbook Medical Publishers, 1990, pp 76–88

Baleydier B, Damsa C, Schutzbach C, et al: [Comparison between Swiss and foreign patients' characteristics at the psychiatric emergencies department and the predictive factors of their management strategies] (French). Encephale 29:205–212, 2003

Baron-Cohen S: The Essential Difference. New York, Basic Books, 2003

Bateman AW, Fonagy P: Mentalization-based treatment of BPD. J Personal Disord 18:36–51, 2004

Bjerre P: Zur Radikalbehandlung der chronischen Paranoia. Jahrbuch für Psychoanalitischen und Psychopathologischen Forschungen 3:759–847, 1912

Boehnlein JK, Tran HD, Riley C, et al: A comparative study of family functioning among Vietnamese and Cambodian refugees. J Nerv Ment Dis 183:768–773, 1995

Bond MH: Beyond the Chinese Face: Insights From Psychology. New York, Oxford University Press, 1991

Cloninger CR, Przybeck TR, Svrakic DM, et al: The Temperament and Character Inventory (TCI): A Guide to Its Development and Use. St. Louis, MO, Center for Psychobiology of Personality, Washington University, 1994

Cloninger CR, Svrakic DM, Bayon C, et al: Measurement of psychopathology as variants of personality, in Personality and Psychopathology. Edited by Cloninger CR. Washington, DC, American Psychiatric Press, 1999, pp 33–65

TABLE 1–1.   Guideline for evaluating treatability factors in personality disorders

Treatability factor	Components	Evaluation
A-1	Ability to think about oneself and others and about one's feelings	
	Introspectiveness	high.................low
	Psychological mindedness	high.................low
	Mentalization	high.................low
	Empathy	high.................low
A-2	Intelligence	above average.....below average
B	Character	
	Uprightness	high.................low
	Likeability	high.................low
C	Spirituality	
	Hopefulness versus despair	high.................low
	Forbearance versus impatience	high.................low
	Humility versus false pride	high.................low
	Other- versus self-oriented	high.................low
	Faith in self versus disillusion	high.................low
	Self-acceptance versus self-pity	high.................low
	Resignation versus bitterness	high.................low
	Serenity versus tormentedness	high.................low
	Forgiveness versus grudge-holding	high.................low
	Compassion versus hard-heartedness	high.................low
	Uncomplainingness versus querulousness	high.................low

TABLE 1–1. Guideline for evaluating treatability factors in personality disorders *(continued)*

Treatability factor		Components	Evaluation
		Self-transcendence versus giving up easily	high............low
		Common decency versus mean-spiritedness	high............low
		Dignity versus lacking in dignity	high............low
		Morality versus moral shabbiness	high............low
D	Candor		high............low
E	Motivation		high............low
F	Perseverance		high............low
G	Life circumstances		favorable............unfavorable
H	Object relations		harmonious............impaired
I	Cultural factors		favorable............unfavorable
J	Symptom disorders		serious....moderate...mild...absent

Note. For the spirituality factors, rate as "high" or "low" the positive factors only; e.g., hopefulness, forebearance, humility.

Damasio AR: Descartes' Error: Emotion, Reason, and the Human Brain. New York, Grosset/Putnam, 1994

Eibl-Eibesfeldt I: Human Ethology. New York, Aldine de Gruyter, 1989

Fonagy P: Attachment Theory and Psychoanalysis. New York, Other Press, 2001

Fonagy P, Higgitt AM: A developmental perspective on borderline personality disorder. Revue Internationale de Psychopathologie 1:125–159, 1989

Fonagy P, Steele M, Steele H, et al: Attachment, the reflective self, and borderline states, in Attachment Theory: Social, Developmental, and Clinical Perspectives. Edited by Goldberg S, Muir R, Kerr J. Hillsdale, NJ, Analytic Press, 1995, pp 233–278

Fossati A, Novella L, Donati D, et al: History of childhood attention deficit/hyperactivity disorder symptoms and borderline personality disorder: a controlled study. Compr Psychiatry 43:369–377, 2002

Frank N: In the Shadow of the Reich. New York, Knopf, 1991

Freud S: On psychotherapy (1904), in The Standard Edition of the Complete Psychological Works of Sigmund Freud, Vol 7. Translated and edited by Strachey J. London, Hogarth Press, 1953, pp 257–268

Freud S: Character and anal eroticism (1908), in The Standard Edition of the Complete Psychological Works of Sigmund Freud, Vol 9. Translated and edited by Strachey J. London, Hogarth Press, 1953, pp 168–175

Gabbard GO: Psychodynamic Psychiatry in Clinical Practice: The DSM-IV Edition. Washington, DC, American Psychiatric Press, 1994, pp 419–448

Gilmore M: Family album. Granta 37(autumn):11–52, 1991

Green A: The effects of trauma in an adolescent who committed murder. Paper presented at the Fourth International Symposium of Adolescent Psychiatry, Athens, Greece, July 1996

Halmi KA, Kleifield EI: Inpatient treatment of bulimia nervosa, in Synopsis of Treatments of Psychiatric Disorders, 2nd Edition. Edited by Gabbard GO, Atkinson SD. Washington, DC, American Psychiatric Press, 1996, pp 925–928

Hare RD: Without Conscience: The Disturbing World of the Psychopaths Among Us. New York, Picket Books, 1993

Harpur TJ, Hare RD, Hakstian AR: Two-factor conceptualization of psychopathy: construct validity and assessment implications. Psychol Assess 1:6–17, 1989

Judd PH, McGlashan TH: A Developmental Model of Borderline Personality Disorder: Understanding Variations in Course and Outcome. Washington, DC, American Psychiatric Publishing, 2003

Kernberg O[F]: Borderline personality organization. J Am Psychoanal Assoc 15:641–685, 1967

Kernberg OF: Object-Relations Theory and Clinical Psychoanalysis. New York, Jason Aronson, 1976a

Kernberg OF: Technical considerations in the treatment of borderline personality organization. J Am Psychoanal Assoc 24:795–829, 1976b

Kernberg OF: Internal World and External Reality: Object Relations Theory Applied. New York, Jason Aronson, 1980

Kernberg OF: Severe Personality Disorders: Psychotherapeutic Strategies. New Haven, CT, Yale University Press, 1984

Klein DN, Schwartz JE: The relationship between depressive symptoms and borderline personality disorder features over time in dysthymic disorder. J Personal Disord 16:523–535, 2002

Kraepelin E: Manic-Depressive Insanity and Paranoia. Translated by Barclay RM. Edited by Robertson GM. Edinburgh, Livingstone, 1921

Leung PWL, Lee PWH: Psychotherapy with the Chinese, in Handbook of Chinese Psychology. Edited by Bond MH. New York, Oxford University Press, 1996, pp 441–456

Lewis CF, Bunce SC: Filicidal mothers and the impact of psychosis on maternal filicide. J Am Acad Psychiatry Law 31:459–470, 2003

Linehan MM: Cognitive-Behavioral Treatment of Borderline Personality Disorder. New York, Guilford, 1993

Lorenz K: Evolution and Modification of Behavior. Chicago, IL, University of Chicago Press, 1965

Maeder A: Psychologische Untersuchungen an Dementia praecox–Kranken. Jahrbuch für Psychoanalitischen und Psychopathologischen Forschungen 2:234–245, 1910

Mailer N: The Executioner's Song. Boston, MA, Little, Brown, 1979

Main M: Recent studies in attachment: overview with selected implications for clinical work, in Attachment Theory: Social, Developmental and Clinical Perspectives. Edited by Goldberg S, Muir R, Kerr J. Hillsdale, NJ, Analytic Press, 1996, pp 407–474

McDonagh M: The Beauty Queen of Leenane. New York, Dramatists Play Service, 1996

McGuire M, Troisi A: Darwinian Psychiatry. New York, Oxford University Press, 1998

Oldham JM, Skodol AE, Kellman HD, et al: Comorbidity of Axis I and Axis II disorders. Am J Psychiatry 152:571–578, 1995

Petrova A, Watson P: The Death of Hitler. New York, WW Norton, 1995

Phillips KA, Kim JM, Hudson JI: Body identity disorder in body dysmorphic disorder and eating disorders: obsessions or delusions? Psychiatr Clin North Am 18:317–334, 1995

Posner GL: Hitler's Children. New York, Random House, 1991

Regier DA, Robins LN: Psychiatric Disorders in America. New York, Free Press, 1991

Reich W: Character Analysis, 3rd Edition. New York, Farrar, Straus & Giroux, 1949

Sar V, Kundakçi T, Kiziltan E, et al: Axis-I dissociative disorder comorbidity of borderline personality disorder among psychiatric outpatients. Paper presented at the 4th Conference of the International Society for the Study of Dissociation, Manchester, England, May 1999

Spillane R: Rhetoric as remedy: some philosophical antecedents of psychotherapeutic ethics. Br J Med Psychol 60:217–224, 1987

Stone MH: Treating the wealthy and their children. Int J Child Psychother 1:15–46, 1972

Stone MH: Treating the children of famous parents, in Basic Handbook of Child Psychiatry. Edited by Noshpitz JD. New York, Basic Books, 1979, pp 382–387

Stone MH: The Fate of Borderline Patients: Successful Outcome and Psychiatric Practice. New York, Guilford, 1990

Stone MH: Abnormalities of Personality: Within and Beyond the Realm of Treatment. New York, WW Norton, 1993

Stone MH: Schizoid and schizotypal personality disorders, in Synopsis of Treatments of Psychiatric Disorders, 2nd Edition. Edited by Gabbard GO, Atkinson SD. Washington, DC, American Psychiatric Press, 1996, pp 953–957

Stone MH: The personalities of murderers: the importance of psychopathy and sadism, in Psychopathology and Violent Crime. Edited by Skodol AE. Washington, DC, American Psychiatric Press, 1998, pp 29–52

Stone MH: Wesentliche prognostische Faktoren für die Borderline-Persönlichkeitsstörung, in Handbuch der Borderline-Störungen. Edited by Kernberg OF, Dulz B, Sachsse U. Stuttgart, Germany, Schattauer Verlag, 2000, pp 687–700

Strachey L: On the theory of the therapeutic results of psycho-analysis. Int J Psychoanal 18:139–145, 1937

Svrakic DM, Whitehead C, Przybeck TR, et al: Differential diagnosis of personality disorders by the seven-factor model of temperament and character. Arch Gen Psychiatry 50:991–999, 1993

Trull TJ, McCrae RC: A five-factor perspective on personality disorder research, in Personality Disorders and the Five-Factor Model of Personality. Edited by Costa PT Jr, Widiger TA. Washington, DC, American Psychological Association, 2002, pp 45–57

Valenstein AF: The psycho-analytic situation: affects, emotional reliving, and insight in the psychoanalytic process. Int J Psychoanal 43:315–324, 1962

van den Bosch LM, Verheul R, Langeland W, et al: Trauma, dissociation, and post-traumatic stress disorder in female borderline patients with and without substance abuse problems. Aust N Z J Psychiatry 37:549–555, 2003

Waldinger RJ, Gunderson JG: Completed psychotherapies with borderline patients. Am J Psychother 38:190–202, 1984

Wallerstein RS: Forty-Two Lives in Treatment: A Study of Psychoanalysis and Psychotherapy. New York, Guilford, 1986

Wiggins JS, Pincus AL: Personality structure and the structure of personality disorders, in Personality Disorders and the Five-Factor Model of Personality, 2nd Edition. Edited by Costa PT Jr, Widiger TA. Washington, DC, American Psychological Association, 2002, pp 103–124

Wylan L, Mintz N: Ethnic differences in family attitudes toward psychotic manifestations, with implication for treatment programs. Int J Soc Psychiatry 22:86–95, 1976

Zheng W, Wang W, Huang Z, et al: The structure of traits delineating personality disorder in a Chinese sample. J Personal Disord 16:477–486, 2002

PERSONALITY DISORDERS MOST AMENABLE TO PSYCHOTHERAPY

Borderline Personality Disorder

If we restrict our attention for the moment to the DSM-IV-TR (American Psychiatric Association 2000) personality disorders, a convincing argument can be made that the patients who are most amenable to psychotherapy are those with Cluster C (anxious cluster) disorders. To this short list should be added patients with depressive-masochistic character and patients with hysteric character or hysterical personality disorder (not a DSM-IV-TR diagnostic entity), as mentioned by Clarkin et al. (1999) in their description of borderline personality organization and its domain.

Borderline personality organization is a much broader concept than borderline personality disorder (BPD). Patients with BPD exhibit the characteristics of borderline personality organization, which include a poorly integrated sense of identity (Erikson 1956) but an intact capacity for reality testing. Other characteristics of borderline personality organization are primitivity of defense mechanisms, reduced ability to handle stressful situ-

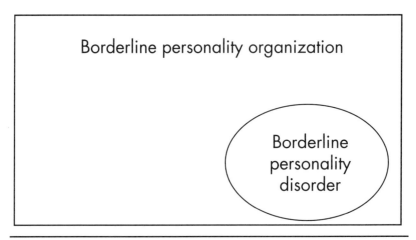

FIGURE 2–1.   The domains of borderline personality organization and borderline personality disorder.

ations, impulsivity, and impairment in the ability to channel anxiety into constructive hobbies and other avocations, such as reading.

Figure 2–1 shows the comparative sizes of the domains of borderline personality organization and BPD in the general population. Kernberg estimated the prevalence of borderline personality organization to be 10% in the general population (O. Kernberg, personal communication, 1975); the prevalence of BPD is approximately 2.5% (Widiger and Frances 1989).

As Figure 2–2 illustrates, some of the other personality disorders often, although not always, overlap conceptually with the characteristics of borderline personality organization. There is far more overlap involving these other disorders—not only overlap with BPD but overlap with each other—than is shown on the diagram. Most patients with histrionic personality disorder, for example, fit within the domain of borderline personality organization and also have comorbid BPD. Many histrionic persons are also narcissistic, and some show paranoid or antisocial traits as well.

As for patients with Cluster C disorders, many function at a higher level than that of patients with borderline personality organization. They show what Kernberg (1977) identified as neurotic personality organization, in which the identity sense is reasonably well integrated. But a proportion of patients with hysteric personality, obsessive-compulsive personality, or depressive-masochistic personality, as well as a proportion of those with dependent personality or avoidant personality, function at the borderline level (that is, they show borderline personality organization). In addition, the more psychologically impaired of those patients may meet the criteria for

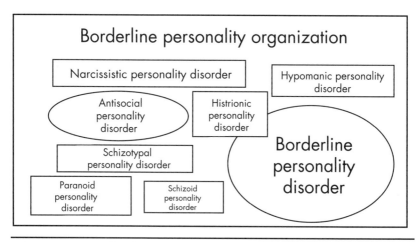

FIGURE 2-2.   The domain of borderline personality organization in relation to borderline personality disorder and other personality disorders.

BPD. To describe these patients, some investigators have coined portmanteau words such as *hysteroid* or *obsessoid* to draw attention both to the coloration of the personality and to the seriousness of pathology (Cornfield and Malen 1978; Easser and Lesser 1965). There is less overlap, both conceptually and clinically, between the Cluster A disorders and BPD, even though patients with paranoid, schizoid, or schizotypal disorder usually function at the level of borderline personality organization. As I mentioned in Chapter 1, some persons with mild paranoid traits function at a higher level, as do certain aloof and markedly reserved "schizoid" persons. Greater overlap exists between antisocial personality disorder and both borderline personality organization and BPD. In addition, a proportion of persons with antisocial personality disorder—the less impulsive or violent ones— have an intact identity sense and function at a high level socially, managing to elude arrest or public censure through their cleverness at conning others.

The focus of this chapter, however, is on the borderline patients who are the most accessible to therapy. I include depressive-masochistic persons in this category, and one could also include the patients Phillips et al. (1998) described under the heading of depressive personality, the features of which are outlined in Appendix B of DSM-IV-TR (American Psychiatric Association 2000, p. 788–789).

Phillips et al. (1998) drew attention to the fact that *depressive personality* (emphasizing cheerlessness, a sense of inadequacy and low self-esteem, self-blame, worrisome and pessimistic attitudes, and a tendency to be critical of others) is not coextensive with *dysthymia*, which has as symptoms poor appetite, sleep disturbance, low energy, and poor concentration, as well as low self-esteem, although one-third of the subjects with depressive personality they studied also had dysthymia.

The *depressive-masochistic personality* (a type more likely to be recognized by the psychoanalytic community than in general psychiatry) may be viewed as a combination of the depressive personality features just described with the features of "self-defeating personality," as described in DSM-III-R (American Psychiatric Association 1987). The attributes of self-defeating personality include choosing people and situations that lead to disappointment or mistreatment, rejection of the help of others, and inciting of angry or rejecting responses from others. This personality type is explicated more fully by Millon and Davis (2000, p. 492ff.). In the older psychoanalytic literature, the concept of masochism was associated with being female (Berliner 1958; Brenner 1959; Deutsch 1965). More recently it has been recognized that masochistic personality is about equally distributed between men and women (Reich 1987).

Patients who meet the criteria for BPD frequently have depressive symptoms—at least at the level of dysthymia, and often with bouts of major depression—and also exhibit many masochistic (in the sense of "self-defeating") traits. The manipulative suicide gestures so common in the histories of BPD patients can certainly be seen in this light, in line with the comment of McGuire and Troisi (1998) that, from the standpoint of evolutionary psychiatry, borderline pathology represents a "failed attempt" to secure attachment to a supportive person. The emotional blackmail involved in manipulative suicide gestures is bound to fail and therefore qualifies as "self-defeating."

Despite this pattern, the borderline patients who show the greatest accessibility to psychotherapy usually have two features in common. First, they have as a secondary personality constellation a disorder in the anxious cluster or a disorder that has the anxious and inhibited traits of that cluster, even though the disorder is not included among the current DSM categories. Patients with *hysteric personality*, for example, whether associated with the neurotic personality organization or borderline personality organization, show fewer of the "dramatic" attributes shown by patients with histrionic personality disorder, at least those enumerated in DSM-III-R (novelty-seeking, egocentricity, tendency to be demanding, and angry outbursts). In DSM-IV (American Psychiatric Association 1994) and DSM-IV-TR, these items were toned down, which made the profile of histrionic personality disorder very similar to that of the hysteric personality of psychoanalytic tradition. The classic hysteric patient was pictured as outwardly somewhat seductive but inhibited and rather timorous sexually, more apt to be ingratiating than to throw tantrums, and more anxious and insecure than impulsive. Likewise, depressive-masochistic persons fit best the criteria for the anxious-inhibited group of disorders.

Second, the borderline patients (with borderline personality organization or BPD) who have the greatest accessibility to therapy are those who show to the greatest degree the *positive* characteristics enumerated in Chapter 1, including a high level of psychological mindedness, good character, high levels of motivation and perseverance, candor, and a good capacity for object relations (that is, a capacity for intimacy).

These considerations provide the background for a discussion of the treatment approaches advocated for optimal results with borderline patients, especially those with the greatest promise of a favorable long-term outcome.

APPROACHES IN THE TREATMENT OF BORDERLINE PATIENTS

By amenability or accessibility to psychotherapy I am referring not just to one type of therapy but rather to the group of currently popular and accepted psychotherapeutic approaches as a whole. These approaches vary over a wide range and reflect a number of psychotherapy training schools and their respective orientations. Among the most important types, each developed for effectiveness in the treatment of borderline patients, are 1) *psychoanalytically oriented therapy*, 2) *cognitive-behavioral therapy*, and 3) *supportive therapy*. Each of these categories represents a family of subtypes. Psychoanalytically oriented therapy, for example, encompasses the exploratory approach advocated by Gunderson (2001), which includes containment and supportive measures that may be needed by many borderline patients in the early phases of therapy; the Self Psychology approach of Kohut (1971), which also contains supportive elements; the method utilized by Masterson (1976); and the transference-focused approach developed by Kernberg (1984, pp. 97–176; Clarkin et al. 1999), in which supportive interventions are kept to a minimum. Cognitive-behavioral approaches include that of Beck and Freeman (1990, pp. 176–207) and the dialectical behavior therapy developed by Linehan (1993). Supportive approaches earmarked for borderline patients were developed by Kroll (1993), who emphasized the relationship between BPD and posttraumatic stress disorder; by Dawson and MacMillan (1993); and by Rockland (1989), who integrated psychodynamic concepts and supportive elements.

Studies of several different approaches have demonstrated comparable results in diminishing the tendency to self-destructive behaviors in BPD patients. Linehan et al. (1994) showed this response in a randomized study of dialectical behavior therapy. Bateman and Fonagy (1999, 2001) in England and Clarkin et al. (2001) also showed this response for psychoanalytically oriented approaches in randomized studies that included a control group. The earlier study by Wallerstein (1986), conducted at the Menninger Clinic, did not use randomization to different treatment methods, but his long-term follow-up data suggested similar effectiveness with either psychoanalytically oriented therapy or supportive therapy. Although the long-term treatment studies of the 1980s did not include control groups, these studies showed that many patients with BPD ultimately did well with any of the three main approaches (Stone 1990a). Some patients started out with a supportive therapy and later moved to a more psychodynamic approach or to one form or another of cognitive-behavioral treatment (McGlashan 1986; Stone 1990b). Although definitive answers are not yet available, these studies provided useful clues for addressing two important questions: 1) Which borderline patients are most amenable to psychotherapy in general? and 2) Are there certain characteristics that predispose patients to optimal results with one approach but that might militate against similar results with other approaches?

Besides the many variables discussed in Chapter 1, several other factors are pertinent to the question of amenability to psychotherapy in general and to the question about which BPD patients might do better with a particular approach. As for why the different psychotherapies all seem to have a reasonable measure of effectiveness, Ryle (1984) suggested that most patients have the capacity to integrate differently located treatment-induced changes into similar revisions of their cognitive systems. A hypothetical example may make this point clearer. Imagine a borderline patient with body dysmorphic disorder who believes that her nose is "not shapely," even though other people regard her as quite attractive. By using a psychodynamic technique, the therapist might succeed in helping the patient uncover key patterns from the past that led to this exaggerated and unrealistic assumption. As this material came to light, the patient might shake off the unrealistic assumption and feel emboldened to confront social situations she had hitherto avoided. Here, dynamic therapy promoted behavioral change. But one could also picture a therapist with a cognitive-behavioral orientation who might put the spotlight on the unrealistic assumption and exhort the patient to enter the feared arena of social gatherings to test whether others did—or did not—shun her because of her "unshapely" nose. With this treatment, the patient might well become convinced that her fears were unfounded and that her self-image had been distorted. This positive change might inspire her to reconsider the pattern of taunting remarks in the past from family members or school acquaintances that had created the distorted self-image in the first place. The unexpected positive feedback from others might gradually overturn her former convictions about being ugly. She might begin to realize that the remarks in the past may have been made because of envy or some other negative attitude and were reflections of psychological problems of others. Here, a cognitive-behavioral change led to more realistic dynamic insight. Wherever one enters the "circle" of interlocking mental schemata—whether at the point of self-conceptions or at the point of behavioral patterns—benefits that develop at one point in the circle tend to induce beneficial responses at other points. This observation begs the question: are there certain patients, or certain symptom patterns, where it would be more efficient to intervene first at the dynamic level or first at the cognitive-behavioral level? And with which patients would it make no measurable difference where the therapist started, so long as the therapist was well trained and highly skilled at one of the main treatment methods? One variable that may hold a key to the resolution of these questions is the patient's cognitive style.

THE PATIENT'S COGNITIVE STYLE

The term *cognitive style* relates to the primary and typical manner in which people process information, think about their internal and external worlds, and deal, by means of various defense mechanisms, with the interpersonal environment. Cognitive style refers also to the perceptual distortions, attentional biases, and appraisal mechanisms according to which people assess their psychosocial environment (Millon and Davis 2000, p. 62). The patterns of distortions, if such patterns form and persist, also constitute cognitive style. Millon and Davis (2000, p. 66) construed each of the major personality disorders—the DSM-IV-TR personality disorder categories plus sadistic, depressive, negativistic ("passive-aggressive"), and masochistic personalities—as being manifested in a particular cognitive style. Paranoid persons, for example, exhibit a "suspicious" style. Borderline persons show a "capricious" style, owing to their tendency to swing arbitrarily from one attitudinal posture to the polar opposite following minor stimuli or provocations.

The topic of cognitive style has been discussed in a number of interrelated contexts, and not all authors assign the same meaning to the term. Some authors focus on the patterns of "coping styles" with which people deal with stressful situations (Bijttebier et al. 2001). For example, the preferred strategy for coping may be a pattern of increased attention or of avoidance. Another manifestation of cognitive style is whether an internalizing (turning against the self) or an externalizing strategy for dealing with interpersonal stress is used (Kwon 1999). Patients exhibiting dysphoria, for example, typically show a turning against the self, including the self-blame and exaggerated guilt that are the hallmarks of the depressive personality. This style has also been called *intropunitive* and may be seen as an exaggeration of an introspective cognitive style (which is not confined to depressed persons and is also seen in bulimic patients) (Phillips et al. 1997) and the tendency to want to *make changes within oneself* to better adapt to the interpersonal environment—that is, an *autoplastic* adaptation (Frosch 1983, pp. 413–418). Paranoid persons, in contrast, try to change the environment to better suit their own needs; this strategy is *alloplastic* adaptation and is accompanied by an externalizing cognitive style. The manipulative threats and suicide gestures of certain borderline patients also represent alloplastic measures.

What are the implications of cognitive style for borderline patients and their relative amenability to psychotherapy? To begin with, it is important to note that not all borderline patients (both patients with borderline personality organization and the more disturbed BPD group) exhibit the capricious cognitive style, and not all are primarily alloplastic in their interactions with others. Some borderline patients are remarkably introspective and autoplastic (especially those with concomitant depressive-masochistic traits), and although they may show rapid shifts between idealizing and devaluing attitudes toward a love object, they may remain attached to that one object—that is, they are not fickle or flighty and are not capricious with respect to object choice. Borderline patients with this profile tend to do well with psychotherapy—probably with psychotherapy of any type but definitely with psychoanalytically oriented (or psychodynamic) approaches. In contrast, borderline patients who demonstrate a "concrete" cognitive style show little introspective capacity and are probably not good candidates for psychodynamic therapy (Weiner and Crowder 1986). The treatment studies thus far, even those with randomization to two or more different therapy types, did not address the cognitive styles of the borderline patients who were followed. These studies found that some patients did very well in therapy and that others did poorly or dropped out, but the correlations between these subgroups and their respective cognitive styles were not examined. It remains a matter of expert opinion that the most introspective and least capricious or impulsive borderline patients are more likely to reap the benefits of psychotherapy, especially of a dynamic therapy.

THE THERAPIST FACTOR

In addition to the patient's cognitive style, variables that pertain to the therapist also affect amenability to psychotherapy, especially for borderline patients. The *therapist factor* is a seemingly hidden set of variables that complicates the task of ascertaining which psychotherapy approach might be best for a particular borderline patient. Therapists obviously differ in personality (which includes their own cognitive style), experience, talent, and sangfroid. Therapists such as Harold Searles (1986), who primarily use intuitive means of relating to borderline patients, experience patients who happen to "click" well with that approach as easily accessible to therapy. In contrast, therapists who rely on a strictly logical approach might find the same patients baffling and hard to reach. Another set of borderline patients, with a different cognitive style, will respond better to a therapist with a logical mind-set and might be put off by intuitive hunches that seem far-fetched.

As for *sangfroid*, therapists often find that their coolness and comfort in dealing with emergencies is challenged severely in working with borderline patients, who have a propensity for making manipulative suicide gestures and, at times, very serious suicide attempts. Therapists who are cool under fire may therefore experience certain borderline patients as not all that difficult to work with and quite amenable to therapy, while other therapists, not blessed with this sangfroid, might see the same patients as nightmarishly disturbing persons whom they would like nothing to do with. An example may make this distinction clearer:

> **A young woman with BPD** had spent her later teen years in special schools for emotionally disturbed children. Along the way she had made a number of suicide gestures, and at age 20 years she had been admitted to a long-term psychiatric unit for intensive therapy. Her therapist over the past 2 years had been finishing his residency training. Shortly before he was to graduate, he let her know he would be away on vacation for 2 weeks. During the last session before he was to leave on vacation, she threatened to jump off a nearby bridge. Given her past behavior, this threat was not to be taken lightly. Pausing a moment, her therapist smiled and said, "Before you do anything, let me have a half hour's lead time." When she asked what for, he replied, "Well, in that time, I could alert the police, and they could get the Coast Guard mobilized to go out and spread a net and catch you!" His mock-serious response had the desired effect. She did nothing to carry out her threat and endured his absence with a minimum of symptomatic behavior. Each participant in the dialogue had a subtext. The patient was saying, in effect, "I can't bear to be apart from you for so long a time, but if I make you worry that I'll kill myself if you leave, maybe you'll lose your nerve and won't leave." The therapist was saying, in effect, "If you threaten me with something so outrageous, after we've worked together for 2 years, and show so little ability to handle a minor stress like a 2-week absence, you can count on me to pull out all the stops to prevent you from coming to any harm." But his actual response was wrapped in wry humor and did not cause loss of

face to his patient. Earlier in her treatment he would not have been able to make light of her threat in that way, because they would not have had enough experience between them to foster the mutual trust that allowed him to speak directly to her unconscious, as it were, in the way that he did. Had the therapist panicked, instead of displaying the sangfroid—the compassionate coolness—that he did, he might have ordered the patient to be on a close suicide watch (which he felt she no longer needed) during the time he was away. This move would have delayed the patient's development of the inner strength to handle separations more calmly and might have marred their relationship by showing her that he didn't believe she was any more resilient now than she had been years earlier. The patient went on to make an excellent recovery and continued to work with this therapist for several years.

Flexibility is another therapist variable that influences whether a borderline patient is regarded as highly amenable to psychotherapy or highly resistant. Even if a therapist has been trained originally in just one form of therapy—psychodynamic, cognitive-behavioral, or supportive—he or she will need to be able to make shifts from time to time, sometimes suddenly, according to the frequent and unpredictable changes in the circumstances of the borderline patient (Stone 1990b). This need to shift approaches is more pertinent in the beginning phases of therapy than in the later phases, although flexibility may be needed at any point in treatment.

The inability to handle ordinary life stresses adroitly is a prominent characteristic of borderline patients; Kernberg (1967) referred to this *lowered anxiety tolerance* as one of the nonspecific criteria for borderline personality organization. Because of this feature, a course of treatment can be going smoothly for extended periods only to be interrupted when the patient shows a storm of affect or outright self-destructive behavior. This abrupt change may catch the therapist by surprise, because the stressfulness of the stimulus seems insignificant to the therapist. Suddenly, there is a need for limit-setting, an extra session, a phone call at an odd hour, an urgent conversation with a relative, a trip to the emergency room—all in the interest of aborting a serious disruption to treatment or a life-threatening episode of acting out. Whatever the main therapeutic modality had been, a shift into another type of intervention may be needed.

Many interventions of this sort have been described by Waldinger and Gunderson (1987) under the heading of *action parameters* in their book *Effective Psychotherapy With Borderline Patients: Case Studies*. As the authors wrote, "The term 'action parameters' is employed…to identify overt behavioral interventions transcending the boundaries of the usual listening position of psychotherapy" (p. 198). Waldinger and Gunderson listed 40 action parameters, including hospitalization, escorting a patient to a safe place, altering appointment schedules, directive remarks (such as exhortations that the patient stop drinking and enroll in Alcoholics Anonymous), focus on practical problems, and arrangement for an interim therapist during an absence. In other respects, Waldinger and Gunderson's book represents a manual of treatment (concentrated on a psychodynamic-exploratory approach) similar to the more recent manuals of Clarkin et al. (1999) for transference-focused psychotherapy, Luborsky (1984) for supportive-expressive therapy, and Linehan (1993) for dialectical behavior therapy. In each of these sets of guidelines, the authors acknowledged the need for occasional modifications from the "purity" of the approaches they describe.

A similar point about flexibility was made recently by Judd and Mc-Glashan (2003), who mentioned, with a wisdom born of many years in the "front lines," that work with BPD patients is not for everyone. In their words, "Flexibility and creativity within an ethical and commonsense frame of reference not only are essential [in the treatment of BPD patients] but make the work challenging and rewarding" (p. 173).

The following example describes the treatment of a borderline patient that began in a predominantly psychoanalytically oriented mode, with an emphasis on the transference manifestations. At critical junctures in the treatment, supportive interventions were precipitated by suicide threats and gestures. At a later point, behavior modification techniques were brought to bear on the peculiarities of the patient's habit patterns. Medications were also used. This multiplicity of approaches was employed in a flexible way to meet the fluctuating demands and priorities of the clinical situation.

> **The patient was a single 30-year-old woman** when I first began working with her. She had been hospitalized twice for suicide attempts, once when she was in her late teens and again in her mid-20s. Her father had died when she was young; afterward, a pattern of mutual dependence had evolved between her and her mother such that neither was comfortable when separated from the other.
>
> The premature death of her father colored her view of life, which seemed to her precarious and fraught with hazard at every turn. She was often agoraphobic and in general led her life along paths that minimized risk as much as possible. In addition, she had an intense preoccupation with germs, which led her to take extraordinary precautions to avoid contact with the myriad things she considered "dirty." The germ phobia and the compulsive measures she adopted to remain "clean" were outgrowths primarily of her fundamentalist religious upbringing. This upbringing had created an intolerable conflict between her longing for intimacy and marriage and her conviction that sex was "dirty" and that sexual activity of any sort was sinful.
>
> She had developed anorexia nervosa during adolescence and was still

underweight, at times dangerously so. In the early phase of our work, the focus was on her eating disorder and the accompanying distortion in self-image. The latter amounted to body dysmorphic disorder, inasmuch as she regarded herself as "fat" even as her weight slipped below 90 pounds. She recounted dreams in which she was walking in the street as a fat woman approached her and she ran in terror from the fat woman, as though the mere proximity of the woman would magically transform the patient into a morbidly obese creature.

Her associations to the obese woman led her to thoughts of pregnancy. She feared pregnancy, partly because of the (in her view) unattractive shape pregnancy imposed on a woman but mostly because she felt herself in no way ready to take on the role of a sexually active woman, let alone to assume the obligations of motherhood. She also feared that her mother would resent any efforts on her daughter's part to lead an independent life, which would upset the comfortable symbiosis that held them together. When the patient expressed any desire to meet men (hitherto studiously avoided), she assumed I would strongly disapprove. Exploration of the transference implications—she saw me as a duplicate of her sternly disapproving mother—led eventually to a lessening of her fears, and she did begin to go to social events where she could meet men. A serious relationship with a man developed some months later, but as the relationship progressed to include sexual activity, she experienced an upsurge of guilt and germ phobia. As she described her activity with her boyfriend in our sessions, she sometimes "tuned out," staring at the ceiling and talking to herself, saying "You're garbage." I could interrupt these brief dissociative episodes by clapping my hands (a supportive intervention), which would break the spell and restore our communication. During the dissociative episodes she would "mix me up" with her mother and assume that I felt she was "garbage" for daring to indulge in sex with her boyfriend.

Some months later she and her boyfriend became engaged. The ambivalence relating to sex intensified; she was at once much happier yet more guilt-ridden and, because of her guilt, more compulsive about germ avoidance. She was already taking fluoxetine in an effort to correct the compulsive cleaning symptoms, but the medication had only limited effectiveness. I had also prescribed small doses of a neuroleptic to control her tendency to cognitive distortions and dissociative experiences. I felt it might be useful to add behavioral interventions such as *flooding*, where she would be forced to handle money or newspapers, objects she was loath to touch because of the germs from other people that they supposedly carried. This maneuver had a favorable result in that she grew less apprehensive about touching many previously taboo objects. But her symptoms flared up again, and she became suicidal once more, during a visit she and her fiancé made to her relatives in California. There, she was caught in a crossfire between various relatives, some of whom thought well of the fiancé and others of whom did not. She made matters worse by stopping her medications, which led to a recurrence of cognitive disturbance and suicidal ideation.

By the time she returned (a day earlier than her fiancé), she was acutely suicidal, and she came for her session simply to "say her goodbyes" to me.

As she prepared to leave, I held her by the wrist and, with my other hand, dialed the number of the emergency unit of the nearest hospital. I took her there by taxi and waited for several hours, after briefing the on-call psychiatrist about her situation and her medication regime. Fortunately, her equilibrium was quickly restored, and her medications were restarted. I later dropped her off at her apartment, with an arrangement to meet the next morning. By then she was in much better spirits. Her fiancé arrived in the evening. He was not aware of what she had been through the day before, and this preserved their relationship for the time being. She got to know him better over the next few months and concluded that he was not the right person for her. She became more stable, worked on the ambivalent feelings concerning her mother, grew less dependent on her mother, and developed insight about her morbid fear of becoming "fat." The dynamics behind that fear related to assuming certain key roles of an adult woman—wifehood, pregnancy, and motherhood. As these fears lessened, she was able to move beyond her first relationship. She left treatment after 4 years of twice-weekly sessions. When I contacted her 10 years later for follow-up, she had been married for several years to a man much more suitable than her earlier fiancé and had a 4-year-old daughter. She no longer showed the signs of BPD. She was still a slow and "picky" eater, but she was now of low normal weight.

I chose to present this patient's case to illustrate the flexibility required of therapists who, in their work with borderline patients, must at times of crisis shift away from the main therapeutic approach with which they are most comfortable. This case also illustrates the attributes of a patient with high amenability to psychotherapy. Besides having considerable psychological mindedness, this patient was also a woman of excellent character. She was compassionate, generous, solicitous of others, and of high moral standards—initially, one might say, of exaggeratedly high standards that prevented her from partaking in aspects of life that she had every right to enjoy. She was highly motivated for therapy and persevered in coming to her sessions and in working diligently on her problems, which were severe at the beginning of treatment. An additional factor that facilitated the psychodynamic aspects of her therapy was her ability to work well with the dreams that she reported. Dream analysis deserves greater attention, given that it may play an important role in the psychotherapy of borderline patients, particularly those who demonstrate optimal amenability to therapy.

DREAM ANALYSIS WITH BORDERLINE PATIENTS

Working with dreams can facilitate the therapist's understanding of the inner, hidden layers of conflict and emotion with which borderline patients struggle, and it can shorten the time it takes for this understanding to come about. As vast as the literature on borderline personality and its treatment has become, the portion addressing dreams is minuscule. I addressed the topic elsewhere (Koenigsberg et al. 2000, pp 207–228; Stone 1979), and it is accorded a few pages in the manual on transference-focused psychotherapy by Clarkin et al. (1999), who wrote, "In the early stages of treatment, dream analysis consisted of selecting an aspect of then manifest dream as an element to be integrated with transference interpretations. [Later] dream analysis may take the more classical form of inviting the patient to free-associate regarding the…manifest dream content, connecting these associations…with the transference dominant at that point" (p. 298). In the books by Gunderson (2001), Kernberg (1984), Kroll (1993), Linehan (1993), and Waldinger and Gunderson (1987), the topic is alluded to only briefly or not at all. A British psychoanalyst of an earlier generation, Michael Balint (1968/1979), who wrote about a "basic fault" in patients who would now be classified as exhibiting borderline personality organization, had a few salient remarks about the dreams of these patients. He explained the basic fault as a "fault in the basic structure of the personality, something akin to a defect or a scar," that leads the patient to feel that "nothing in the world can ever be worthwhile unless something that was taken away or withheld—usually something unattainable in the present—is restored to him" (p. 88). Balint illustrated this feeling through one of his patient's dreams: "She was walking in a wood; suddenly a large flesh-coloured bird swooped down, hit her violently, and made a gash in her forehead. The patient was stunned and fell down unconscious. The terrible thing was, the bird never looked back; it was quite unconcerned about what it had done" (p. 89). Balint did not mention the patient's associations in detail, but we get a picture here of a patient who may have been traumatized in her earliest years by a harsh, neglectful parent—one who never had a passing thought about the impact of such treatment and never apologized to the patient for the hurt that had been inflicted. I say "may have been" because those were my associations, not the patient's. Had she told me that dream, those are the ideas that would have sprung up in my mind about the manifest content, and my inquiry would have taken that direction. I would, in other words, have found the patient's dream communication very useful in suggesting the dominant emotion and dynamism in that session.

The opinion of the French psychoanalyst André Green (1977) about the utility of dream analysis with borderline patients is quite different. He went so far as to say: "As many workers in the field have realized, dream analysis in the treatment of the borderline is, as a rule, unproductive" (p. 38). Green explained that "in borderline cases, even though the dream barrier is effective, the dream's purpose is not the working through of instinct derivatives, but rather the unburdening of the psychic apparatus from the painful stimuli" (p. 39). Further, he added that one can observe dream failures in these patients; they may awaken to prevent dreaming or to prevent finding themselves surrounded by a strange, disquieting atmosphere. I believe Green is quite correct in this last point. Nightmares that awaken the dreamer can be seen as "dream failures," and many borderline patients sometimes report these terrifying dreams, especially patients whose past was marred by sexual abuse or brutal physical abuse. Dreams of being dead—which Freud thought were impossible (as if the Ego could not conceive of its own death)—do occasionally occur in borderline (and in psychotic) patients. I will address this topic in a later section in this chapter.

I am not in accord, however, with Green's point about the lack of utility in pursuing dream analysis with borderline patients. To the contrary, there are many occasions when a report of the manifest content by itself, even without the subsequent associations, unlocks material in borderline patients that demystifies a previously incomprehensible issue, allowing the therapist to make interventions that are not only useful in unearthing the central dynamics, but that bring quick relief from intolerable feelings in the very session in which the dream is reported. I am willing to acknowledge that a "therapist factor" is operating here—I am almost alone among my colleagues in stressing the utility of dream analysis with borderline patients, and so I may be somehow neurologically "wired" to show this preference and to take particular enjoyment in this approach in my work with these patients. Thus, borderline patients who, besides showing many of the favorable factors enumerated in Chapter 1, recall dreams easily and work well with them strike me as more amenable to psychotherapy than they might appear to another therapist less attuned to this form of communication. One should keep in mind that Balint and Green designated patients as "borderline" by using criteria that were different both from the DSM-IV-TR criteria for BPD and from Kernberg's criteria for borderline personality organization. Thus, their observations about dream analysis in "borderlines" may be valid for the patients they treated, although not necessarily for other borderline patients. The usefulness of dream analysis in a *variety* of clinical conditions (apart from BPD) was highlighted recently by Rosalind Cartwright (2005), who also mentioned several reasons why this technique has lately fallen into desuetude. For example, she wrote that dream content "is inherently subjective and not open to objective observation, the heart of scientific methods" (p. 20).

The caveat about differing criteria for "borderline" applies to the extensive comments by Searles (1986) concerning psychotherapy with borderline patients, because he too was using a different diagnostic schema from those of Kernberg or DSM. Searles described certain borderline patients who seemed to exemplify Green's assertion about the lack of utility of dream analysis in this domain—although for a different reason. Searles was treating a man in his 30s who told him, "I had a dream last night. I have *lots* of dreams; my trouble is that I can't *remember* my dreams. It's an uncooperative part of me that I resent, because my dreams say things more clearly and succinctly than *I* do when I digress throughout my sessions" (Searles 1986, p. 121). Searles felt that this man was unconsciously jealous of his dreams, as equivalent to persons "more articulate" than himself.

One could add that this patient may have at the same time taken a secret pleasure, as part of a passive-aggressive personality, in frustrating Searles by promising so much (dream material) and giving so little. I had occasion years ago to work with a passive-aggressive man (with borderline personality organization rather than DSM BPD) who had grown up terrified by his extraordinarily irascible and menacing father. The patient reported dreams only very rarely and seldom had any associations to them—one of many attributes of his meager amenability to psychotherapy. Yet the dreams he did report were revealing nonetheless. In one of his dreams, which came after a day when his father had upbraided him mercilessly for some minor failing, a Roman general, probably Caesar, was leading a legion of spear-carrying troops rushing on horseback toward the cowering patient, who awoke with a start just before the hurled spears were about to penetrate his backside. How much skill does it take to decipher this dream? Even the patient, ordinarily loath to admit how frightened he was of his father, agreed that there was "probably a connection" between his father's screaming at him the day before and the furious Caesar bearing down on him, poised to strike a fatal blow.

Heinz Kohut (1971), the founder of the Chicago psychoanalytic school of Self Psychology, mentioned the dreams of his borderline patients more frequently, but he too used the term "borderline" in a way that differed considerably from current standards. Furthermore, unlike Searles, who worked extensively with both hospitalized and ambulatory patients, Kohut concentrated on ambulatory patients in his private practice. For Kohut, "borderline" was not so much a diagnosis made at the time of an initial evaluation as it was a label to designate patients who proved, after a period of some months, refractory to the techniques of conventional analysis.

I can find nothing in the manifest content of the dreams Kohut mentioned that suggests the kind of primitive, grotesque imagery that would set them apart from the dreams of better-integrated neurotic patients capable of classical analysis. Nor does Kohut provide enough clinical material about the patients in his examples to allow them to be placed with any accuracy along the spectrum of patients with BPD, let alone borderline personality organization. A hint of the "sicker," more primitive quality I have noted in the dreams of many borderline patients can be found in the dreams that Kohut mentioned in connection with an introverted patient he described in a later book (Kohut 1977). This patient had dreams throughout his life "in which he experienced himself as a brain at the top of a substanceless body" (p. 126). As I discuss later in this chapter, this kind of fragmentation of the body image occurring in a dream is, if not actually a neurophysiological "marker" of borderline (in the current sense) psychopathology, at least a phenomenon more often associated with this psychiatric disorder. Even the sense of danger and impending doom that characterized a dream reported by a patient described in a casebook edited by Kohut's colleague Arnold Goldberg (1978) is not materially different from the frightening quality of dreams occasionally reported by ordinary people. In that dream, the male patient saw himself looking out the window of a high-rise building as a tornado approached; at the end of the dream "he is hanging by his fingertips onto a ceiling beam across the bottom of a staircase, waiting for the tornado to hit" (p. 412).

The most useful comments about dreams in psychosis, some of which apply with equal relevance to borderline conditions, are those of John Frosch (1976, 1983), a psychoanalyst who taught at Bellevue Hospital a generation ago. Frosch had wide experience with hospitalized patients, including those with schizophrenia and with "psychotic character," a term he coined for a syndrome comparable to the current definition of BPD (Frosch 1964, 1970). Frosch cited a study in which the manifest dreams of patients with schizophrenia and persons without schizophrenia were submitted "blind" to a panel of analysts to see whether they could distinguish between the two groups. The correlation was not high, yet it was noted that "the presence of unusual, strange, uncanny and bizarre qualities was more common for the schizophrenic than for the non-schizophrenic dream" (Frosch 1983, p. 37).

Patients with lifelong nightmares, as opposed to the rare emergence of such disturbing dreams, tend to be quite disturbed, and some have a "borderline" diagnosis. The extreme vividness and scariness of certain dreams, especially when the dreamer cannot readily distinguish between the sleeping state and the waking state, are indications of a more serious psychiatric disorder and are in keeping with a vulnerability to psychosis, although they are also compatible with BPD. Frosch described such states in both psychotic and borderline patients, who may reveal that they "are still inside the dream." One of his borderline patients, for example, reported a vivid dream in which her mother was on top of her, having intercourse with her (Frosch

1983, p. 40)—a dream so vivid that she wasn't sure whether such an event had really taken place or not. Dreams that reflect ego disintegration or fragmentation may be prodromal of a psychotic break, and such dreams in borderline patients may come in the wake of acute, overwhelming stress and may be the first indication of the patient's fragility. Examples are offered in the next section. As to whether these terrifying dreams presage psychotic breakdown just because of their manifest content, Frosch (1983) cautioned that therapists must take into account what is happening in the therapy at the time and also whether the patient showed previous examples of ego defect (p. 47).

DREAMS OF FRAGMENTATION AND DREAMS OF BEING DEAD

Although most dreams of borderline patients do not point to serious psychopathology and are similar to the dreams of better-integrated persons, some of these patients' dreams do have the eerie quality alluded to by Frosch. All dreams, whatever their manifest content, are helpful in highlighting the patient's underlying psychodynamics, but the dreams with special significance are of two main types: 1) dreams in which the dreamer's body is mutilated or fragmented in a serious way that would imply dire or fatal consequences (not just the loss of a tooth or some hair, which would not affect one's overall health) and 2) dreams of being literally dead. Judd and McGlashan (2003), in a description of the sickest of four former BPD patients from Chestnut Lodge, mentioned that this patient, who was the most severely traumatized, abused, and neglected of the four, reported fantasies and dreams of people being dismembered (p. 135). Perhaps a third variety of significant dreams can be identified: one in which terrible things are about to happen either to the dreamer or to someone of importance in the dreamer's everyday life. An example of the latter can be seen in the dream of a hospitalized borderline patient I treated during my residency training. The dream occurred the day before I was to take a week's vacation. The patient reported: "I dreamed you were flying back from Europe. As the plane was about to land, it crashed into thousands of pieces and your body was reduced to splinters from all the broken glass." This dream included both mutilation and death—of the dreamer's therapist rather than of herself. Shortly thereafter, however, she reported another dream in which she was the victim: "I dreamed I was hooked up to the electric chair. Someone pulled the switch, and I died. When I awoke, I was surprised that I was still alive."

Dreams of being dead—in seeming contravention of Freud's dictum—constitute a phenomenon that I have noted in many borderline patients over the years, and only once in a better-integrated patient who was functioning at the neutral level of organization, according to Kernberg's model (Kernberg 1977). That patient, however, had severe obsessive-compulsive personality with narcissistic traits, coupled with the symptoms of bipolar II disorder, along with a family history of affective disorder.

The first dream a patient reports in therapy is often considered to contain the kernel of the most important psychodynamics, alerting the therapist to the path that will prove most fruitful in the ensuing exploration of the patient's primary conflicts. If that dream happens to bespeak a fatal mutilation, it may be an indicator of a borderline (or psychotic) condition, the other features of which may not yet have become apparent. This point is illustrated by the following dream, which was the first dream mentioned, in the second session, during my work with a outwardly well-functioning woman in her mid-20s who was in the grips of severe and apparently irresolvable marital difficulties. She reported, "I am in the recovery room of a hospital. On the gurney all my internal organs had been placed, some to the left, some to the right: the heart, lungs, kidneys, spleen. The surgeon who operated on me comes in to reassure me, saying, 'Don't worry, lady; everything's going to be all right.' Only he is drunk, and his speech is quite slurred."

The patient did not experience herself as "dead" in the dream, yet death would be the inescapable result of such mutilation, which one would associate with an autopsy. Her father, as it happened, had been a surgeon (he had died a few years before) and had also been an alcoholic. The manifest content told me two things right away: she had a more fragile ego structure than I had initially thought and, from the standpoint of the transference, she saw me as a replica of her unreliable father. I was about to analyze her—that is, "take her apart"—but she had no great confidence I would be able to put all the pieces back together, let alone cure her illness. Subsequent work with this patient made it clear that she would have met the DSM-IV-TR criteria for BPD, although the case is from the era before DSM-III (American Psychiatric Association 1980) first included BPD. She was easily able to grasp the importance of this initial dream and indeed showed most of the characteristics of patients who are highly amenable to psychotherapy. After a stormy period lasting about 2 years, she eventually divorced, married a much more supportive and affectionate husband, and has now remained well for the past 26 years.

The following dream came during the early months in my work with a married woman in her late 20s. She would qualify for a diagnosis of mixed personality disorder with histrionic and obsessive features; she met Kernberg's criteria for borderline personality organization but fell one item short of the DSM-IV-TR criteria for BPD. She showed identity disturbance, stormy relationships, lability of affect, and inordinate anger, although the latter was displayed only with her husband. She had begun to realize that her marriage could not be salvaged, but she had great worries about what would become of her after a divorce. She reported this dream: "I was trying to swim across a river. Before I got to the other side, I encounter a shark, and it bites off my left leg. So I end up stranded and bleeding to death in the middle of the water. I was just about to faint when I woke up, frightened."

As to her associations, she likened the shark to her husband, who constantly "nibbled" at her, in the sense of criticizing her and humiliating her as if she were stupid. During the first year of therapy, she obtained a divorce and overcame her fear of not being able to get safely to the "other side." By the time her treatment ended 2 years later, she had remarried. The new relationship was much more harmonious than the first marriage. She later on obtained a doctoral degree and became a college professor; she is now (40 years later) a grandmother and continues to teach. She has not been in treatment in the intervening years, but when she was in therapy, she worked assiduously, was highly motivated and introspective, and showed all the attributes of *good character* that conduce to a favorable outcome.

A 38-year-old man with borderline personality and concomitant schizotypal personality often had dreams that were notable for the absence of the usual "censorship" mechanism that operates in better-integrated persons to shield the dreamer from various potentially alarming connections. His dreams had a kind of "nakedness" that is common to the dreams of more fragile persons. The following dream was the first dream this man reported in therapy: "You are in bed with me—only you're dead. I wonder, 'What'll I do now?' I decide I'll just keep you with me; I'd feel safer that way."

Healthier, neurotic-level patients simply do not incorporate a new therapist into their dream lives after the first meeting. One senses a desperate hunger for attachment in patients who dream of their therapists right off, undisguised, as though their need is so urgent that it overwhelms the usual wariness about a stranger that makes ordinary people wait for several weeks or months before they feel comfortable enough to see others (including therapists) undisguised in their dreams. This man's dream had the added bizarre feature that I was "dead," which raised the question of what good I could be to him, even if so close by, if I were dead. In his elaboration of the dream, he acknowledged that as a corpse I wouldn't be as useful to him as I would be alive, but there would be the advantage that *I couldn't leave him—*

as so many other key people in his life had done. This example brings to mind people who engage the services of a taxidermist to perpetuate a beloved cat or dog that has died or, more to the point, the London serial killer Dennis Nilsen (Masters 1986), a schizoid, lonely man who brought men to his apartment for sex, killed them, and kept their bodies under the floorboards until they became rank—a practice that allowed him to maintain his fantasy that he had "company."

Dreams of being (literally) dead may occur in nontraumatized borderline patients with marked depressive features, but sometimes such dreams point to a highly traumatic background. The following dream was reported by a suicidal, and subsequently hospitalized, woman with BPD whose father had involved her in an incestuous relationship throughout her early adolescence: "I take a thin strand of electrical wire and wind it around my leg. Then I pull the wire as tight as I can till it goes right through the flesh down to the thighbone. I then lie on my back and bleed to death." This woman was tormented by the ambivalent emotions concerning her father, which included hatred for his having misused her sexually, side by side with the pleasure of being his "favorite" and the enjoyment she experienced during the sex. Her guilt over the latter was overwhelming and was the primary motive for her suicidal behaviors and her conviction that she deserved to die for having been a willing partner to the incest. As for the wire imagery, she recalled having helped her father do electric wiring around the house during the years the incest took place.

SIGNIFICANT DREAMS IN PATIENTS WITH OTHER PERSONALITY DISORDERS

Many patients with personality disorders other than borderline personality who are excellent candidates for psychotherapy (as judged by the amenability factors discussed in Chapter 1) report dreams early in their treatment that point the way to the crucial dynamics with great clarity. The following vignettes reflect my work with patients exhibiting a variety of personality disorders:

> **A college student with avoidant personality** sought treatment for his shyness with women and his overdependence on his parents. When he was away from home, he would often experience episodes of anxiety and depersonalization, which he referred to as the "dream feeling." These uncomfortable states could be relieved if he returned home and slept in his old bed. His father was a supportive and generally positive figure in his life, but his almost totally deaf mother was an acid-tongued and querulous woman who ruled the household with her demands and criticisms. He had recently given

his mother a Christmas present consisting of a hairbrush and comb set. She screamed at him that it was "junk" and threw it on the floor. The patient tried hard to maintain an image of his mother as a cherished and loving parent, whose interactions with him were unrelated to his inability to form an intimate relationship with a woman. Shortly after his mother's rejection of his present, he reported a dream in which he was mountain climbing. As he reached a particular point near the top of the mountain, he placed his hands on the ledge from which he could then hoist himself to the summit. But his mother, who was wearing ski boots, stepped on his hands, crushing his fingers and sending him plummeting to the bottom. After this dream, he could begin to grasp that his attitude toward his mother was hardly one of unalloyed affection. He began to recognize her cruel side as well.

A young woman with a depressive-masochistic personality had just graduated from a university. She had a flair, as she called it, for falling in love with men who ended up making her feel miserable; some were harsh, others were jealous, and still others, rejecting. When she was 12 years old, her mother, while in the midst of divorce, died in a car crash, leaving the patient in the role of mother to her younger sister. Their father, a successful businessman, was cordial to everyone else but humiliated both his daughters with senseless criticisms and insulting demands. He would dump garbage on the kitchen floor, for example, and make the patient gather up the pieces. If he crossed her path as she emerged from the shower, he would tell her she "smelled awful." Yet at other times he behaved seductively toward her, ogling her in a sexual manner or walking in front of her clad only in his underwear. The first dream the patient reported when she began therapy was as follows: "I'm in bed and little spiders are crawling on me: baby spiders. There is a big spider on the wall that is about to explode, and more little spiders would burst forth. I figure that if I pour honey on the big spider, I can placate it." The big spider was "pumping like a heart." The year before, the patient had become pregnant by her boyfriend and had the pregnancy terminated. She had always been frightened of spiders. This imagery led her to think about her father, of whom she was also always frightened. The "explosion" of the big spider she equated with a man's orgasm and ejaculation. Her father had never molested her sexually, but she felt he often struggled with himself to rein in such an impulse. As her therapy progressed, she began to realize that his contemptuous behavior and remarks were part of a defense to deny that he was attracted to her (a kind of "negative" incest). In time, this interpretation helped her accept him for who he was and to form attachments with men who were less abusive and inconsiderate than were her previous boyfriends.

A man with obsessive-compulsive personality and obsessive-compulsive disorder was referred by his doctor in Haiti to come to the United States in hopes of finding a French-speaking psychiatrist who could help him. He was a successful businessman who had shortly before become engaged to a woman who was divorced. He lived with his mother, who held very rigid religious beliefs and who regarded it a sin for her son to marry a divorcée. Devoted as he was to both women, he was in a state of great conflict. He developed a compulsion in which he had to walk with extreme care in the street, lest he step in dog feces. In addition, he developed an obsession in which he would begin thinking of the Virgin Mary just as he and his fiancée were about to make love, and these thoughts would cause him to lose his erection. This case occurred in the 1960s, long before the era of selective serotonin reuptake inhibitors, so there was little that could be done for the man psychopharmacologically. He was very hesitant to express any negative feelings about his mother, the more so because his father had died the year before and the patient was quite dependent on his mother. Not long after our twice-weekly psychodynamic therapy sessions began, he reported the following dream: "I am walking down a long corridor in my house, when I suddenly encounter my mother. She is angry at me and hurls at me a roll of toilet paper that had been used." The significance of the dream was transparent, and he grasped it immediately: his preoccupation with stepping in feces was linked directly with his awareness that his mother regarded his fiancée in much the same light as that material and was willing to humiliate him any way she could to ensure he did not marry. He began to see that in this respect his mother was being unfair—the fiancée was a lovely and estimable woman, of whom his mother was jealous, lest in her loneliness, she would lose her hold on her son. Once he realized that he had a right to marry his fiancée and that the real "problem" lay with his mother more so than with him, his symptoms subsided. Sometimes the vision of the Virgin would recur as he was having intercourse (now that that had become possible once more), but he could now wave to her as a friendly spirit, rather than fear her as a figure scolding him for being "sinful."

A married woman in her early 30s began therapy in hopes of resolving tensions with her husband. She was a successful stockbroker in a large firm and was an obsessive-compulsive "workaholic," in contrast to her easygoing and less ambitious husband, who worked in the same field. He was keen on having a child; she was just as eager not to. Her younger sister already had two small children. The patient was contemptuous of her sister, referring to her as a "broodmare," and spoke of her two nieces as "mice." Yet she also felt guilty toward her sister and recognized that it was unpopular to be so "down" on traditional feminine values. She began to feel that her marriage was unworkable, given the strength of her sentiments. These sentiments came through in the following dream: "My husband and I are in my folks' home for the holidays. It's stormy outside. My mother lets the cat in, but as she does, squirrels and bears come in, as do some chipmunks and raccoons. All the animals seemed nice at first, but then it got much too crowded. I try to chase them out, except for the cat; I wasn't able to, and then the squirrel attacks the cat." In her associations, the "Noah's ark" of animals (as she called it) represented babies. Her mother was urging her to start a family, symbolized in the dream by the mother letting all the animals in. The patient identified with the cat (the pet she grew up with), which in the dream is being challenged by a smaller animal (the squirrel), just as she would be overwhelmed by the burdens of having a small child. After working on this dream, she no longer felt torn in the conflict about whether to have a child. She was now determined that if she could not have control over the path of the marriage and thus avoid getting pregnant, she would have to end the marriage, which she did several months later.

A young woman with schizotypal personality had recently graduated from college, where she had majored in art. She was uncertain what direction to take in life—whether to pursue a career in art or to work in a different field—because she was unsure if her paintings were good enough to be marketable. Her mother had been chronically depressed. Her father was an executive in a large corporation but was alcoholic and eventually lost his job. He had been abusive physically toward her mother, although he never laid a hand on the patient. Her mother openly favored her brother. The patient had grown up feeling "left out" and had spent much time daydreaming and living in a private world of her own creation. What led her to seek therapy was that she had felt herself attracted to another young woman whom she had gotten to know while at college. She felt conflicted about these feelings, because she had dated men, although she had never formed a satisfying relationship with any of them. As she was struggling with the decision about "which way to go," she had the following dream: "My friend and I had been vacationing together in the islands off Spain. We had to go through Paris on our return to America. In the Paris airport, people were divided into two lines: those who were going to stay in Paris and those who were not. In the larger line of those staying were many women in skirts and fancy frocks. My friend and I were in the shorter line; we were wearing just T-shirts and jeans and were carrying backpacks." The dream, as she associated to it, underlined the shift that was taking place in her sexual orientation. She could not identify with the traditional and conventional feminine stereotype of ladies in skirts and frilly clothes, happy to be in Paris, the center of *haute couture*. She and her friend had to make their lives elsewhere. In the months that followed, she not only firmed up this change by moving into an apartment with her friend, but she also changed fields, going on to graduate school in English, which she eventually taught.

RELATIONSHIP BETWEEN AMENABILITY TO PSYCHOTHERAPY AND PROGNOSIS

The patients described in the brief vignettes just presented would all meet the criteria for borderline personality organization, and most would also satisfy the DSM-IV-TR criteria for BPD. I regarded them all as highly amenable to therapy because of their better-than-average ability to become involved with the process of psychotherapy. Their capacity for introspection was good, as was their psychological mindedness and their ability to understand symbolism. Likewise, their ability to "mentalize"—Fonagy's term—was good; that is, they had to a sufficient degree acquired the abstract reflexive and implicit awareness of the mental states (beliefs, feelings, attitudes, desires, etc.) of other people (Fonagy 2001, pp. 165–168) and of their own mental states. These attributes correlate with attachment, in the sense that optimal parenting fosters successful containment of affects, setting the stage for the development of secure attachment. Only a few of the patients in these vignettes showed secure attachment at the beginning of therapy, and the others showed an entangled form of insecure attachment at the outset, but most progressed to a more secure form after a period of many months to several years in treatment. They were highly motivated to seek and obtain help for their conditions.

These variables are important in establishing amenability to therapy, but they do not by themselves guarantee a good outcome. It would be nearer the truth to say that the *absence* of adequate mentalization, motivation, psychological mindedness, and introspection makes for poor amenability to therapy of whatever sort and conduces to a poor prognosis. Overwhelming abuse and neglect can so hamper the development of mentalization and attachment as to cripple amenability to therapy altogether. In the group of patients depicted in the vignettes, an incest history—but not neglect—was present in two; of the three who had experienced parental neglect, only one had also been physically abused. The patients with secure attachment from the beginning had childhoods that were free of both abuse and neglect. The prognosis in borderline patients, as tested in long-term outcome studies, depends on a multitude of variables, including intelligence, talent, self-discipline, attractiveness, hobbies, and the ability to refrain from abuse of alcohol or drugs (McGlashan 1986; Stone 1990a). Some borderline patients ultimately do well even without much gift for introspection, or even much ability to "click" with a therapist. Yet others possess the favorable amenability factors in abundance, work well in therapy, become attached to their therapists, and come to understand "everything," and yet, as the following case illustrates, improve only a little.

> **Kristen** (not the patient's real name) had just had her thirtieth birthday when I began treating her. Her parents had divorced when she was 6 years old. She was an only child, conceived before her mother was married and born when her mother was 17 years old. Her maternal grandfather, a minister of a rigid and paranoid personality, insisted that her parents marry, so as not to cause a scandal. In her earliest years she spent much of her days with her maternal grandmother, a warm and gentle person. She described her father in similar terms. But her mother was consistently cruel, alternating between verbal or physical abusiveness and outright rejection. Her mother had never wanted a child in the first place and lost no opportunity to remind Kristen of that fact. Child rearing interfered with her mother's

ambitions for college and a career in government, which she pursued to the neglect of her daughter. Prone to migraine headaches, her mother would lock herself in her bedroom, posting a "Do Not Disturb" sign outside the door. Kristen was yelled at constantly by her mother, although she could not recall the reasons; as she put it, "I was timid and well behaved and never gave my mother any real trouble." At times her mother would shake her strenuously in a fit of anger and then leave her alone in her crib.

When Kristen was 9 years old, her mother married a passive man who took verbal abuse from his wife without protest and never intervened to protect Kristen from her mother. In recent years her mother verified certain memories and stories about her own treatment of Kristen. She mentioned, for example, that she had often struck Kristen about the head during her first year of life (for crying or making too much noise) and was in general cold and rejecting, as her own father had been toward her. Her mother also told her that when Kristen was 3 months old and was with her mother on a train, she held Kristen down and put her hand over her mouth to stifle her crying. At times, Kristen would be sent to bed without supper, or her mother would snatch her plate away when her dinner was only half eaten and she was still hungry. On other occasions her mother would lock her in the bathroom until she had a bowel movement, which might take 3 or 4 hours. She repeatedly called Kristen a "filthy devil."

Studious, bright, and intensely lonely, Kristen was always a top student, and she won a scholarship to a prestigious university. She graduated as valedictorian. Her success earned her a scholarship to graduate school, where she planned to take a degree in history. None of these accomplishments elicited any compliments from her mother, who once reacted to Kristen's telling her that she had been nominated for a fellowship by saying that it was probably a "printing error." Around that time, Kristen discovered a lump in her breast, benign as it turned out, but when she mentioned this to her mother, the reply was "Don't you think I have enough worries in my head already?"

The men Kristen chose treated her shabbily in various ways; as she put it, "I keep getting involved with cruel arbitrary people." This tendency was a manifestation of her depressive-masochistic personality, with marked obsessional traits. The main problems confronting her when she entered therapy were two general issues—her inability to complete her doctoral thesis and her indecision about whether to have a child—and one specific situation concerning her previous therapist, a psychoanalyst who had made sexual advances toward her and to whom she had become romantically attached. She realized the relationship was wrong and hopeless, and that realization was her motive for changing therapists, but it took almost 2 years before she could finally bring herself to stop seeing the former therapist in secret meetings that she would tell me about weeks afterward.

Her perfectionistic and overdetailed approach to her thesis led to extraordinary delays in finishing the project. Her adviser at the college was indulgent and let her have one extension after the other, until his own advancing age led him to prompt her gently to finish, if possible, before he died. Her procrastination with the thesis, which took her all of 16 years to complete, was inextricably bound up with her ambivalence about having a child. She often stated she didn't want to think about getting pregnant until the thesis was done, so delaying the former put the idea of pregnancy permanently on hold. She would complain about her thesis in language that made the connection clear, saying at one point, "I can't seem to *produce* anything. I worry about imperfections. The writing is such a *labor*. I can't start it up." She would see at once the parallel between her words and the concepts of producing a baby and the delivery room labor. She would then express her anxiety that she might behave toward a child in the same way that her mother behaved toward her.

She reported two terrifying dreams that occurred while she was working on her feelings about having a child. In one dream, she saw her mother as fat, having become so because she had gorged on human flesh. In another, she and her mother were in a restaurant, eating a dish her mother had recommended. The meat tasted bitter and had an odd shape. She then realized it was a penis, whereupon she threw up and then left the table and refused to come back. These dreams reminded her of an earlier dream in which her stepfather pushed her off a bridge and she died. Her body was then cut up and packaged in various pieces for sale in a supermarket, with the packages labeled "meat may be infectious." The major themes of these dreams, which are reminiscent of the dreams of fragmentation and of being dead alluded to earlier in this chapter, included cannibalism, ingesting foul material, and becoming herself foul material, as well as being poisoned or killed. All this material made her think about the poisonous relationship with her mother, who had wanted her dead. Kristen could not separate her own self-image from the one she "ingested" from her mother—that of being a bad, disgusting baby, and now a bad and disgusting woman contemplating giving birth herself to a baby she was ill prepared to care for.

Kristen did finally obtain her doctorate when she was 38 years old. She felt she now had to "show cause" why she was not trying to get pregnant. She and her husband bought a puppy, as a kind of experiment in taking care of a small creature. In a dream at this time she saw herself running toward a train that was the last train for the day; she just managed to board it, and she was uncomfortable because the cars were so mobbed. She likened this discomfort to the feelings she had when she realized that, at her age, she was nearing her last chance to have a baby but that the birth of a baby would create a situation of "three's a crowd"—herself, her husband, and the half-desired, half-dreaded child. She said she anticipated feeling irritated at the idea that the baby would need her so much, yet she also worried that somehow she would become too dependent on the baby.

In the end, the conflict was decided in an indirect way, which was characteristic of the ways she dealt with other major issues in her life. She felt humiliated to acknowledge that she didn't want a child, but she believed she would feel overwhelmed if she pretended she did want a child and got pregnant. So she did what she so often did to get her husband riled—she bought some very expensive designer suits and dresses from a fashionable boutique and put the charges on his credit card. Kristen was ordinarily frugal and self-effacing, but excessive spending on clothes was her one indulgence and was

guaranteed to anger her husband. Their relationship had always been fragile, and this behavior strained his defenses beyond their flexibility. He said
he wanted a divorce. She quickly packed her bags and moved to a different
city, away from both husband and mother.

Kristen's story is that of a borderline patient at the higher-functioning
end of the borderline spectrum. She was intelligent, attractive, motivated,
psychologically minded, and introspective. She had a depressive-masochistic
character style, and she persevered in her involvement in therapy. Her amenability to treatment was of a very high order, but her degree of improvement in therapy was only modest. She did complete her advanced degree,
but she was unable to use it to the fullest extent, and she was not able to
transcend her fears about motherhood. She made some progress in getting
past her original view of herself as a bad, undeserving child—a view that was
the legacy of her mother's cruelty—but was unable to discard this unrealistic image entirely. In these respects, Kristen's course was like that of many
other borderline patients who have excellent amenability to the process and
demands of psychotherapy, and whose long-term outcome can be considered good, although not outstandingly so. Some borderline patients, with
greater genetic risk for mental illness and experience of even worse degrees
of brutalization, lead no better than marginal lives, even if their ability to
"click" with therapy is very good. Still others with different sets of variables
and early life experiences are able to make the most of their amenability
level, overcome every adversity, and eventually have highly successful lives.

REFERENCES

American Psychiatric Association: Diagnostic and Statistical Manual of Mental
Disorders, 3rd Edition. Washington, DC, American Psychiatric Association,
1980

American Psychiatric Association: Diagnostic and Statistical Manual of Mental
Disorders, 3rd Edition, Revised. Washington, DC, American Psychiatric Association, 1987

American Psychiatric Association: Diagnostic and Statistical Manual of Mental
Disorders, 4th Edition. Washington, DC, American Psychiatric Association,
1994

American Psychiatric Association: Diagnostic and Statistical Manual of Mental
Disorders, 4th Edition, Text Revision. Washington, DC, American Psychiatric
Association, 2000

Balint M: The Basic Fault: Therapeutic Aspects of Regression (1968). New York,
Brunner/Mazel, 1979

Bateman A, Fonagy P: Effectiveness of partial hospitalization in the treatment of borderline personality disorder: a randomized study. Am J Psychiatry 156:1563–1569, 1999

Bateman A, Fonagy P: Treatment of borderline personality disorder with psychoanalytically oriented partial hospitalization: an 18-month follow-up. Am J Psychiatry 158:36–42, 2001

Beck AT, Freeman A: Cognitive Therapy of Personality Disorders. New York, Guilford, 1990

Berliner B: The role of object relations in moral masochism. Psychoanal Q 27:38–56, 1958

Bijttebier P, Vertommen H, Steene GV: Assessment of cognitive coping styles: a closer look at situation-response inventories. Clin Psychol Rev 21:85–104, 2001

Brenner C: The masochistic character: genesis and treatment. J Am Psychoanal Assoc 7:197–226, 1959

Cartwright R: Understanding dreams: tapping a rich resource. Current Psychiatry 4(5):15–21, 2005

Clarkin JF, Yeomans FE, Kernberg OF: Psychotherapy for Borderline Personality. New York, Wiley, 1999

Clarkin JF, Foelsch P, Levy K, et al: The development of a psychodynamic treatment for patients with borderline personality disorder: a preliminary study of behavioral change. J Personal Disord 15:487–495, 2001

Cornfield RB, Malen RL: A multidimensional view of the obsessive character. Compr Psychiatry 19:73–78, 1978

Dawson D, MacMillan HL: Relationship Management of the Borderline Patient: From Understanding to Treatment. New York, Brunner/Mazel, 1993

Deutsch H: Neuroses and Character Types. New York, International Universities Press, 1965

Easser R, Lesser S: Hysterical personality: a reevaluation. Psychoanal Q 34:390–402, 1965

Erikson EH: The problem of ego identity. J Am Psychoanal Assoc 4:56–121, 1956

Fonagy P: Attachment Theory and Psychoanalysis. New York, Other Press, 2001

Frosch J: The psychotic character: clinical psychiatric considerations. Psychiatr Q 38:81–96, 1964

Frosch J: Psychoanalytic considerations of psychotic character. J Am Psychoanal Assoc 18:24–50, 1970

Frosch J: Psychoanalytic contributions to the relationship between dreams and psychosis: a critical survey. Int J Psychoanal Psychother 5:39–63, 1976

Frosch J: The Psychotic Process. New York, International Universities Press, 1983

Goldberg A (ed): The Psychology of the Self: A Casebook. New York, International Universities Press, 1978

Green A: The borderline concept: a conceptual framework for the understanding of borderline patients: suggested hypotheses, in Borderline Personality Disorders: The Concept, the Syndrome, the Patient. Edited by Hartocollis P. New York, International Universities Press, 1977, pp 15–44

Gunderson JG: Borderline Personality Disorder: A Clinical Guide. Washington, DC, American Psychiatric Publishing, 2001

Judd PH, McGlashan TH: A Developmental Model of Borderline Personality Disorder: Understanding Variations in Course and Outcome. Washington, DC, American Psychiatric Publishing, 2003

Kernberg OF: Borderline personality organization. J Am Psychoanal Assoc 15:641–685, 1967

Kernberg OF: The structural diagnosis of borderline personality organization, in Borderline Personality Disorders: The Concept, the Syndrome, the Patient. Edited by Hartocollis P. New York, International Universities Press, 1977, pp 87–121

Kernberg OF: Severe Personality Disorders: Psychotherapeutic Strategies. New Haven, CT, Yale University Press, 1984

Koenigsberg HW, Kernberg OF, Stone MH, et al: Borderline Patients: Extending the Limits of Treatability. New York, Basic Books, 2000

Kohut H: The Analysis of the Self: A Systematic Approach to the Psychoanalytic Treatment of Narcissistic Personality Disorders. New York, International Universities Press, 1971

Kohut H: The Restoration of the Self. New York, International Universities Press, 1977

Kroll J: PTSD/Borderlines in Therapy: Finding the Balance. New York, WW Norton, 1993

Kwon P: Attributional style and psychodynamic defense mechanisms: toward an integrative model of depression. J Pers 67:645–658, 1999

Linehan MM: Cognitive-Behavioral Treatment of Borderline Personality Disorder. New York, Guilford, 1993

Linehan MM, Tutek DA, Heard HL, et al: Interpersonal outcome of cognitive behavioral treatment for chronically suicidal borderline patients. Am J Psychiatry 151:1771–1776, 1994

Luborsky L: Principles of Psychoanalytic Psychotherapy: A Manual for Supportive-Expressive Treatment. New York, Basic Books, 1984

Masters B: Killing for Company: The Case of Dennis Nilsen. New York, Stein and Day, 1986

Masterson JF: Psychotherapy of the Borderline Adult. New York, Brunner/Mazel, 1976

McGlashan TH: The Chestnut Lodge follow-up study, III: long-term outcome of borderline personalities. Arch Gen Psychiatry 43:20–30, 1986

McGuire M, Troisi A: Darwinian Psychiatry. New York, Oxford University Press, 1998

Millon T, Davis R: Personality Disorders in Modern Life. New York, Wiley, 2000

Phillips KA, Gunderson JG, Triebwasser J, et al: Reliability and validity of depressive personality disorder. Am J Psychiatry 155:1044–1048, 1998

Phillips L, Tiggemann M, Wade T: Comparison of cognitive style in bulimia nervosa and depression. Behav Res Ther 35:939–948, 1997

Reich J: Prevalence of DSM-III-R self-defeating (masochistic) personality disorder in normal and outpatient populations. J Nerv Ment Dis 175:52–54, 1987

Rockland LH: Supportive Therapy: A Psychodynamic Approach. New York, Basic Books, 1989

Ryle A: How can we compare different psychotherapies? why are they all effective? Br J Med Psychol 57:261–264, 1984

Searles HF: My Work With Borderline Patients. Northvale, NJ, Jason Aronson, 1986

Stone MH: Dreams of fragmentation and the death of the dreamer: a manifestation of vulnerability to psychosis. Psychopharmacol Bull 15:12–14, 1979

Stone MH: The Fate of Borderline Patients: Successful Outcome and Psychiatric Practice. New York, Guilford, 1990a

Stone MH: Treatment of borderline patients: a pragmatic approach. Psychiatr Clin North Am 13:265–285, 1990b

Waldinger RJ, Gunderson JG: Effective Psychotherapy With Borderline Patients: Case Studies. New York, Macmillan, 1987

Wallerstein RS: Forty-Two Lives in Treatment: A Study of Psychoanalysis and Psychotherapy. New York, Guilford, 1986

Weiner MF, Crowder JD: Psychotherapy and cognitive style. Am J Psychother 40:17–25, 1986

Widiger TA, Frances AJ: Epidemiology, diagnosis, and comorbidity of borderline personality disorder, in American Psychiatric Press Review of Psychiatry, Vol 8. Edited by Tasman A, Hales RE, Frances AJ. Washington, DC, American Psychiatric Press, 1989, pp 8–24

3

PERSONALITY DISORDERS MOST AMENABLE TO PSYCHOTHERAPY

The Anxious Cluster and Related Disorders

If we leave aside the issue of how few "pure types" exist among the personality disorders—that is, how few personality-disordered patients manifest *only* the traits described for just one of the DSM-IV-TR Axis II categories (American Psychiatric Association 2000)—we can create a list of disorders that correlate best with the concept of amenability to psychotherapy. The categories on this list represent the *main* trait collection of the patients who meet this amenability criterion, granted that each such patient almost surely exhibits several traits that we associate with other categories. In Chapter 2, the characteristics of amenable borderline patients were examined; in this chapter, the emphasis is on the other personality disorders, with two provisos.

First, a few of the disorders that are generally most amenable to psychotherapy fall outside the narrow list encompassed in Axis II of DSM-IV-TR.

Now that the label "histrionic" in Axis II has replaced the older term "hysteric," two types of interrelated personality disorders—one mild, the other more severe—have been conflated, at the cost of considerable confusion in the field of personality. *Hysteric character*, the milder condition, found currency mainly in the psychoanalytic literature. As Kernberg (1980, p. 68) pointed out, Oedipal conflicts were central to the psychopathology of hysteria in the view of Freud and later of Fairbairn. From the standpoint of psychosexual health, hysteric character was long thought to represent the least pathological disturbance of personality. Freud and the psychoanalytic pioneers put credence in a developmental track according to which infants and children passed through stages—oral, anal, and genital—with each succeeding stage being an advance over its predecessor in personality integration and each being associated with ever "healthier" levels of adjustment: depressive, paranoid, schizoid (oral manifestations), compulsive (anal), narcissistic (phallic-narcissistic), and finally hysteric (nearest to full "genitality"). This developmental path now seems simplistic, because clinical experience shows that each of these personality (or "character") types encompasses a spectrum. There are fairly healthy depressive persons, mildly paranoid persons, and profoundly ill obsessive-compulsive persons as well as healthier ones, and so forth (Stone 1980). Therefore, the various personality types cannot be well ordered with the same ease as was the custom many years ago.

But in the list of *generally* more amenable disorders, we would want to include hysteric personality, as well as the three anxious cluster (Cluster C) disorders: avoidant, obsessive-compulsive, and dependent. I am purposely using the term *hysteric personality* for what had been called *hysteric character*, to minimize the confusion that might result from speaking now of personality, now of character, when a label for a disorder of personality is meant. The term hysteric personality is also used to distinguish this disorder from its decidedly less healthy cousin, Axis II *histrionic* personality disorder, because most patients exemplifying the latter disorder function at the *borderline level* of mental organization in Kernberg's (1967) nosology. Patients with hysteric personality, in contrast, function at the *neurotic level* of mental organization, insofar as their *identity sense* is well developed. It so happens that patients with hysteric personality are usually anxious in ways and degrees similar to those of patients with the anxious cluster disorders, such that if hysteric personality *were* to be included in Axis II, it would be placed in Cluster C. The same can be said for depressive-masochistic personality. The intropunitive, anxious qualities of patients with depressive-masochistic personality would also earn them a berth in the anxious cluster. As for hysteric personality, Mardi Horowitz et al. (1984) mentioned specifically that persons exhibiting this personality "style" (which they refer to as *hysterical*) "may seek attention in an imperative way, but do so through passivity, shyness, and displayed vulnerability, rather than through flamboyant dramatics" (p. 70). In contrast, *flamboyant dramatics* is one of the characteristics that signal the more pathological adaptation of histrionic personality.

The second proviso concerns the *spectrum* concept of personality types. Most of the personality labels span a spectrum from near normalcy, through mild disturbance, to clear-cut disorder, even on to a disabling, psychotic extreme. We do not assign a new name to these variations in functional level, except in the case of "hysteric"; as this dimension increases in severity, it becomes "histrionic." In addition, some categories of personality disorder scarcely accommodate "mild" variations. We don't ordinarily speak of *mildly* sadistic or *mildly* psychopathic personalities, although some persons manifest only one or two of the traits that are said to compose these disorders. Amenability to psychotherapy is seldom good even in the mild forms of sadistic or psychopathic personalities, so they will not be discussed in this chapter. The remainder of the personality disorders—narcissistic, paranoid, schizoid, schizotypal, hypomanic, passive-aggressive, antisocial, and irritable-explosive—are usually associated with intermediate levels of amenability to psychotherapy at best. These personality types will be discussed in subsequent chapters. In this chapter, the spotlight is on hysteric, obsessive-compulsive, dependent, avoidant, and depressive-masochistic personalities.

The anxious cluster and the related disorders are most often spoken of as shading into the personalities found in the normal population. By analogy, although in the opposite direction, paranoid, schizoid, schizotypal, hypomanic, and irritable-explosive disorders shade into the major psychoses.

Depressive symptoms, as well as depressive traits, accompany the anxious cluster personality disorders. As Trull and McCrae (2002) wrote, "If personality disorders are understood as variations of normal personality dimensions, then…comorbidity data [pertaining to depression] suggest that personality traits may themselves be linked to Axis I syndromes of anxiety and depression" (p. 47). Widiger and Trull (1992) emphasized that personality disorder and depression can interact in a number of ways: personality disorder can predispose the patient *to* depression, abnormal traits can arise *from* preexisting depression, both can arise independently and then interact, or both can arise from one etiological source. Depressive-masochistic personality, viewed in this light, can be seen in some instances as the personality component of a complex condition, after the depressive symptoms have been brought under control. Something similar can be said for depressive personality, as described by Phillips et al. (1998). Likewise, avoidant personality can be understood as what is "left over" in certain persons after their severe anxiety has been brought under control, either through treatment or by purposeful absence from the anxiety-engendering arena of social interaction. As long as people with agoraphobia stay home, they show only avoidant personality.

One by-product of these interrelationships is that the personality disorders that appear to be the most amenable to psychotherapy often overlap in their clinical expression with symptom disorders involving anxiety or depression. Conceptually, with respect to Axis I and Axis II, these disorders have a foot in both boats. Although this chapter focuses on amenability to psychotherapy associated with the *personality* aspects of these disorders, it remains true that in certain patients, alleviation of the *symptom* aspects leads to amelioration of the personality component (Gorenstein et al. 1998), just as, *mutatis mutandis*, in other patients, successful therapy for the personality traits leads to relief of the anxious or depressive symptoms.

It is not surprising that the anxious cluster and related disorders show generally good amenability to psychotherapy. Although personality traits are customarily spoken of as ego-syntonic, in contrast to symptoms (which are, by definition, ego-dystonic), many patients with anxious cluster disorders experience considerable discomfort with their personalities. Avoidant persons are painfully shy, for example; dependent persons are clingy and often wish that they were more independent and autonomous. Obsessive-compulsive persons often get bogged down in unimportant details, such that their work goals become like mirages in the desert—seemingly almost attainable, yet somehow still beyond reach. Hysteric persons crave intimacy but find sex anxiety-provoking. Depressive-masochistic persons long for the "right" mate, yet keep ending up with lovers or spouses who disappoint, betray, or even injure them. Persons with these characteristics tend to blame themselves harshly for their shortcomings and are often of an introspective bent—and, to that extent, are likely to seek treatment.

Patients with anxious cluster and related disorders in general show what Heath et al. (1999) called *harm avoidance*, a temperamental quality believed to be mediated by the serotonin system. Harm avoidance is a key tendency from an evolutionary standpoint, because it conduces to appropriate socialization: children, to the extent they are harm avoidant, prefer to *behave* (that is, to conform) when remonstrated or punished by parents, rather than to *defy*, at the risk of being punished further. By the same token, harm-avoidant people, if they experience psychological difficulties, are usually motivated to take whatever steps would be most likely to alleviate their distress. If they enter therapy, they are likely to persevere until their goals are accomplished. This quality makes for good "patienthood." As for patients whose main traits are obsessive-compulsive, they are often moralistic and overly scrupulous—the very opposite of antisocial—and suffer intensely because of the temptation to do things that they consider questionable or wrong but that most people would do without giving a second thought.

The following three clinical vignettes all involve men with obsessive-compulsive personality disorders who were functioning at the neurotic level of personality organization as depicted by Kernberg (1967).

A single man in his mid-20s sought treatment for mild depression and fears concerning work. He was not particularly ambitious, and he supported himself by means of a family trust, yet he felt he should get a job, if for no other reason than that women seemed to prefer men who were good earners and could support a family. His fears had to do with his father having died at an early age when the patient was 6 years old. Hard work became equated in his mind with premature death. In addition, he was an only child and was the chief companion of his mother, who had never remarried. He came from an upper-class and very law-abiding, conservative background. Therapy was concentrated in the beginning on helping him overcome his fear of early death.

Many relatives were attorneys in high positions in government. He eventually secured a government post himself, where he displayed admirable attention to detail and vigorous pursuit of his assignments, well above the levels shown by his co-workers. The patient's scrupulosity could be seen as an exaggeration of attitudes already common throughout his family. He agonized, for example, over his income tax return, fearing that he had put down too many miles in the deduction for work-related driving, as though he drove 40 miles to and from work instead of the 36 miles his odometer usually indicated. He was about to submit an amended return and to speak with a lawyer to make sure he would not be dealt with severely by the Internal Revenue Service (IRS). It took great effort for me to convince him of the legal adage *de minimis non curat lex* ("the law does not concern itself with trifles"), meaning, in his case, that the IRS was not about to hire an agent to check out the actual mileage, at a cost of several thousand dollars, to prove that he really owed the government an additional $15 in taxes.

The next hurdle involved finding the perfect girlfriend. He was eager to settle down and raise a family, but he could consider only women who had never smoked. An unusually handsome and eligible man, he had many brief relationships and a few near engagements, but he turned down all the women he had dated because they had all smoked, some recently, others just a few times years earlier. He also turned down the one woman who had never smoked, because, as beautiful and highly educated as she was, she spoke with a "lower-class" accent that he felt sure his mother would find unacceptable. He had strong motivation to conquer this problem, which nevertheless proved all but intractable. Based on his dreams and other indications, I felt he was extremely conflicted about leaving his lonely and aging mother, to whom he was very, albeit ambivalently, attached. For several years he remained unable to see the positive side of this attachment.

Clearly, his stringent "no-smoking rule" preserved this attachment. I told him he was looking for a needle in a haystack. Worse, he was looking for one needle in two haystacks, and he was paying attention only to the haystack that didn't have the needle. No woman could pass muster with his rigid requirements.

Fortunately his strong motivation compensated for his low level of psychological mindedness. He seldom recalled dreams, and he was slow to grasp their symbolism. But after a time, he reported a dream in which the woman he was in bed with bore many of the features of his mother. He became more cognizant of the conflict he had hitherto been unable to resolve. Also, he realized that his mother's happiness at having a grandchild would be greater than her sadness at his pursuing an independent life. At this point he met a woman who was "99% perfect" (she had smoked a few cigarettes in her teens), married her, and had the child he always wanted—and his mother had the grandchild she had just about given up hope for.

A single 26-year-old man came for treatment of two main problems. One concerned whether he should marry his current girlfriend. The other related to his addiction to adult female pornography accessible through the Internet, about which he had considerable anxiety. He had been raised in a well-to-do French family in Lyon, where his father was a manufacturer of textiles. Until he went to college, he had been in "all boys" schools and had had little contact with girls, apart from his female cousins. He had always led a sheltered existence. His mother was a warm and caring person who tended to pamper him, seemingly because he was her firstborn. His father was often away on business but was easy to get along with and enjoyed taking the family for outings at their weekend home. Both parents were modest in dress and habit, and neither discussed sexual matters with the children.

Unlike his practical-minded father, the patient was artistic, spiritual, rather passive, and at times "dreamy." For a time he considered becoming a priest. Lacking the drive that had made his father a successful entrepreneur, he had thoughts of being a writer, although he seldom put pen to paper. He wanted to marry and raise a family, but he knew of no way to implement such a plan unless he were to work at his father's factory, which had little appeal to his artistic sensibilities. While he was in college, he began to peer through binoculars at the people in the house across the street from his house. After this period of voyeurism, he switched to the Internet and looked for adult pornography sites. This activity bothered him tremendously, because it violated his sense of what was morally correct and also because, as he put it, it troubled his serenity. He started dating late and had his first serious girlfriend at age 22 years. They had a good sexual relationship, yet that did not dampen his compulsion to access the Internet pornography sites. He had done brilliantly at college, majoring in languages, but he did not feel equipped for any particular line of work. At that point, at age 22 years, he moved to the United States to work for a relative.

When he began therapy, he was in the midst of a 2-year relationship with a woman he contemplated marrying, and he worried that she might discover his preoccupation with pornography and sever their relationship.

In the first week of therapy he reported a dream: "I am in my girlfriend's apartment, in bed with her, when a man breaks into the apartment. He has a gun, and I somehow manage to disarm him. This happens three times, until finally the police take him away. Yet I was still afraid he might return." The intruder seemed to be an older man, whose features the patient couldn't make out. One of his associations was "Maybe it's my father? No, no, that can't be!" This dream was followed by another dream in which, the patient reported, he is driving in the mountains with a girl sitting next to him. He feels he is going too fast. A van careers down the road in the opposite direction and smashes into his car. Looking into the other vehicle, he sees a girl inside, but when he tries to pull her out, he realizes that she is dead. He feels, "All this tragedy for nothing; we were just being careless!" But then the dead girl comes back to life.

In discussing this dream, he said that the car going too fast and out of control made him think that he wasn't ready to marry and had been forcing himself into that decision ahead of his emotional "schedule." He spoke about his strong attachment to his mother: "Maybe my love for her is excessive, and if things don't work out with my girlfriend, I'd end up being like a kid again, clinging to my mother." During an argument with his girlfriend (about whether he was going to give her a ring), she said: "Well, go love your mother!" He was enraged by this outburst. He calmed down after his girlfriend apologized, but the incident did point up the conflict of loyalties he struggled with—his mother versus his prospective fiancée. In a number of subsequent dreams, he finds himself in a room with his girlfriend while he looks out the window to buildings nearby, where he can make out the silhouettes of beautiful dark-haired women. He feels disloyal to his girlfriend yet drawn to these unknown beauties. Working on this recurring theme, he eventually concluded that the unattainable women, with their dark hair (like his mother's), are "stand-ins" for his mother and that the attraction to pornography must be serving the same purpose: permitting vicarious access to forbidden woman or at least to the woman he must grow less emotionally dependent on if he is to make a successful attachment to a woman he can marry.

Highly motivated and perseverant about his therapy, this man was eventually able to suppress the desire to use the Internet pornography sites, except for occasional lapses. He became engaged to his girlfriend, whom his parents warmly accepted. A new fear surfaced that he would have less access to his mother, whom he always regarded as his "confidante" (although he never spoke to her about his pornography interest). As a married man, he would have less time to spend with her, because his major obligations and time would revolve around his wife. These thoughts made more clear than ever before the connection between his use of pornography and his constant turning to his mother as the woman who was always "there" for him.

Thanks to his high level of psychological mindedness, he was able rather easily to translate the symbolic overtones in the dreams he reported, many of which centered around protecting a woman—seen sometimes as a beautiful stranger, sometimes as his fiancée—from an older male assailant. He began to understand that the assailant rival stood for his father, who naturally had a closer relationship with his mother than he could ever have. In real life, there had never been any significant unpleasantness between father and son, and the patient's casting of his father as the dangerous rival had primarily to do with his hidden resentment of his father's privileged position vis-à-vis his adored mother, on whom the patient had been so dependent.

After 2 years of twice-weekly sessions, the patient married his fiancée and made the decision to return to France and work in an administrative capacity at his father's factory. The decision to work in his father's factory was clearly a wise one from a practical standpoint, because he did not have skills or experience in another field that would have allowed him as comfortable a livelihood. When I contacted him 6 years later, I learned that he and his wife now had a child and were living contentedly in his native city.

A 51-year-old man was referred for treatment because of difficulty deciding whether to marry the woman he had been dating for the past year. He had been divorced for several years and had a son and a daughter by the earlier marriage. For the past 20 years he had been working as a philosophy professor at a university. The divorce had been bitter, the more so because his daughter sided strongly with her mother and now rarely spoke with her father except to vilify his new friend, a respected business executive, as a "tramp" and a "Jezebel." There was some difficulty at the university as well, owing to his being considered "unconventional" in some of his views and approaches to teaching philosophy. This experience had led to his feeling unaccepted by some of his colleagues.

Highly adept at deciphering the symbolism of his dreams, he understood with little prompting the "message" of the first dream he reported, in which he saw himself in his former house as a realtor was taking prospective buyers through. He was apprehensive because the basement was a "disaster," which he tried hurriedly to straighten up. As he did so, the sides caved in on him and he was buried up to his waist in rubble, just as the realtor came down to show that part of the house. He likened these images to his feeling that things were "closing in" on him and that he felt trapped. He wanted to marry the woman he had been seeing, but he worried that he might, in effect, lose his daughter in the process. The basement he analogized to the lower depths of his psyche, a layer "full of garbage and stuff" whose exposure would spell embarrassment for him. The transference implication was clear to him also: I was the "realtor" who was making him "show all parts of the house."

In a dream a few days later, he was driving from the house where he used to live to the one he now shared with his new friend. But something happened to the car's transmission, and it would only go backwards. He ended up traveling against the traffic and was almost cut off by a red sports car. He had been thinking the day before about his conflictual feelings about the woman he hoped to make his fiancée and about his life during the previous marriage—as unhappy as he was with his former wife, at least he had not been estranged from his daughter. He had some nostalgia for the early days of that marriage, when the family was still harmonious.

As he gradually overcame his guilt for leaving the unhappy marriage and transferring his affections to his friend, they became officially engaged. The Christmas holidays were nearing, and he received an unexpected call from his daughter, still angry, who complained that she felt betrayed and couldn't trust him anymore. He wondered whether she chose this time to get in touch to put a damper on the holidays.

After that call he reported a dream in which a Korean terrorist was firing at people with an automatic rifle. The patient was afraid he'd be targeted too. Oddly, the terrorist handed him a gun and said, "Join our group!" The patient took the gun and turned it on the terrorist, but there seemed to be no bullets in it. He was given another rifle, which he test-fired into the air, but it too was empty when he tried to shoot at the terrorist. After relating this dream, the patient mentioned that his sexual life with his fiancée had been fine, but, because he was older than she was, he was concerned about whether it would continue to be so after they were married. As for the enemy who seemed at some moments to be on his side, he compared the figure to his daughter—she was his flesh and blood, yet hostile, and lately "alien."

For a long time, the main thrust of therapy with this meticulous man, who felt it was important to have everything in his life "just so" and who was so prone to guilt if these conditions were not achieved, was on the relationship with the estranged daughter. He made a number of efforts to regain her affection, but all were rebuffed. He was putting his future with his fiancée on hold, reluctant to set a wedding date until he could count on both of his children's accepting the marriage. A year went by, and still he had the support only of his son. This delay was taxing the patience of his fiancée. I made interpretations that his daughter was being rigid and unreasonable, which meant that his attempt to win her over was destined to fail. If he hesitated about a wedding date, it suggested that he was postponing the possible in hopes of gaining the impossible or that he had misgivings about his fiancée or about marriage and was using the recalcitrance of his daughter as an excuse.

He had a dream around this time that heralded a resolution to the dilemma. He saw himself in my office, where there was an unfinished Oriental rug spread out before him. I give him colored pens and rulers for him to complete the design. He protests that if he made drawings on the rug, it would be ruined. I tell him, "It's yours to do with it what you want." He responds, "Even if I mess it up?" I reply, "Who cares?" He makes some careful drawings with the ruler, but even so there are a few irregularities. However, he finds that I don't mind and am not as judgmental as he expected. As he worked on this dream material, it became clear to him that the dream had to do with the course of his life in the future. He had the right to draw in the unfinished spaces as he saw fit. There would inevitably be a few mistakes along the way. But his conscience was less punitive now (less directed, in a manner of speaking, by his judgmental parents or by his overly critical daughter), having become less harsh under the influence of our work together. He knew something about Oriental rugs—that irregularities were woven in on purpose, as a sign that perfection is the province only of the Deity. After this time, it became easier for him to depart from his perfectionistic goal. He set a date for the wedding, accepting the fact that his son but not his daughter would attend.

The three clinical vignettes in this section center on women with a de-pressive-masochistic character structure, a combination of depressive and self-defeating personality traits that is usually associated with good amena-bility to psychotherapy. These women, too, functioned at the neurotic level in Kernberg's schema.

A 36-year-old woman sought therapy ostensibly because of "trouble find-ing the right man." She was a successful stage actress whose roles were mainly in tragedies or serious dramas. The eldest of three sisters, she had grown up in Montana and considered herself a very "outdoors" person. Her parents' marriage was not happy; during the patient's teenage years, her fa-ther had been unfaithful, often coming home late at night and under the in-fluence of alcohol. Yet as her father's favorite, the patient had for years been closer to him than to her mother, until, in her teenage years, she became aware of his infidelity. Her allegiance then switched to her mother. Attrac-tive and popular, she had many boyfriends, but she gravitated toward those who ended up disappointing her in various ways. As for her personality, her main traits were those of the hysteric and depressive-masochistic personal-ity types. On some days she was exuberant and outgoing, and on other days she was tearful and sad. These mood changes became much more marked in her early 20s, after she was raped by a stranger as she was returning home from a theater where she had been acting. The man was apprehended and given a long sentence, but this outcome did not reduce her fear that one day he would be released and would harm her again.

This incident colored her subsequent relationships with men, whom she now placed into either of two categories: the dangerous and the safe. Those who were strong, virile, and ambitious she saw as "dangerous"; those who were passive and submissive and who were not "go-getters" in the workplace she viewed as "safe" but uninteresting and poor marriage pros-pects. She had never married, although she had once gotten pregnant by a boyfriend and had terminated the pregnancy. Her career was just taking off at that time, and being an unwed mother would have been a great burden. However, she had regrets about this decision, and she wondered what the child might have been like.

She had sought treatment because of the turmoil she was experiencing in her current relationship. The man she was seeing worked "on and off" at odd jobs and was much less successful than she was, to the point of depend-ing on her financially. As her story unfolded, it became clear that she grav-itated toward men who were handsome and socially presentable but unreliable and passive. The advantage to her was that they would be un-likely to leave her or reject her, and she was guaranteed of not ending up alone, a fate that she dreaded. The disadvantages were that she could not respect these men and did not look forward to being the sole breadwinner.

These cost-benefit factors were themselves related to an underlying is-sue of greater magnitude: she was fiercely jealous and had become so after discovering her father's cheating. The rape experience aggravated the jeal-ousy, by souring her view of men all the more and further diminishing her trust even in the best of them. Ironically, her current boyfriend, because he was so dependent on her, grew increasingly anxious that her success would prompt her to reject him and to search for a man nearer her level of success and income. Knowing that she had a jealous streak, he would taunt her with talk of previous girlfriends or with threats of going out with other women, in the hope that he could bind her to him (through marriage) so that she would be less disposed to leave him. She meanwhile would twit him about his fecklessness in the work sphere. Their mutual taunts led to arguments in which both of them ended up apologetic and crying.

Her jealousy and fears that her boyfriend would leave her for a "more desirable woman" were highlighted in a dream she reported early in therapy. In the first part of the dream, she sees a green snake. In the next sequence, she sees her boyfriend in the company of a homely girl. Even so, she feels jealous. Her boyfriend says, "Well, she and I are together, and after we have sex we're going out to shoot us some snakes." In discussing the dream, she likened the *green* color to envy or jealousy, and the *snake* to her own jealous self that her boyfriend seemed intent on getting rid of. The same theme recurred in most of her later dreams, including one she reported a few months later in which she is with her boyfriend in the dining room of a luxury train. In the midst of the meal, she vomits, and she does so repeatedly until the dining car fills up with vomit. Finally, she tells him to go away; he is both mad and sympathetic, but he does leave. In discussing the dream, she said, "I know the vomit meant my jealousy." The jealousy is "disgusting" and spoils everything; it drives her boyfriend away.

In therapy she began to grapple with the fact that her feelings toward her boyfriend were tilting—she was growing more eager to be rid of him than to hold on to him, even though it caused her great anxiety to be alone. She clung to the relationship, although a few months later she reported a dream in which she herself cheats on her boyfriend with another man who is in love with her. Her boyfriend ends up crying. This dream was the harbinger of their breakup. She felt there was no future for the two of them, although she was still reluctant to make a definitive split—until she received an excellent offer for an acting job in another part of the country.

She was very adroit at working with symbolism, as she was at grasping emotions (which contributed to her professional success). She was also highly motivated and earnest about working hard on her jealousy in therapy. Psychological mindedness, good character, and perseverance all made for excellent amenability to psychotherapy. The treatment had to be interrupted because of her job offer, which was realistically "too good to turn down." In the 12 years after she left treatment, she continued to be a success in her career. She remained single, although she had a few long-lasting and more gratifying relationships with men who were closer to her level of success. Toward the end of our work, she acknowledged that she was still apprehensive about marriage, because "motherhood is the tin can attached to the honeymoon car." She dreaded ending up like her mother—humiliated and emotionally abandoned by her father—even though she understood that such a fate was not inevitable. Picking a man who would prove to be neither an alcoholic nor a philanderer seemed too risky a gamble.

A 23-year-old woman was referred for therapy because of mild depression that had occurred within the context of an ungratifying romantic relationship. Having graduated from college the year before, she was now working as an editorial assistant. She was the eldest of three children in a family where the father had been, before his retirement, in the upper-level administration of a large corporation. Although she was quite attractive, she had only limited experience in dating, which she attributed in part to her height. She was 6 feet tall, and she felt that most boys—except for those who were taller still—avoided asking her out. But the main reason for her sparse dating, in her opinion, was her face: she was convinced she was ugly.

Throughout her teenage years, she had been the butt of disparaging remarks by her father, who had something negative to say about each facial feature, besides being critical and unsympathetic toward her in general. He favored her two brothers in ways that made her feel cursed to be female. That she outperformed her brothers—and indeed most students in her classes—scholastically was little consolation; in fact, her academic success had the reverse effect, in her view, because to be tall, ugly, *and* very smart meant she had three strikes against her. Who would ask such a woman out? As for her current boyfriend, they had been together for about 8 months, the longest relationship she had sustained. Earlier, she had had three or four brief affairs with men who seemed content to take advantage of her sexually but who were "wrong" for her in numerous ways. One was hypercritical, like her father; another was stingy; and a third was ill-mannered and from very different social circumstances. All of these doomed choices gave a depressive-masochistic cast to her personality. She seemed drawn as if by a perverse magnetism to men destined to disappoint her. In this respect her new boyfriend was no different. He came from a well-to-do background like hers, but he had been disowned by his father, a prominent judge, for having refused to enter the father's profession. Embittered, her boyfriend took out his disgruntlement on her.

Her treatment consisted of thrice-weekly psychoanalysis, using the couch. During her sessions, she was often tearful as she recounted stories of maltreatment by her boyfriend, punctuated by similar stories concerning her father. Every few months, for example, her parents would travel from the Midwest to spend a few days with her, always camping out in her tiny apartment on air mattresses, although they could easily have afforded to stay in the best hotels. Much of their time together was taken up with her father's bickering and casting aspersions on either her décor or her appearance. She was much too timid to suggest a more convenient arrangement. A few months after she began treatment, she moved in with her boyfriend. This arrangement turned into a battleground not so different from early years at home. She worked as hard as he did, but unless she had a hot meal on the table when he came home at 6 o'clock, he would fly into a rage. Once he threw a coffee cup at her, fracturing one of her fingers. After this incident, her sessions included serious discussion of why she put up with such indignities.

Fortunately, she had in abundance every quality that accounted for amenability to psychotherapy, including the ego strength to picture herself surviving the dissolution of this love relationship. She could begin to see, for example, that the suffering she endured from life with her boyfriend paralleled in many ways the suffering she endured from her father. She thought at first that the boyfriend, a good deal older than she was, would prove to be the "good" father she always longed for, only to discover that he was like her ambivalently loved real father. As she became more convinced of the hopelessness of the relationship, she was able after some months to sever it.

The focus of therapy then shifted to her father. She began to recall that, during her adolescence, her father would walk in on her while she was dressing in her bedroom and he would, while naked, pass her in the hallway, as if unaware she was still at home. He began making slips of the tongue, introducing her to guests as "my wi...I mean, my daughter." Because these incidents were occurring at the same time that he was becoming outwardly critical and dismissive toward her, a revised picture of her father began to emerge. She saw it as nearer the truth that he had harbored a secret attraction to her, against which he defended himself through denial and by converting his feelings into their opposite. Presumably this process was not a conscious one on his part but rather an unconscious mechanism that allowed him to repudiate the incestuous impulses against which he struggled. Obviously, we could get no corroboration on this interpretation from him, but it made sense. We took to calling his behavior "negative incest." She drew the conclusion that far from viewing his daughter as "ugly," her father was doing his best to cope with what to him were unacceptable sexual feelings. Three benefits accrued from this part of her analysis: she felt much better about her appearance, realizing that her self-image had been shaped by a father who saw her, if anything, as too attractive, not too ugly; she became more forgiving toward him; and she was able to shake off her masochistic tendency to seek out men who would treat her shabbily.

A woman in her late 40s had recently divorced after a marriage of more than 20 years. She became depressed and came for therapy not only for the immediate distress of the divorce, but also for the lifelong pessimism, self-defeating choices, and bad luck that made her current loneliness all the harder to bear. She had been a brilliant student and gifted writer in her college days and had married a writer whose descendants had come to America on the Mayflower. More snobbish than talented, he never had any financial success from his writing. The patient ended up as the breadwinner and also assumed the burden of caring for their one child. She took a job as an editor at a publishing house, a task she performed well, albeit with regrets that she scarcely had time for any creative writing of her own.

As to her amenability for therapy, she brought to our work an acute psychological mindedness and introspective turn of mind, as well as a highly developed reflective capacity, and she was self-effacing and moral almost to the point of scrupulosity. She had an excellent, wry sense of humor and was well aware of the "tonnage of Weltschmerz," as she put it, that she carried into all her life's activities. Motivation and perseverance were also high; her only failing was in the domain of ego strength or perhaps in the will to *change*. She wanted to make certain changes in her life, but she felt hopeless about putting any such changes into effect. The depressive-masochistic nature of her personality expressed itself with especial poignancy in a vignette she told me a few months into our work. When her baby was born, she tried to juggle three tasks: her job, motherhood, and some creative writing during the wee hours. After fashioning some short stories, she chanced to place the typed pages near the changing table where she was diapering the baby. She then carelessly tossed out the short stories along with the disposable diapers. She took this as an evil omen and made no more attempts as a fiction writer. The episode itself had the makings of a short story, but when I encouraged her to take up her pen again and use this experience as the basis of story, the idea made her sad all over again, and she did nothing with it.

At this point she had a dream in which she wrote me a check while drinking coffee in my waiting room. She spilled the coffee on my chair and was embarrassed. She then wrote something with a pencil, which she thought was mine. I asked her to return my pencil, which she felt was mean-spirited on my part. Her first association was to a cousin who once spilled Coca-Cola all over her rug, sofa, and compact disc collection. She felt like "murdering" him at the time, although she realized she identified with him in his carelessness—after all, she was the one who threw her "novel-baby" out with the diapers. She equated the pencil she borrowed in the dream with the "penis," concluding that men can write and do what they want because they're blessed with that organ. It was not that she envied the penis per se—she felt Freud went a bit over the top with the notion of women's "penis envy"—but she envied the cultural advantages that men, such as her husband, possessed. He wrote while she slaved away at work and motherhood. She had a number of close male friends, several of whom had ditched their first wives, as her own husband had done, to be with much younger women—another enviable male prerogative, according to her experience. There were women to envy, too. Her son had a college friend who became a protégée of the patient because of her writing talent. While still in her early 20s, this young woman won a coveted writing prize, and her work was then published in a prestigious magazine. The patient felt it was her destiny to be the key to everyone's success but her own.

As she turned 50, she saw many doors closing in her life; she felt it was too late to meet another man and too late to return to creative writing, plus she now had to live alone and forfeit the social status of being a married woman, even though in all other respects she was glad to be rid of her husband. She found many comparatively minor situations in her life to be overwhelming. She noticed that mice had begun to invade her apartment. Although she knew they were harmless pests, they frightened her tremendously. She couldn't seem to master the trick of setting traps and was anyway horrified at the prospect of having to remove a dead mouse. My suggestion that she get a cat was rejected, because she was afraid of cats as well. During the third year of therapy, she began to overcome the pain of divorce and her loneliness. She resumed contact with old friends she had rarely seen while married, and she even began thinking about writing creatively again. But at this point she developed a cancer that cut short her ambitions to write and, 11 months later, ended her life.

The last clinical vignette concerns a young man with what would currently be called an avoidant personality disorder—a term that replaced the older psychoanalytic term *phobic character*. As it happens, this man was actually much more phobic in the classical sense (he was afraid of water and of flying) than he was of social situations. Far from avoiding social situations or feeling uncomfortable in new social settings or in crowds, he was quite comfortable and effective in these settings. It was the accompanying phobic symptom of intense anxiety in certain specific situations (being in an airplane, especially) that lowered the ceiling of his potential—making long-distance trips, for example, was necessary for advancement at work—until he was able, through the psychotherapy, to overcome his fears.

A **26-year-old man** entered treatment because of indecision about marrying and also because of a fear of flying, which was a problem because his occupation required frequent plane travel. He had graduated from a university with a degree in mathematics and a specialty in statistics, and he had been hired by a large insurance firm because of his talents in actuarial analysis. With his co-workers and even with his superiors, he was self-assured and forceful to the point of being abrasive. With women, he was demanding and critical. He chose women who were submissive and not very broad in their education, whom he would berate for their ignorance. This narcissistic edge to his personality—one could call it arrogance—was oddly discordant with his fearfulness about planes, itself a part of a larger preoccupation with death and dying that had permeated his existence since his early years.

Initially he did not show much psychological mindedness. He was not introspective, rarely recalled dreams, and was not particularly empathic. Despite these drawbacks, however, his amenability was raised to a high level because of the strength of his motivation, which was fueled by the urgency of his work situation. He had already advanced beyond his years to a middle executive position, but his ambition could carry him no further unless he conquered his plane phobia. The treatment regimen consisted of twice-weekly sessions of psychoanalytically oriented psychotherapy.

He viewed his mother as overprotective. He attributed this tendency in part to her having lost her father to a traffic accident when she was young. There was some suspicion that he may have been pushed into the path of the car that ran him over, in what might have been a murder. She would never allow any member of her family to visit the city in which she had grown up. In addition, his mother was asthmatic and allergic—*deathly* allergic, as she liked to emphasize—to many common food items and animals. When the patient was at summer camp at age 12 years, he had a traumatic experience, nearly drowning when he caught his foot on an object while underwater. He was soon rescued, but he had avoided the water ever since and had never learned to swim. As for airplanes, he knew quite well, as an actuary, how safe commercial flights were, but the idea of "not being in control" he found intolerable.

Thanks to the family atmosphere, charged as it was with worries about car crashes, drownings, plane crashes, murder, and other disasters, thoughts of death were never far from his mind. Wherein death had its sting was, in large measure, the idea that he would be totally forgotten—unless perhaps he had children who would remember him. This thought put him in a hurry to marry and create heirs, a desire that had a higher priority than whether he was in love with the woman he chose to bear these children.

In my experience, he was one of the very few neurotic-level patients who had a dream of being dead. Some years earlier he dreamed he was flying in a balloon. He fell out, crashed to the earth, and died, although he could hear people say: "Oh, he's dead!" After he had been in treatment for a few months, he began to recall his dreams before almost every session and began to show a sincere interest in reflecting on them. His psychological minded-ness noticeably increased. The theme of death cropped up in unexpected places. Without any evidence of infidelity on his father's part, he found himself thinking that if his father were to cheat on his mother, "my father would be dead to me." This extremity of attitude we later concluded was a projection of his own concerns about how faithful he could be throughout all the years of a marriage. Thus far he had a long string of "conquests"; some-times, he maintained relationships with two women at the same time.

Water was an ever-present accompaniment in his dreams. In the second year of therapy, for example, he reported a dream in which he saw himself in a large church-like room that contained a rock formation at one end; the place was filling up with water, such that he had to climb the rocks to the top, where he could still breathe. There was no exit, and some people had already drowned. The dream came at a time when his company had given him an assignment that involved flying across country for a meeting in a few weeks, and he had become increasingly anxious as the date approached. Two days later he had another dream, in which he was flying a plane near his of-fice building and was hovering over a river. He had to make an emergency landing but didn't think he could do it safely. The Coast Guard then radioed him that there was no room to land in the water. Meantime, the plane was running out of fuel. This dream pointed up something worse than not being in control while in a plane under the command of a pilot—he himself was the pilot, and he still felt fatally out of control.

His worries were not just about the upcoming flight but also about the woman he was dating. He felt that this woman was the one he wanted to marry, but he had a great deal of anxiety about whether he could be a good provider and a good father and, if he had children, whether he would live long enough to launch them into a comfortable adulthood. Of the two problems, the one about flying was the easier to deal with. I recommended a behavioral intervention that consisted of his taking several short flights, each one a little longer than the previous one. He was to take one-half mil-ligram of alprazolam before the first flight and, if that flight went well, to simply carry a few tablets of the medication in his pocket during the other flights just in case he needed them. This strategy worked very well. By the time he had to fly across country on business, he was scarcely anxious at all. A month later, he proposed to his girlfriend. They married 6 months later and had their honeymoon in Rio de Janeiro, a trip that required a 10-hour flight, which he managed without difficulty.

Looking back over our work, we were able to dissect his fear of flying into its major component parts. The psychodynamic interventions unearthed the psychological meanings of his fear, and the supportive and behavioral interventions speeded up the conquering of the fear. His amenability to therapy extended, fortunately, to all these approaches. Being a mere passenger on a plane meant submitting control to someone else—the pilot. His fear of not being in control while at 35,000 feet in the air ushered in the second fear—the fear of crashing and dying in obscurity, without children to remember him. Like most persons with a marked fear of flying, he could drive a car without a twinge of apprehension, despite the staggeringly greater risk attached to that means of transportation—he was, after all, the "pilot" of his own car.

As these clinical vignettes illustrate, the patient's capacity to work well with one mode or another of psychotherapy—that is, the patient's *treatability* or amenability to psychotherapy—is not a guarantee of *curability*. By "curability" I have in mind only the ability to progress, after a period of time, to a distinctly improved level of overall function and adaptation. This level is not normalcy or perfection, unless we define "normal" in a counterintuitive way. To be perfectly "normal" is not part of the human condition, insofar as one is always struggling with conflicts that are seldom completely resolved. Normalcy might be thought of instead as a state in which one feels adequate to the task of dealing with the main problems of one's life and content to resign oneself (as is emphasized in the 12-step program of Alcoholics Anonymous) to those aspects of one's life that one cannot change. Some people do manage to find contentment and happiness, but persons we consider normal also have the capacity to bear a certain measure of being unfulfilled with equanimity and without too much regret. Happiness is more apt to be the unexpected by-product of this type of adaptation, rather than a quality one strives for directly. Einstein is said to have asserted that happiness was "the ambition of a pig." By this I think (or I hope) he meant that a life where one's only goal is to be "happy," without recognizing the misery that is all around us and without attempting to contribute in some small way to *tikkun olam* (the Hebrew phrase for the *restoration of the world*), may be enjoyable but would ultimately be empty.

The relatively healthy patients in these vignettes, all of whom functioned at the neurotic level, for the most part did eventually use their treatability to achieve a "cure." They made significant strides in their intimate lives and resolved certain key conflicts, accepting a good that was possible in favor of a good that was unreachable. This process was illustrated in the case of the professor who went ahead with a reasonable marriage at the sacrifice of a rapprochement with his daughter. The man with the fear of flying represents a comparative rarity: a person whose tendency to panic could be reduced almost entirely by means of dynamic psychotherapy. A similar case was reported by the Danish psychoanalyst Thorkil Vanggaard (1989), whose patient was a well-integrated and highly esteemed physician.

The editor who years ago threw her short stories out with the diapers had greater amenability to treatment than most of the other patients in these vignettes, but she derived only limited benefit from her therapy. Perhaps the main benefit from her treatment was a lessening of her loneliness and sense of failure, simply through the relationship with a therapist who admired her wit and intelligence and who was "there" for her throughout her divorce and during her final illness. The dream analysis and the work on her dynamics, in other words, became the medium through which this comforting relationship was brought about. I realized early on, for example, that she was not likely to *do* all that much with the therapeutic work: she wasn't going to write the book she had given up on when her son was born; she wasn't going to meet Mr. Right; she wasn't even going to do anything about the mice. But it eased her depression to know that I understood and liked her and that the understanding and liking were genuine. Freud (1910/ 1957) imparted a similar message in his essay on the future prospects of psychoanalysis, where he wrote: "Let us remember that our attitude to life ought not to be that of a fanatic for hygiene or therapy. We must admit that the ideal prevention of neurotic illnesses which we have in mind would not be of advantage to every individual.... Is there one of you who has not at some time looked into the causation of a neurosis and had to allow that it was the mildest possible outcome of the situation?" (p. 150)

The patient who made the most gains was the man who showed the least psychological mindedness at the outset (although this quality improved over time) and who started out with the most rigid character structure. He grew less compulsive and less judgmental about smoking, and he finished treatment at a time when he had a job he enjoyed, a marriage that was fulfilling, and a child to whom he was devoted. The man with the pornography addiction, whose psychological mindedness was substantial to begin with, did almost as well. He gave up his dreams of being a writer (with no secure income), settling for a lucrative but not so satisfying post in his father's factory, which made marriage and fatherhood possible. The rewards he reaped from his new family made this a most reasonable compromise.

The two younger women—one masochistic, the other hysteric—whose relationships with men had proven so miserable both found increasing satisfaction in their careers and in a widened circle of friends. They grew less apprehensive about whether the more traditional goals of being a wife and mother would be a part of their lives.

REFERENCES

American Psychiatric Association: Diagnostic and Statistical Manual of Mental Disorders, 4th Edition, Text Revision. Washington, DC, American Psychiatric Association, 2000

Freud S: Future prospects of psychoanalysis (1910), in The Standard Edition of the Complete Psychological Works of Sigmund Freud, Vol 11. Translated and edited by Strachey J. London, Hogarth Press, 1957, pp 141–151

Gorenstein C, Gentil V, Melo M, et al: Mood improvement in "normal volunteers." J Psychopharmacol 12:246–251, 1998

Heath AC, Madden PA, Cloninger CR, et al: Genetic and environmental structure of personality, in Personality and Psychopathology. Edited by Cloninger CR. Washington, DC, American Psychiatric Press, 1999, pp 343–367

Horowitz M, Marmar C, Krupnick J, et al: Personality Styles and Brief Psychotherapy. New York, Basic Books, 1984

Kernberg OF: Borderline personality organization. J Am Psychoanal Assoc 15:641–685, 1967

Kernberg OF: Internal World and External Reality: Object Relation Theory Applied. New York, Jason Aronson, 1980

Phillips KA, Gunderson JG, Triebwasser J, et al: Reliability and validity of depressive personality disorder. Am J Psychiatry 155:1044–1048, 1998

Stone MH: Traditional psychoanalytic characterology re-examined in the light of constitutional and cognitive differences between the sexes. J Am Acad Psychoanal 8:381–401, 1980

Trull TJ, McCrae RR: A five-factor perspective on personality disorder research, in Personality Disorders and the Five-Factor Model of Personality, 2nd Edition. Edited by Costa PT Jr, Widiger TA. Washington, DC, American Psychological Association, 2002, pp 45–57

Vanggaard T: Panic. New York, WW Norton, 1989

Widiger TA, Trull TJ: Personality and psychopathology: an application of the Five-Factor Model. J Pers 60:363–394, 1992

PERSONALITY DISORDERS OF INTERMEDIATE AMENABILITY TO PSYCHOTHERAPY

Borderline Personality Disorder

In a fairly lengthy therapy of a patient with neurotic-level personality organization, as defined by Kernberg (1967), the therapist sometimes becomes the repository of the patient's unfulfilled wishes. This phenomenon may be more evident in a psychoanalytic therapy, where a greater emphasis is placed on uncovering and resolving unconscious strivings than would be the case in a more practical therapy oriented to the here and now. Often, the intensity of such wishes to "actualize" the transference is comparatively mild in better-integrated patients. An example is mentioned in the textbook of Thomä and Kächele (1992), who recount an episode from the analysis of a female patient: "Her sexual curiosity had been stimulated in the transference.... Finally I interpreted her unconscious wish to have a child with me and from me. She said that this made sense to her *although she had never consciously had such a wish*" (p. 45, emphasis added). In the case of this patient, one could surmise that if she *did* have such a wish, it was probably rather muted and by no means all-consuming.

The situation with borderline patients is quite the opposite. It is a regular and predictable feature of any extended therapy with borderline patients that they seem considerably more interested in *actualizing the transference* than in reflecting on and exploring the transference. This situation occurs irrespective of the therapeutic approach, including dynamic, cognitive-behavioral, and supportive therapies. Furthermore, the more ill and the less reflective the borderline patient, the stronger is the effort to actualize the transference, or convert the therapist into the person who is most sorely missing in the life of the patient. Depending on the dominant conflict and most distressing emotion in the patient, this effort may take the form of making the therapist into a friend (someone to share a meal with or go to the movies with), a lover, a parent, or, conversely, a figure to vilify and "get back at" for wrongs inflicted long ago by a parent or someone else who occupied a central role in the interpersonal life of the patient.

If a patient feels that his or her main caretakers were remarkably unkind or consistently untrustworthy, compared with those of more fortunate persons, the patient may have a sense that something essential was missing as he or she grew up. This sense is in part what Balint (1968/1979) meant when he spoke of the "basic fault" in persons whom we would designate as borderline. This phenomenon is so common that it would not be incorrect to state that therapists begin to label certain patients "borderline" when they try with such insistence to actualize the transference. In other words, a patient who behaves in this manner *is*, by that very fact, "borderline." Balint (1968/1979) mentioned in this regard that "[p]atients begin to know too much about their analysts...their interest gets centered more and more on divining the analysts' 'real motives' for saying this, for behaving that way...and this is perhaps the reason why patients in this state apparently lose a good deal of their drive to get better, of their wish, and even their ability to change....Their expectations from the analyst grow out of proportion to anything realistic" (p. 85).

Harold Searles (1986), who worked with borderline patients who were generally sicker than those described by Balint, gave an example of a man who would ask at the end of each session, "Time to go?"—but with an intonation that conveyed, "Time for *us* to go?" Or he would often begin his sessions by saying that "we" did such-and-such over the weekend or "we" had a nasty argument last night or "we" had sex the other night, in a way that Searles felt "contained unconscious references to me as his symbiotic-identity partner. In the transference, I represented mainly aspects of his symbiotically related-to mother" (p. 86). Minde and Frayn (1992) described this phenomenon as a process that occurs at a level more often encountered in intensive therapeutic work with schizophrenic patients. They wrote that in clinical work with borderline patients, "[t]here may also be a blurring of psychic boundaries so that patients experience their wished-for ideals or feared deficiencies through their subjective experience of the therapist" (p. 105). They added that very archaic longings may be invoked in this process, to the point where the therapist may be cast in "strangely different transference roles than [he or she is] accustomed to." The therapist may become viewed not as an incestuously unavailable father or a nurturing mother, but "as a corpse, a supernatural force, or an inanimate container for unwanted affects." This phenomenon is reminiscent of the importance of the nonhuman environment in understanding the dynamics of certain schizophrenic patients, some of whom, as Searles (1960) described, vastly preferred a tree in the garden of their home or the family dog, which seemed to them a more reliable source of consolation and warmth than either parent.

These eerie phenomena are more likely to surface in work with borderline patients who are particularly lacking in some of the treatability factors I outlined in Chapter 1. They inhabit the *intermediate* realm of access to therapy, which is the focus of this chapter. Many patients in this realm were traumatized so severely in their earliest years that they cannot articulate with any ease or accuracy what befell them. They may instead manifest only *bodily* memories of the sort studied intensively by Bessel van der Kolk (1996). A smell, a sound, or a sight may make available to consciousness what could not be accessed by words. One such patient of mine described the attempt to recall these painful memories by telling me, "I can't really get at it; it all happened before speech." Other borderline patients, particularly those who were victims of incest by an older relative (father, stepfather, uncle), make it clear that they do remember various facets of what happened to them, but they dare not speak aloud the words that accompany the traumatic memories, at least until therapy has progressed considerably and sufficient trust has been established. They remain still engulfed in magical thinking that the offending parent can somehow "hear" the critical remarks, even though the patient and the parent may now be separated by a continent or an ocean, and will surely "kill" the child for divulging the secret.

Among borderline patients showing intermediate levels of treatability, an incest history is neither a necessary nor a sufficient precondition for diminished accessibility to therapy. Many borderline patients who have been traumatized in this way have a high level of accessibility to therapy, and there are other, particularly "difficult" borderline patients (as defined by

Colson et al. [1986]) who owe their marginal treatability to entirely different factors. These factors cannot easily be generalized, because they occur
in many complex combinations. Factors that singly or in combination compromise treatability include the following:

- Parental cruelty, whether in the form of physical abusiveness or chronic
  verbal humiliation
- Parental neglect
- An attachment style that is distinctly dismissive (and that will become
  manifest in the therapist-patient relationship) (see Diamond et al. 1999)
- Comorbid paranoid, narcissistic, passive-aggressive, schizotypal, or
  schizoid personality (Conklin and Westen 2005)
- Marked impairment of self-reflective capacity
- Marked paucity of avocational pursuits (described by Kernberg [1967]
  as poor sublimatory channeling), with correspondingly heightened in-
  tolerance of being alone
- Meager occupational experience or success; inadequate training for any
  kind of work that would facilitate self-support
- Severe genetic or constitutional risk for affective disorder, even in the
  presence of adequately sensitive and nurturing parents
- Low levels of motivation and perseverance
- Chaotic life circumstances, with continual crises and disruptions
- Anger and hostility that is intense, chronic, and pervasive
- Severe and disruptive symptoms, such as drug abuse, anorexia/bulimia,
  dissociative identity disorder, relentless self-mutilation, or suicidal
  threats
- Exquisite vulnerability to relatively minor stresses, which may lead to the
  continual crises mentioned earlier

Many of these factors can be understood as severe versions of the criteria by which borderline personality disorder (BPD) is defined in DSM-IV-
TR (American Psychiatric Association 2000). Others relate to particularly
adverse early environmental circumstances or to adverse constitutional givens. Although the matter has not been studied systematically, borderline
patients who possess any or several of these negative factors might be over-
represented among the ranks of those who drop out of therapy prematurely.
Waldinger and Gunderson (1984) estimated the dropout rate to be about
40% in patients with BPD. The rate may be substantially higher in the
group of patients with intermediate accessibility to psychotherapy and may
be even higher for those with the most guarded prognosis.

Poverty should probably be added to the list of factors that limit treatability. Patients in economically straitened circumstances are often unable to keep appointments, have little means with which to improve their education or work skills to afford better and safer housing, and are often embroiled in tumultuous and often dangerous relationships. Their lives are a concatenation of crises that far exceed their adaptive capacities, and they have few opportunities to escape their present condition.

A corollary to the factor of exquisite vulnerability is *lack of courage*. Some borderline patients of intermediate accessibility to therapy are kept from solidifying their gains and from working consistently in therapy by a certain want of courage. (This quality might be placed among the "spirituality" factors, because of its similarity to lack of self-transcendence.) Faced with stressful situations that most persons—even most borderline patients—cope with adequately, those with a lack of courage may buckle under the stress, give up, and resort to self-destructive behaviors. The latter need not be extreme behaviors such as self-mutilation or suicide gestures—they may include quitting a job, walking out of a needed and previously sustaining relationship, abusing alcohol or drugs, neglecting one's physical health, and quitting treatment.

The combination of *marked antisocial traits* with borderline personality creates a gloomy prognosis and constitutes a condition that is barely treatable or even untreatable. The presence of a milder degree of antisociality, however, may be compatible with an intermediate level of accessibility to therapy. At this level, the patient may show *impulsivity carried to an extreme*. This quality in turn is a cause of chaos with continual crises and disruptions in the patient's life. Extreme impulsivity may lead, for example, to driving while intoxicated, a lovers' quarrel that ends up in violence or destruction of property, harassment following a romantic breakup, street fights over trivial matters, shoplifting, and a host of other spur-of-the-moment behaviors that may land the patient in trouble with the law, if only briefly. Sometimes these behaviors may be manifestations of the acting out of a conflict that was being examined in therapy. If the acting out results in an injury or a jail stay, however, the behavior becomes more difficult to explore and smooth out in ensuing sessions, because the therapy may be interrupted for a few days or weeks. Momentum is lost, and when therapy resumes, it may be difficult to recapture the essence of what spurred the patient to the reckless behavior.

This behavior amounts to what, in the calmer waters of therapy with steadier patients, is called *resistance*. But the resistance encountered in highly impulsive, action-prone borderline patients is obviously much more formidable. These patients put greater effort into actualizing the transference than do their less impulsive counterparts, and this tendency may account partly for the extraordinary lengths of time necessary to effect an adequate result in treatment with such patients.

These borderline patients show *alloplastic* adaptation. They do not view the therapist as someone to help them discover what has gone wrong inside them. They wish, instead, to "correct" the problem by coercing changes in the external world. In the treatment situation, they attempt to manipulate the therapist into becoming the friend, protector, parent, punching bag, or whatever "vital" object is missing from their lives and would, if present, make their lives all right, without any need for the laborious exploration that therapy entails.

The highly impulsive borderline patient and the therapist do not start out on the same page. Even where treatment ultimately succeeds, a good deal of extra time is needed at the beginning of therapy to convince such patients of the value of looking *inside* themselves as a prelude to making *internal* changes. Treatment must be aimed at altering two sets of habits instead of just one: first, the habit of dealing with conflict very rapidly by means of behavior unaccompanied by thought, and second (after the first tendency is minimized), the habit of thinking about the interpersonal world in stereotypic, unrealistic ways, with splitting as a primary defense.

Strictly speaking, "acting out" refers to behaviors of a patient who is currently in therapy and who is indulging unwittingly in behaviors that express feelings generated through the therapist-patient relationship. Because the behaviors are occurring in the patient's external world, they are in effect being acted *out*—that is, outside the therapist's office. Acting out that meets this definition can be distinguished from other actions that are typical of the patient's behavior before entering therapy, that keep happening during treatment, and that have little or nothing to do with any feelings toward the therapist. The following case example concerns a patient who showed both kinds of behavior:

> **A 40-year-old man** entered treatment with the hope of resolving problems that kept cropping up in his relationship with his girlfriend. He was a moderately successful public relations executive in a large company. Married briefly in his 20s, he had subsequently been in a number of relationships lasting 2 or 3 years. His most striking personality features, aside from the anger, storminess, impulsivity, and intolerance of being alone that defined him as borderline, were hypomanic, narcissistic, and (mildly) antisocial elements. He was a problem drinker, but he did not abuse other substances. Thrill-seeking was another facet of his personality. He enjoyed "living on the edge."
>
> His latest choice of girlfriend partook of what psychogeneticists like to call "assortative mating": her personality was strikingly similar. She was fiery, tempestuous, volatile, manipulative, and just as prone to creating scenes

as he was. Their life together oscillated between days of frantic lovemaking and days of vicious arguments that usually ended in physical fights or in the destruction of each other's belongings. Sometimes the police were summoned. I was "hired," so my patient quipped, to help him smooth out the relationship. He was drawn to her because she was very attractive and only 23 years old. Although he complained about their frequent scenes, this storminess was the oxygen that kept the fire of passion burning and supplied the thrills without which he would have become bored and restless.

It rapidly became clear he did not want the relationship made smooth. He would have lost all interest if it were smooth; he simply wanted the temperature turned down a little, with less destructiveness. After an argument, for example, his girlfriend would sometimes burst into his office and hurl things at him in front of the other employees. This behavior threatened his job. Both were pathologically jealous, and any hint of infidelity or waning interest led to recriminations and a pitched battle. Each such battle would be followed by a breakup that lasted no more than a few days, but during that time, he would have a one-night stand with a woman he met in a bar— a permissible action, in his mind, because the relationship with his girlfriend was "over and done with." Three days later, there would be a tearful call from the girlfriend and a torrid resumption of the affair. A little later, however, rifling through his wastepaper basket, she would discover the champagne cork from the night he had spent with the woman he'd met during the breakup. She might confess that during that brief interlude she had sex with a former lover. They would both became enraged, she would "key" his car, he would punch her for defacing his car, and she would barge into his office—and the cycle would repeat. So far, none of this behavior constituted acting out his transference, although one could argue that both he and his girlfriend were reenacting patterns that related to their respective families. The *true* acting out was to come later.

After he had been in treatment for 2 years, he could begin to understand that marriage with someone like his girlfriend would be like continuing a bad movie. He was reaching an age when a day without sex was not as bad as a day without peace. The breakup this time was definitive. But after finally severing their relationship, he was at first intensely lonely and depressed, and his abuse of alcohol became worse. At my urging, he went to Alcoholics Anonymous but found it "boring" and quit after a few meetings. One evening, on a day when no session was scheduled, he called me when quite inebriated and demanded to see me. I was unable to accommodate him, to which he reacted angrily. Several hours later, the doorman at my building called, informing me that my patient had staggered to the lobby and had then urinated into the large flowerpot that graced the entranceway. *That* was acting out.

This man had been well motivated to bring the problematic relationship with his girlfriend to a reasonable conclusion, one way or the other. He showed a number of other favorable treatability factors, most notably candor and likeability. As with many hypomanic persons, he was outgoing, cheerful, humorous, and engaging. But I find that persons with this personality configuration oftentimes are not very psychologically minded or introspective. If he benefited at all from therapy, it had to do more with the feeling that I was his ally than with my remarks about the futility of the relationship with his girlfriend or about his self-destructiveness.

The man just described had fairly good ego strength and functioned well at his job, although he had little aptitude for making psychological connections. In contrast, the patient in the following vignette had excellent psychological mindedness but was overwhelmed with symptoms that clearly stemmed from a shatteringly abusive childhood and adolescence. Her motivation for psychotherapy was keen, but her perseverance was adversely affected by the many disruptions in her treatment, owing primarily to frequent suicide gestures. These negative factors reduced her amenability to psychotherapy to the intermediate level, as the unfolding of her story makes clear:

In her late 30s when she was referred to me, this woman, who had been employed as a nurse on a pediatric unit of a hospital, had been in a dynamically oriented therapy for a number of years before I undertook to treat her. The psychopathology in her family was extreme. Her father had manic depression. Both maternal grandparents were alcoholic; the grandmother committed suicide. The grandfather had carried on an incestuous relationship with the patient's mother. The paternal grandfather had committed incest with a granddaughter (the patient's cousin).

When the patient was 10 years old, her father began an incestuous relationship with her, forcing her into oral sex. The incest lasted until mid-adolescence. She kept the memory of it suppressed until she was in her 20s, but in the meantime she experienced depression and periods of dissociation for which, at the time, she had no explanation. When she began to recall the incest, she felt she could tell no one. In line with Searles' remarks about the importance of the nonhuman environment (Searles 1960), she felt she could speak of the incest only to a tree outside her house. She had worshipped her father as a "god" when she was young, when he doted on her and lavished her with attention, but then she grew to hate him after the incest began. Her father took to walking around the house naked. She would have many angry outbursts at him during those years, for which she would be reprimanded by her submissive mother, who kept telling her "your anger will kill your father."

In the months before I became her therapist, she had grown increasingly symptomatic. This increase in symptoms coincided with her having taken a new job as a pediatric nurse at a hospital where many of the children had histories of severe abuse. Their stories reawakened her memories of her own traumatic past. She experienced dissociative episodes, depression, flashbacks of the incest scenes, and aggravation of her symptoms in the days before her menstrual period. She reported several highly disturbing dreams. In the first of these dreams, she saw herself as a 14-year-old girl who had something "horrible" to reveal to some people, perhaps to her family. No one seemed to want to hear what she had to say. She then emitted "poisonous rays" that would kill those around her. She felt that she was "evil." Later she dreamed that she was a member of a doomed religious group, the leader of which said, "The time has come, and we must all die together." These dreams followed evenings when she attempted sex with her fiancé, which she found disturbing because his advances triggered memories of her father. She equated her inability to respond with any pleasure during sex as a kind of being "dead," and she worried that she would remain "stuck" in this emotionally deadened state, despite the therapy.

Although her fiancé was nurturing, patient, and not sexually aggressive—very different from her father—she found it difficult to keep separate her image of him from that of her father. In her dreams, she always pictured her fiancé as different from his real self; in one such dream there were snakes in his bed. She continued to feel guilt toward her mother, whom she imagined would be crushed if she knew about the incest. Besides, her father often told her she was "better in bed" than her mother, which increased her guilt further.

Her work as a nurse made it easy to obtain drugs, and she began to abuse benzodiazepines. Hostile fantasies of injuring men in their genitals began to dominate her mind, especially before her menstrual periods. She would become angry even at her fiancé, who had done nothing, as she recognized, to provoke such a reaction. Half a year after I began working with her, she became seriously depressed and discouraged about the future. She made a serious suicide attempt with a mixture of psychoactive medications and was briefly hospitalized. When she resumed therapy afterward, she insisted that I prescribe the same medications for her. Because of concern that she might misuse the medications and make another attempt, I refused to prescribe them, and as a result she quit therapy at that point.

This patient experienced *dissociative episodes* when confronted in the course of her work with children who had been victimized in ways similar to those in her background. This aspect of her case raises the question of why some persons subjected to serious abuse (especially sexual abuse) in early life develop dissociative symptoms and others do not. A genetic predisposition appears to be present in many such persons who develop dissociative symptoms. Others describe the mental effort they made to distance themselves emotionally from what was happening to them at the moment the abuse was taking place—a kind of *willed* dissociation. The patient just described certainly made this mental effort. After she regained memory of the incest, she began to recall how, when her father was performing sexual acts on her (such as intercrural rubbing of his penis), she would make a conscious effort to divorce the lower half of her body, where the "bad things" were happening, from the upper half. The "she" that she was then willing to acknowledge was the "unaffected" upper half of herself. The lower half was no longer "her."

The distinction between dissociation related to genetic predisposition and consciously willed dissociation may be more arbitrary than real. The "choice" to engage in willed dissociation may be made mostly in persons who were born with a brain whose "wiring" facilitates this symptom selection. This relationship would presume an interactive model of causation. Anthony Ryle (2004) endorsed this dual concept when he wrote, "in genetically predisposed individuals exposed to severe abuse, the experience or anticipation of such unmanageable emotions provokes dissociation....Some patients describe how this originated in the deliberate absenting of the self from unmanageable experience of abuse" (p. 12). In any event, incest victims and other severely abused or neglected persons often show only intermediate levels of amenability to psychotherapy because of the gross interference with therapist-patient dialogue imposed by the dissociative tendencies.

The patient of the next example owed his reduced amenability to psychotherapy to distractibility stemming from attention-deficit/hyperactivity disorder (ADHD). Characteristic of many persons with ADHD, he found it difficult to persevere at tasks of any length, from brief errands to long-range tasks such as staying with a job or finishing courses at school. His personality traits were confined mostly to the dramatic cluster and primarily to those of BPD. He showed a few other traits of this cluster, including preoccupation with power and success (a narcissistic trait), irresponsibility, and failure to plan ahead (the latter two, antisocial traits). He did not have an introspective turn of mind. His motivation for treatment shifted from fairly high (when he was experiencing depression) to meager (when his mood was brighter). Further details concerning his treatment are given in the following vignette:

> **The patient was a 21-year-old** college student when he first came for treatment. He had just broken up with a girlfriend he had been with for 2 years. She was the first girl with whom he had felt intense passion, and he had hoped to marry her after graduation, but she had become distant toward him and had eventually severed the relationship. He felt devastated and began to abuse a variety of drugs, including marijuana, alcohol, heroin, and cocaine, to assuage his depression. He contemplated suicide and on several occasions took small overdoses of hypnotics, but he experienced no serious consequences. Because his depression disrupted his academic life, he dropped out of college and returned to live with his parents. Even while at college, he had difficulty concentrating on his studies, grew easily bored, and often skipped classes. At home, he got into frequent arguments with his parents, most of which centered around their urging him to do something productive—take a few courses at another school, get a job, pursue a hobby. But he had no enthusiasm for these activities. He came faithfully to his

twice-weekly sessions while he was still depressed and derived some benefit from a combination of antidepressant and mood-stabilizing medications.

Some months later, as he began to improve, his attendance at sessions became more erratic. He would sometimes skip a session without calling beforehand. His restlessness and boredom became more noticeable. When he did finally get a job, he complained that it wasn't challenging enough and that he deserved more pay and a better position, despite his having no special training for the kind of work he was doing. He showed up late and was surly with his boss—and got fired. Finding himself now with nothing to do, he became more bored and restless and went back to abusing drugs, which further interfered with his ability to do anything productive. Sometimes he pilfered small sums of money from his parents to pay for drugs, and he was reprimanded when he was caught. He then complained about his parents treating him "like a kid" and could not grasp that he brought their reprimands on himself through his immature and irresponsible behavior.

When, at my urging, he enrolled in a 12-step program to help him conquer his drug problem, he went begrudgingly to a few meetings, made disparaging remarks about the other attendees, and soon quit. He returned to barhopping with his friends because, as he said, "that's where the action is." Absent any hobbies and too restless to read, he was at the mercy of whatever activities put some "drama" in his life: racing his motorcycle, picking up girls at bars, getting "smashed" on liquor, and so on. For a time, he maintained a facade that everything was fine. He had a breezy affability that helped to underscore this impression. Yet inwardly, as he could occasionally acknowledge, he felt lost and directionless. The situation grew more serious, and his attendance at sessions poorer, until I found it necessary to meet with his parents. An agreement was reached that he needed residential care, with a focus on stopping the drug use, and this plan was quickly put into effect. He made an excellent adjustment to the rehabilitation center. Once in the drug-free environment, he became goal oriented and looked forward with enthusiasm to resuming course work at college.

The way this patient's life had unfolded over the past few years, however, pointed to another problem—that he was still too dependent on an external locus of control. So long as he had a girlfriend, a job he liked, and a 12-step program with people looking after him, he could function well. But his situation was inherently fragile, because he was overly dependent on favorable circumstances. As Foon (1987) emphasized, persons with an external locus of control respond better to highly structured forms of therapy that impose limits and can ensure that the participants remain involved in growth-promoting activities. Many borderline patients have an external locus of control, especially those in whom mentalization (Fonagy 2001, p. 165) and introspectiveness are not well developed. Optimal response to psychodynamic therapies depends on an internal locus of control and adequate measures of introspectiveness and mentalization.

Fortunately, having an external locus of control does not in itself relegate a patient to a poor outcome. The long-term follow-up study of BPD patients, for example, has made it clear that some of the best outcomes, one or two decades later after treatment, belonged to those who did not have much aptitude for introspection but who responded well to supportive or other interventions (Wallerstein 1986). Some patients improved because of their perseverance and "true grit," with very little subsequent therapy, except perhaps enrollment in a 12-step program, for those who had abused substances. And some patients who were introspective, insightful, and quick to grasp the symbolic overtones of what they said and what they dreamed did not do well years later.

As for the reliance of this patient on alcohol, marijuana, cocaine, and (to a lesser extent) heroin, it is noteworthy that all four of these agents enhance, either directly or indirectly and through different mechanisms, the amount of dopamine-signaling dopaminergic pathways in the nucleus accumbens (Chao and Nestler 2004; Nestler and Malenka 2004) and medial forebrain bundle (Wise 1996). They all, in other words, spike the brain's pleasure centers (Grigsby and Stevens 2000, p. 181). There would appear to be a correlation between dopamine levels, attraction to these drugs, and the personality attribute of *novelty seeking* (see Cloninger 1986), an attribute common to BPD and to the other disorders of the dramatic cluster. One of the most noticeable characteristics of borderline patients from the standpoint of behavior is their inordinate *craving*—whether for drugs, alcohol, food (as in bulimia), sex, or (less often) gambling and other forms of risk-taking behavior.

These activities are believed to be related to what some researchers call a "reward deficiency syndrome" (Blum et al. 1996). A variant for a normal gene (i.e., an allele) that prevents dopamine from binding to cells in the "reward" pathways may be a contributing factor (Carter 1998, p. 64). Persons with this allele may be driven to seek out, to an excessive degree, the objects of their craving. The more imperious the craving, the less amenable the condition is to psychotherapy alone, although the chance of success may be better with behavioral therapies. This view is echoed by Koenigsberg et al. (2000), who wrote, "For some borderline patients, a particular behavior, such as drinking..., self-mutilation, risky sexual behavior, spending money, provides such a ready solution for painful feelings that psychotherapeutic examination of such feelings is practically impossible" (p. 252). These authors acknowledged that some addictive behaviors compromise cognitive functioning to such an extent that exploratory psychotherapy is useless. The pathological craving may be seen as a *symptom disorder*, which is a factor influencing treatability (see Table 1–1). If the symptom disorder is severe, it can get in the way of amenability to psychotherapy unless other means are brought to bear to reduce the intensity of the craving. For the patient in the previous clinical example, treatment of his substance abuse in a residential center devoted to that task became a necessary step in his recovery.

The patient in the following example had an intermediate level of amenability to psychotherapy because of her marked impulsivity and lack of introspectiveness, despite her high motivation to change, and her tendency in the early phase of treatment to show manipulative behavior and deceitfulness:

> **The patient was age 26 years** when she began treatment. All four grandparents had emigrated to the United States from Taiwan. Her father was a successful entrepreneur. She was raised with many advantages. She grew up in a large and comfortable home, attended private schools, dressed stylishly, and had a circle of friends consisting mostly of Chinese Americans like herself. She received a new car as a gift for graduating from high school. Her parents were gentle and attentive with her and her brother, both of whom were well behaved and did not require much discipline. There was no hint of abuse or traumatic experiences during any phase of her upbringing. The family traveled as a foursome on vacations and visited Europe on several occasions.
>
> Her parents placed enormous importance on education and spent many hours helping her and her brother with their homework. This emphasis led to a cloistered existence during her adolescence, with the result that she postponed dating boys until well beyond the age when her friends began dating. Even her carefully reared Chinese American girlfriends were more venturesome in this respect. Some of those friends were also accepted by more prestigious colleges than the one she went to, and this difference made her feel that they were somehow better than she was.
>
> She did not have her first boyfriend until age 25 years. By this time she was working in an advertising firm and earning a good salary. She was at first enthusiastic about the boyfriend. She felt she was in love and that he was a good marriage prospect because he was ambitious, was already on the fast track at his job, and seemed able to handle any situation. But he began to treat her shabbily, making depreciatory comments about her knowledge, her cooking, and her sexual inexperience. She endured these cruelties, partly because her self-confidence was destroyed and she imagined she could do no better; partly because she assumed if she made certain improvements in herself, all would be "wonderful" again. Hence she clung to a hopeless situation. A year later, after he humiliated her in a particularly painful way, she made a suicide attempt with an overdose of hypnotics and was hospitalized briefly. He then terminated their relationship.
>
> In ways similar to the borderline patient described by Ryle (2004, p. 19), she manifested three distressing states: *victim, rage,* and *revenge.* The revenge consisted in her calling him frequently at his office or home, disrupting his work. Having been submissive and polite to the point of

obsequiousness all her life, she now began to engage in behaviors that were out of character. She would send letters to his family chastising him for his cruelty, but writing them as if they came from someone else, as if a whole chorus of people were eager to denounce him to his relatives. Other hate mail was sent to his superiors at work. In the meantime her own work was compromised because so much time was taken up creating the vengeful letters or crying uncontrollably over the loss. Her boyfriend threatened to go to the authorities.

Her vengeful behavior was becoming as self-destructive as her suicidal attempt. To point this out to her proved treacherous: she took my comments as a sign that I was "taking his side." Her mind admitted of no gray areas. It took many months to convince her that my efforts to check her self-destructiveness meant that I was indeed "taking sides," but not with her former boyfriend. She had, as a consequence of severe splitting, become two people: one half was her generous, polite, considerate self (the self she grew up with), and the other half was the self-denigrating, vengeful self lacking in self-confidence that surfaced much of the time since she had begun the disastrous relationship with the boyfriend.

It puzzled me that her capacities for mentalization and for introspection were so meager, given her nurturing family and the absence of any trauma. In our 3 years of work, she almost never recalled dreams, and when she did, her associations to them were sparse. In one, in the aftermath of the breakup, she envisioned her boyfriend riding in a fancy car with a beautiful Chinese actress. She tries to catch up with the car, but he speeds away. Her only thought about it was a jealous lament that "it could have been me." A week later she reported another dream, in which a war was going on between soldiers from the Chinese mainland and those of the small island of Taiwan where her ancestors came from. Her boyfriend reassures her that "no one can conquer us," but a bomb falls nearby, and they perish. They disintegrate, and the pictures of her decaying body are shown on TV to her relatives in the United States. The dream mirrored her sense of hopelessness about ever being able to recoup the loss of her first love, even though he had made her miserable. Furthermore, the dream expressed her feeling that his rejection had destroyed her world altogether. In her mind, this feeling justified her rage and the vindictive acts she directed against him.

During the second year of therapy, she began dating other men. Some she rejected for various reasons, and these breakups were not upsetting, because in these situations she was the one in control. But with others the original pattern repeated itself: desperate clinging to a seemingly admirable but self-centered man who treated her shabbily, followed by depression, rage, suicidal thoughts, and vindictive reprisals. Rage swept away reason, and she would turn to suicide gestures (with small overdoses of pills) that were meant to humble the man who had hurt her feelings, upbraiding him by in effect saying, "Look what you made me do!" Or she would make calls or write angry letters that were intended to make the man suffer so she could "get even." Her impulsivity was limited to these actions, which were, in effect, tantrums; there was no substance abuse, no promiscuity, and no acts of vandalism. At the same time, she had no relief from books, sports, hobbies, or other useful activities that could distract her from the alternating rage and crying spells.

Gradual changes for the better occurred during the third year. By this time, she had enough awareness of her vulnerabilities that she was able to count to 10 when disappointed or angry—and then *not* do whatever she might have done in the past that would have gotten her into trouble. Her improvement came about through a kind of behavioral training; introspection and insight had little to do with it. She found it useful to make lists of her main problems and possible solutions. Her therapy took on the characteristics of Ryle's Cognitive Analytic Therapy (Ryle 2004), although his treatment method is more systematized, including, for example, patient homework, writing of angry letters that are not sent, and a time-limited format (a 24-week program). Toward the end of the third year, she met a much more suitable man from her own background and got married. By now, she was much calmer. The cheerful, outgoing, and considerate self resurfaced and gained the ascendancy.

DISSOCIATION: A SEVERE SYMPTOM INTERFERING WITH TREATABILITY

Dissociation, one of the many paradoxical situations in work with borderline patients, occurs regularly in those who also exhibit *dissociative disorder* or the rarer *dissociative identity disorder* (the latter formerly called *multiple personality disorder*). The interrelationship between BPD and these disorders is complex. Some researchers have argued that a considerable number of patients with dissociative identity disorder—approximately 60% or more—also have BPD (Horevitz and Braun 1984; Ross et al. 1990). Fink (1991) noted that dissociative identity disorder can occur with any of the DSM personality disorders, although much symptom overlap exists between dissociative identity disorder and BPD. He emphasized, however, the distinction between the *splitting* defense of the borderline patient and *switching* (from one personality to another) in patients with full-blown dissociative identity disorder or *depersonalization* in patients with dissociative disorder (who do not exhibit "alters").

Patients with dissociative identity disorder need not function at the borderline level of mental organization. Some may show either a higher (neurotic) or a lower (psychotic) level. A separation between the observing and experiencing ego is "crucial to insight therapy" (Kluft 1991, p. 697), yet may not be available to the patient with actual alters, because, as Kluft wrote, they are "cut off from full memory and pensive self-observation…remain prone to react in their specialized patterns…and find it difficult to learn from experience" (p. 697). Important memories are kept apart in logic-tight compartments. Until the "multiple" personality is converted into a unitary

personality (through specialized methods for this task), conventional psychotherapies may remain ineffective.

Common to both BPD and the whole group of dissociative disorders is
a history of childhood trauma, especially sexual trauma (most notably, incest by an older relative that occurs when the child is 10 years old or
younger [Stone 1990]). From the standpoint of amenability to psychotherapy, the paradoxical aspect is that borderline patients with the milder dissociative disorder, let alone the more dramatic dissociative identity
disorder, may contain within themselves an abundance of positive treatability factors, yet may be unable to access them or make use of them, at least
initially. They may dissociate during the stressful moments in therapy sessions, disrupting the train of dialogue between therapist and patient with
alarming frequency, a pattern Kluft (1991) described in discussing the treatment of patients with dissociative identity disorder. The dissociations give
a disjointed quality to the flow of treatment, as though one were trying to
make sense of a novel where every fourth word had been scratched out. One
such patient, a woman who had begun to broach the painful subject of incest with an uncle, would suddenly "tune out," fall into a near sleep, and
mumble words that had nothing to do with what was being discussed, such
as lists of ingredients for recipes or items to be sent to the laundry. Sometimes minutes, or even the remainder of the session, would be forfeited to
this detour. In other borderline patients entering treatment, dissociation is
so marked that psychotherapy in any meaningful sense cannot get under
way until measures are taken to remedy the dissociative state and restore
the patient's accessibility to therapy, as illustrated in the following case example:

> **In the 1960s** a patient was transferred from a general psychiatric hospital
> to one specializing in intensive psychotherapy. The patient was a young
> woman who was uncommunicative, at times seemingly mute, and who had
> made a number of suicide gestures and self-mutilative acts. She was able to
> reveal little more than that she felt inordinately guilty and bad; she could
> give no coherent account of the reasons for these intolerable feelings.
>
> In that era, the diagnosis of schizophrenia was applied to almost any in-
> patient, and drastic treatments were administered to these "schizophrenic"
> patients. Electroconvulsive therapy (ECT) was then popular as a remedy for
> otherwise treatment-resistant psychoses. Accordingly, this woman received
> many courses of ECT, with the result that her short-term memory was im-
> paired for a long time, making awareness of her past and of her "dynamics"
> even less accessible than it had been originally.
>
> Because she derived no benefit from ECT, the decision was made to try
> a different approach at a different hospital. In the first year at the new hos-
> pital her symptoms were not alleviated; she remained largely uncommuni-

cative and self-destructive. The importance of the therapist factor became clearly demonstrable in the second year. Assigned to a different therapist, she felt understood and accepted in ways she had not felt before. She attributed these feelings to the new therapist's quiet strength, emotional availability, and ability to listen. The material locked away in the dissociated state did not emerge all at once, and many details were not to surface for years. But she began to recall the severe and protracted abuse she had experienced during her early years at the hands of several relatives. This recall was the first step in a long process of reintegration.

The unfolding of this case illustrates what happens with disturbing frequency in patients with borderline personality. Their recovery often depends on chance occurrences, such as the luck of being assigned to a therapist to whom they can relate comfortably (or with whom they "click"). Failing this good luck, the result may be a tragic death by suicide. The woman in the previous example went on, within a few years with that same therapist, to a spectacular recovery that included a successful professional career, marriage, and children. In addition, she was able in time to recall more precisely the nature of the abuse she had experienced, such that the dissociative tendency dissipated and she achieved the integration that had for so long eluded her. This patient started out with no better than an intermediate level of treatability, or even worse, but ended up with a high level of treatability, once the positive factors could be mobilized—in this case, her candor, spirituality, and good capacities for introspection and mentalization.

REFERENCES

American Psychiatric Association: Diagnostic and Statistical Manual of Mental Disorders, 4th Edition, Text Revision. Washington, DC, American Psychiatric Association, 2000

Balint M: The Basic Fault: Therapeutic Aspects of Regression (1968). New York, Brunner/Mazel, 1979

Blum K, Cull JG, Braverman ER, et al: Reward deficiency syndrome. Am Sci 84:132–145, 1996

Carter R: Mapping the Mind. Los Angeles, University of California Press, 1998

Chao J, Nestler EJ: Molecular neurobiology of drug addiction. Annu Rev Med 55:113–132, 2004

Cloninger CR: A unified biosocial theory of personality and its role in the development of anxiety states. Psychiatr Dev 3:167–226, 1986

Colson DB, Allen JG, Coyne L-F, et al: Profiles of difficult psychiatric hospital patients. Hosp Community Psychiatry 37:720–724, 1986

Conklin CZ, Westen D: Borderline personality disorder in clinical practice. Am J Psychiatry 162:867–875, 2005

Diamond D, Clarkin J, Levine H, et al: Borderline conditions and attachment: a preliminary report. Psychoanalytic Inquiry 19:831–834, 1999

Fink D: The comorbidity of multiple personality disorder and DSM-III-R Axis II disorders. Psychiatr Clin North Am 14:547–566, 1991

Fonagy P: Attachment Theory and Psychoanalysis. New York, Other Press, 2001

Foon AF: Locus of control as a predictor of outcome of psychotherapy. Br J Med Psychol 60:99–107, 1987

Grigsby J, Stevens D: Neurodynamics of Personality. New York, Guilford, 2000

Horevitz RP, Braun B: Are multiple personalities borderline? An analysis of 33 cases. Psychiatr Clin North Am 7:69–87, 1984

Kernberg OF: Borderline personality organization. J Am Psychoanal Assoc 15:641–685, 1967

Kluft RP: Hospital treatment of multiple personality disorder: an overview. Psychiatr Clin North Am 14:695–719, 1991

Koenigsberg HW, Kernberg OF, Stone MH, et al: Borderline Patients: Extending the Limits of Treatability. New York, Basic Books, 2000

Minde K, Frayn D: The contributions of infant studies to understanding borderline personality disorders, in Handbook of Borderline Disorders. Edited by Silver D, Rosenbluth M. Madison, CT, International Universities Press, 1992, pp 87–120

Nestler EJ, Malenka RC: The addicted brain. Sci Am 290:78–85, 2004

Ross CA, Miller SD, Reagor P, et al: Structured interview data on 102 cases of multiple personality disorder from four centers. Am J Psychiatry 147:596–601, 1990

Ryle A: The contribution of cognitive analytic therapy to the treatment of borderline personality disorder. J Personal Disord 18:3–35, 2004

Searles H: The Non-Human Environment in Normal Development and in Schizophrenia. New York, International Universities Press, 1960

Searles H: My Work With Borderline Patients. Northvale, NJ, Jason Aronson, 1986

Stone MH: Incest in the borderline patient, in Incest-Related Syndromes of Adult Psychopathology. Edited by Kluft RP. Washington, DC, American Psychiatric Press, 1990, pp 183–204

Thomä H, Kächele H: Psychoanalytic Practice, Vol 2. Translated by Wilson M. Berlin, Springer-Verlag, 1992

van der Kolk B: Trauma and memory, in Traumatic Stress: The Effects of Overwhelming Experience on Mind, Body, and Society. Edited by van der Kolk B, McFarlane AC, Weisaeth L. New York, Guilford, 1996, pp 279–302

Waldinger RJ, Gunderson JG: Completed psychotherapies with borderline patients. Am J Psychother 38:190–202, 1984

Wallerstein R: Forty-Two Lives in Treatment. New York, Guilford, 1986

Wise RA: Addictive drugs and brain stimulation reward. Annu Rev Neurosci 19:319–340, 1996

5

PERSONALITY DISORDERS OF INTERMEDIATE AMENABILITY TO PSYCHOTHERAPY

Other Personality Disorders

Although borderline patients have the reputation of being difficult to treat, patients in this group vary considerably with respect to the treatability factors, as discussed in the preceding chapters. Patients with optimal treatability factors have a general tendency to be rewarded eventually with good outcomes, but some who inspired initial pessimism also ultimately do well. The reverse is true as well: some with a promising array of positive factors do poorly. Those with few positive factors usually prove extremely difficult to treat and often have a discouraging life course, but even in this group, favorable outcomes are sometimes obtainable. Much the same can be said for the remaining personality disorders, except for those with the most malignant characteristics—antisocial, psychopathic, and sadistic personality—where positive treatability factors are in short supply and outcome is predictably poor. This latter group is the focus of a later chapter. At present, the spotlight is on intermediate levels of treatability among certain patients with DSM-IV-TR (American Psychiatric Association 2000) Cluster A and Cluster C disorders and others with narcissistic, histrionic, and depressive (or depressive-masochistic) disorders.

The extensive literature devoted to the treatment of specific personality disorders describes a variety of treatments, including psychodynamic, cognitive-behavioral, supportive, group therapy, and combined "eclectic" approaches. Advocates for long-term therapy are in the majority, although several authors have devised and opt for short-term techniques. Table 5–1 lists references for some of the books and articles focused on particular personality disorders. Materials on borderline patients, discussed in Chapter 2 and Chapter 4, are not included in the table. A proportion of patients with any of the remaining personality disorders exhibit intermediate levels of treatability, but the literature seldom distinguishes between recommendations for patients who are readily amenable to the therapy that is being discussed and recommendations for those who are much less accessible. References for sadistic and psychopathic personality are not included in the table, because persons with those personality configurations almost invariably show either the lowest level of treatability or outright nontreatability.

In the clinical examples that follow, it will become clear that personality-disordered patients who occupy the realm of intermediate accessibility to psychotherapy fit into two main groups. In one group the motivation for treatment is good, but psychological mindedness and other related factors, including conscious attributes such as introspection and unconscious ones such as empathy or mentalization, are not well developed. In the other group, those psychological attributes are operating at reasonable levels, but motivation and perseverance are lacking. Occasionally a patient may have adequate psychological mindedness and motivation, but other factors, such as paralyzing anxiety or entrapment in unfavorable life circumstances, may interfere. For these patients, the fear of change overwhelms the desire to change.

The first two case vignettes concern patients with Cluster A personality disorders: in the first, schizotypal personality disorder; in the second, schizoid personality disorder.

A 42-year-old woman came for treatment because she felt her life lacked direction. She was mildly depressed much of the time and lonely. She had only a few friends, had minimal contact with a sister, and had never married or had any significant intimate relationships. Moderately overweight, she dressed in a frumpy manner, creating an uninviting appearance. She did not

TABLE 5–1. Psychotherapy of various personality disorders: relevant literature

Personality type	Psychodynamic psychotherapy	Cognitive-behavioral therapy	Other psychotherapies (including short-term)
Schizotypal	Vanggaard 1979		Stone 1996
Schizoid	Grinberg and Rodriguez-Perez 1982; Liberman 1957	Eidelberg 1957	Leszcz 1989
Paranoid	Meissner 1976; Modlin 1963; Salzman 1960	Beck and Freeman 1990	
Narcissistic	Cooper 1986; Goldberg 1989; Kernberg 1974, 1989; Kohut and Wolf 1978	Beck and Freeman 1990; Young et al. 2003	
Antisocial (mild)		Barley 1986; Black 1999; Meloy 1996	
Histrionic	Easser and Lesser 1965		
Hysteric	Chodoff and Lyons 1958; Easser and Lesser 1989	Fleming 1988	Horowitz et al. 1984
Obsessive-compulsive	Salzman 1973	Guidano and Liotti 1983	Davanloo 1986; Horowitz et al. 1984; Sifneos 1997
Avoidant	Gabbard 1994	Brown et al. 1995; Emmelkamp and Scholing 1990; Marks and Marks 1990	Alden 1989; Barber et al. 1997; Winston et al. 1994
Dependent		Overholzer 1987	Winston et al. 1991
Depressive and depressive-masochistic	Brenner 1959; Jacobson 1971; McWilliams 1994		Millon and Davis 2000, pp. 452–471, 493–511
Passive-aggressive			Millon and Davis 2000, pp. 471–491

work, existing on a fairly liberal trust fund from her deceased father. After finishing college, she toured Europe, roaming the countryside. She was surprised that she had spent one-half of her life as a college graduate but was unable to account for all the years that had gone by.

She had two interests that sustained her: music and astrology. She aspired to be a "great" violinist, although she had taken up the instrument only in the last few years. Her one close friend, a devotee of astrology, took the patient under her wing, instructing her in this pseudoscience by which she attempted to guide her life. This interest was only one of the many eccentricities that alerted me to the schizotypal nature of her personality. Other members of her family were more seriously affected. A brother had received a diagnosis of paranoid schizophrenia. The patient had been raised primarily by nannies on the large estate owned by her father and bordered by a still larger estate belonging to a cousin. She was 12 years old before she was permitted to go into the nearest town and chat with children in more ordinary circumstances. She had little contact with her mother, who, she was told, spent many months "traveling" abroad. Three years after I began working with the patient, she learned, at age 45 years, from an aunt, that her mother had been institutionalized frequently in psychiatric hospitals for paranoid schizophrenia. Her father, while not seriously mentally ill like his wife and son, was irascible and given to violent outbursts, from which her nannies had tried to shield her during her early years.

It was clear that she was strongly motivated to make something of her life and to discover her true calling. But she had little awareness of her limitations and no insight into the ways she avoided the possible by striving after the will-o'-the-wisp. She had developed a strong crush, for example, on her neighbor, to whom she sent numerous "mash notes," slipping them under his door; she would bake him cookies and leave them outside his door in the morning. This man was a famous musician who happened to be homosexual and had been living for more than 20 years in a stable relationship with another man. No matter how delicately, albeit firmly, I pointed out to her that her hopes for this man were unrealistic (and that he had become a fantasized mother-substitute in her mind), she persisted in this fixed action pattern—the way a squirrel paws at the ground continuously to retrieve an acorn that isn't there.

She expressed a desire to return to college to take courses that would prepare her for a career. But her trust fund, having been invested only in stocks, did not afford her enough income to pay tuition. I suggested repeatedly that she call the manager of the trust and have him switch the securities to bonds that would yield her about three times what she currently lived on. Three years went by before she finally took this step. She began taking courses in music history. Her spirits lifted now that she was doing something productive, although she still entertained hopes she could become a professional violinist. I suggested she might find some satisfaction in a related way: she had enough money now to sponsor a scholarship in her name for an aspiring young violinist, and she could become one of the judges who would award the prize. Thus she could be a "factor" in the musical world, helping someone else develop the virtuosity that she at her age could not achieve. This course seemed to me a reasonable and achievable compromise. It did not seem so to her.

Her preoccupation with astrology, another manifestation of her entrenchment in a world of unreality, was of concern to me. I once attempted to challenge her faith in the stars by presenting her with two times of birth just minutes apart. She claimed her friend could tell how the two persons differed and developed. One piece of paper contained the birth time of a woman who was the most brilliant psychiatric resident on the inpatient unit where I worked. The other piece contained the birth time (by coincidence, 9 minutes later on the same day in the same year) of a profoundly schizophrenic woman on this unit. I believe she and her friend suspected the nature of the test, and they did not respond. (This situation occurred 35 years ago; now I would not try to undermine the faith of such a patient, for whom it could be a source of strength.)

I found it difficult in general to enlist her interest in discovering through our work how she had developed as she did and what factors interfered with her finding that "sense of direction" she had so long sought. Symbolism eluded her. She once had a dream in which she was in her bedroom, as a child living in the manor house where she grew up. She could hear her father yelling as he was stomping about in another part of the house. A hole suddenly opened up in the ceiling of the room, and dozens of violins fell down on her as she lay in bed, injuring her. The dream seemed to spell out with great clarity some of the central themes of her life. Her father had forbidden her to take music lessons, because he considered them a frivolous activity. The dream expressed her fear of his violence (materialized through the pun: violins–violence) and her avoidance of attempts to acquire skills in a pursuit that would earn his contempt. Now that she was taking graduate courses, she was more content with her life; she finally accepted the hopelessness of her love for her neighbor, and at this point she gradually drifted away from treatment.

The previous therapist of a woman in her late 20s referred her to me because she seemed distraught about a boyfriend. She felt more and more dissatisfied with him, yet she was unable to break off the relationship. This was one of her two main problems. Born in South Africa, the patient was now an English teacher in a public school. She had difficulty getting along with her supervisors and an inability to fit in with or to be accepted by her peers. These troubles had made her discouraged about her future, and she expressed to me the intention, if she were not married and settled by age 30, to commit suicide. This deadline gave me about 15 months to get her "all better."

The Herculean nature of this task rapidly became clear. Despite her high motivation to get her life in order, she was markedly paranoid in personality and tended to offend half the people she knew and to misunderstand all of them. Her empathic skills were meager at best, and she constantly misread the intentions of other people. At school, for example, a vicious circle took shape. She often scolded her pupils in a harsh way, which came to the attention of her supervisors, who made criticisms about her

work. She then felt picked on and cast racial epithets at some of the supervisors or spoke to them in contemptuous language. These interactions made
her angrier about her job and even more prone to get cross with her pupils.
She spoke in a highly stilted manner, which put off the other teachers whenever she tried to join them for lunch. She then felt isolated and rejected,
which further fueled her distrust and dislike of people in general. As for her
boyfriend, he lived a marginal existence, was out of work, did not maintain
good hygiene, and depended on her financially, yet he was often argumentative and at times physically abusive. She so dreaded being alone, however,
that she clung to this unrewarding relationship despite its obvious drawbacks.

        She could make little use of the therapy as a way of gaining insight and
of mastering her problems through such insight. She had no aptitude for introspection or mentalizing. We initially met twice a week, which may have
helped her feel less alone. After a few months she was able to insist that her
boyfriend leave. But she then frequented bars after work and would have
one-night stands with men who offered no prospect of a lasting relationship. These experiences, temporary anodynes for her loneliness, made her
feel degraded, especially because some of the men were rough characters.
In the hope of improving her social skills and manner of speaking, I advised
her to enroll in a Dale Carnegie course and in another course where people
were taught how to dress to better advantage. She pursued these courses
with enthusiasm, but after a half year of meetings she was no more at ease
socially and no more relaxed in her speech than she was at the start; she did
pass her thirtieth birthday, however, without committing suicide. At that
time she returned to South Africa, where she spent the next 15 years in a
similar teaching job. She lived with her sister and brother-in-law but rarely
dated, continuing to lead the same sort of isolated life she had led while in
the United States.

        At age 45 years, she returned to the United States and to the same
school where she had worked before. We now met for only one session per
week. Her personality was quite the same. She was quick to find fault with
her superiors and co-workers and still made others ill at ease with her
strange speech and confrontational manner. She alienated her few remaining friends with her fastidiousness and critical remarks. But she also blamed
herself for having "ruined" her life by having permitted a black man she'd
met in a bar years ago to have sex with her.

        Some of this grossly unrealistic thinking came through in a dream she
mentioned shortly after her return to the United States: "A boy was doing
voodoo as a way of doing evil; he then changed into a brown wooden statue.
I touched the evil that was in the statue, which made me evil too. I had to
fly away as fast as I could." The day before, she had been reprimanded by
the school supervisor, who was a black woman, for yelling at one of her pupils. When I tried to point out that yelling at a student meant that she was
not in good control in the classroom and that the supervisor could hardly
be faulted for admonishing her about this, she upbraided me, saying: "You
Jews always stick up for the blacks!" When I asked her whether she would
have been completely surprised if the supervisor had been a white Presby-

terian like herself and had still scolded her for yelling at a pupil, she could at least acknowledge that she wouldn't have been surprised.

Now that she was nearing age 50 years, with her life no less lonely and her ability to connect with people no better than when I first saw her, she had grown more embittered, more envious of people whom she saw as better off economically and socially, and more mistrustful of others. She showed highly polarized attitudes toward me. I was someone she could talk to, and she felt less lonely thanks to our long years of working on her problems, yet she also felt I had let her down and failed to turn her life around, even that I had failed "deliberately" because I didn't like her and considered her "white trash." When I remarked that the attitudes she ascribed to me were like the ones she often voiced in criticizing herself, she did show a little insight. She recalled how she continued to berate herself as a "defiled woman" for having once slept with a black man almost 30 years earlier. I had pointed out on innumerable occasions that if she had had this liaison despite her own prejudices, it must have been an expression of her desperate loneliness, which no one would regard as an unforgivable sin. People might, however, be less forgiving about her racial prejudices, even though I could understand them as shallow defenses she had erected against her feelings of unworthiness.

She was impervious to these interpretations, as though her self-hatred had become a cherished part of herself and she was loath to part with it. She returned once again to South Africa after retiring from her job at age 60. Her bitterness, stilted speech, loneliness, and isolation had hardly changed in all the 32 years I had known her. Her main source of consolation was music. I had encouraged her to take up an instrument during the first phase of her treatment, and by now she was a competent flautist who played in ensembles with other musicians. These musicians were as close as she came to having friends, but they seldom met except to play music. Thanks to this hobby, her life felt less barren than it had before, and suicide seemed less beckoning as a "solution." The hope was that she could find another group of musicians in her native city.

In retrospect, this patient might have met the criteria for a DSM-IV-TR diagnosis of Asperger's disorder (diagnostic code 299.80), because she manifested several of the social impairment qualities associated with this diagnosis. She did not, however, show the restricted, repetitive, and stereotyped patterns of behavior that constitute the other important element of this condition. She could be seen as having a kind of Asperger's syndrome manqué, in that her personality attributes—primarily a handicap in grasping the unspoken rules of social interaction—resembled those of patients with the full-blown disorder.

The following vignette concerns a patient with a disorder from Cluster B other than borderline personality disorder (in this case, narcissistic personality disorder).

A 40-year-old man was referred to me for therapy because he had been experiencing severe problems in his marriage. His personality configuration was predominantly narcissistic, as he made apparent with his opening comment. When asked what had prompted his seeking treatment, he replied that he had grown quite concerned that his hairline was beginning to recede, as a result of which he feared it would become more difficult to pick up teenage girls at the beach, which had been his major source of satisfaction. This "chief complaint" seemed a good deal less serious than the suicidality or panic states that figured more prominently among my other patients. I imagined at first that his complaint was the top layer covering a deeper problem of insecurity about his masculinity and his attractiveness. This interpretation would make it easier for me to sympathize with his plight. Sympathy is an important ingredient in a therapist's initial attitude, and a patient who elicits little or none of this response is not easy to work with.

My capacity for sympathy was strained a short while later, when it emerged that he was married. His wife was an attractive woman in her late 20s who worked as a middle-level executive in a large corporation. Her salary was their sole source of income, because he had been out of work for 6 years. In addition, she had recently given birth to their first child, who was now 7 months old. Because he was unemployed, most of the time he stayed at home to take care of their child. He was bitter about this situation, because the obligations of parenthood impinged uncomfortably on his ability to arrange days at the beach. In any case, he found it distasteful to care for an infant. He was equally bitter about work. Although he had worked for some years as a magazine editor, he felt that his true calling was that of photographer. But he had had no success in that field. He complained that his portfolio was every bit as good as the "competition" but that he couldn't break into the business because it was a "closed field," the bosses only bought the pictures submitted by their favorites, and so on.

He had sought treatment, however, not so much because of the receding hairline or his being unappreciated as a photographer but rather because of a blowup between him and his wife when she discovered him phoning one of the young women he had met at the beach. This incident happened when she returned unexpectedly to their apartment one morning because she had forgotten the keys to her office. She threatened divorce, which would have had disastrous consequences for him, given that she was the sole breadwinner in the family.

I felt that this crisis at least provided me with some leverage in the therapy. Several changes had to be made—and fast—to resolve the crisis and preserve the marriage, but the patient was reluctant to contemplate these changes. He mostly wanted reassurance that he was still attractive to women and that his skills as a photographer were as outstanding as he preferred to believe. Most worrisome was his sense of entitlement that he could somehow eat his cake and have it too by holding on to the marriage while continuing to cheat on the wife who was supporting him. I chose to rely on some of the interventions Larry Rockland (1989) mentioned in his book on supportive psychotherapy, including limit-setting (to curb acting out) and exhortation (i.e., suggestions put forth in a forceful way). I told him that economic dependence aside, he owed it to his wife to pursue an honest course: either to remain in the marriage and to try to make it work or to divorce. The first alternative required that he not be unfaithful. The divorce alternative would allow him other partners, but if he opted for divorce, he would have to find a job to support himself, because he could hardly expect alimony under the circumstances.

The crisis in his marriage was the crucial issue. His concern about getting older was a distant second in importance. He was not without motivation, and he came to his twice-weekly sessions regularly for a number of months. But his motivation was not so much to change as to find an ally who would sanction his patterns of behavior and agree with him about the unfairness of the photography business. He nevertheless decided to make a go of the marriage. This course meant apologizing to his wife for the infidelities and promising not to seek out other women. I was able in time to persuade him that it was better to work at something than to remain idle while nourishing fantasies of a greatness that was not likely to be realized.

This man, who finally did get his marriage and his work life back in order, represents an exception to the usual situation with narcissistic personalities. Ordinarily, successful narcissists remain impervious to therapy, because they feel in total control of their world and assume that they are above everyone else. As they see it, they have no problem that would require the services of a psychiatrist. Many politicians and heads of large corporations fit this picture. But if for some reason they fail, they become vulnerable and, at that point, amenable to treatment. This patient started out as a failed narcissist, yet was barely amenable to treatment, mainly for reasons of false pride. Also, he had no compunctions about taking advantage of others. Because of this amorality, he elicited strong countertransference feelings that lowered his likeability. Therapy becomes more difficult in such an atmosphere. He was able eventually to understand the hidden factor behind the false pride—that thinking of himself as a superior photographer who was "simply not appreciated in my own time" shored up his self-esteem and served as a good rationalization for not working. It did not occur to him that if he took a job that was less prestigious but that brought him some income, people in general (and certainly his wife) would think better of him. Once he began to have some success in work (in a field less glamorous than fashion photography), he felt less pressure to prove himself through his attractiveness to young women. He left treatment at that point. Thirty years later, I learned that his marriage and his life in general had gone satisfactorily and that he was content to pursue photography as a hobby rather than as a vocation.

The next two vignettes concern patients with anxiety-related personality disorders: in the first, obsessive-compulsive personality disorder; in the second, depressive-masochistic personality. The latter is not a diagnostic entity in DSM-IV-TR but is composed of a combination of depressive and self-defeating personality traits.

A man in his mid-30s was referred for treatment of a paraphilic disorder. He lived alone and worked as an inspector of automobiles, testing their roadworthiness before they were sent to dealerships. Extraordinarily meticulous about his work and to a marked degree obsessive-compulsive in personality, he alienated many of his co-workers and superiors because he would turn down a car for the slightest defect. He was never fired, however, because his perfectionism was valued, and any car that he did stamp as "OK" could be sold with absolute confidence. He had only one or two friends and had never had an extended relationship with a woman, although he casually dated a few women once or twice and then dropped them. Occasionally he would have sex with a prostitute.

A month before beginning treatment he had exposed himself to some teenage girls in a park. They voiced a complaint, and he was ordered by the court to undergo therapy for his exhibitionism. We met twice a week in what was to be a psychoanalytically oriented treatment. He showed little aptitude for this approach, but I persisted, mostly because, at the time, this method was the only one I knew. (His treatment occurred more than 35 years ago, when the behavioral approach to paraphilia was not as well developed as it is now.) The patient came to sessions with the regularity and promptness one would expect from a perfectionistic person. He sat rigidly in his chair, wore a masklike expression, and seldom radiated emotions of any sort. He showed no spontaneity in bringing forth memories or other material. If I did not ply him with questions, there would have been interminable silences.

Little by little he revealed some episodes from his early years that had significant bearing on his symptom. He was the youngest child in a large family and the only boy. His older sisters picked on him and made fun of him, to the point of his developing a cordial dislike of all of them. But his mother's treatment of him was more humiliating still. The memory that stood out as the most painful concerned the time he was walking with his mother in the downtown section of the city where he grew up. He felt an urge to urinate and asked his mother where there might be a bathroom. She pointed to a space between some parked vehicles near the sidewalk and told him: "Go pee between the cars—you got nothin' to hide!" This seemed to be the wellspring from which his exhibitionistic symptom had sprung. He felt driven in his adult life to show (to the girls in the park, for instance) that he indeed did have something to hide. After the incident with the cars, however, he also became preoccupied with what others—especially his sisters—had to hide. When he was a little older, he would rig mirrors in such a way that he could catch glimpses of his sisters as they undressed.

In his therapy, he did begin to experience some relief from the exhibitionistic urge, once we made the connection between his mother's forcing him to expose himself and his voluntary exposing of himself later on. Some credit must be given to the court, because he knew he faced incarceration if he were caught exposing himself again. This incentive, one might say, was the behavioral component of his treatment. He rarely reported his dreams, but the few he did report were of a gruesome nature. In his first dream, he pictured a huge volcano that was erupting and dumping tons of hot lava on vast populations—in effect, destroying the world. In a later dream, he saw himself as a concentration camp commandant who was hurling women, one after the other, into the ovens. In still another dream, women were being tortured by sadistic authorities. These dreams had an impersonal quality in that he was always the witness, simply viewing terrible things happening to people (mostly women) he didn't know. Occasionally, his face would betray a subtle smirk, as if to signal that he took pleasure in the spectacle of these disasters, where (for the most part) it was "payback time" for the women in his life who had belittled him.

The patient remained in therapy for 2 years altogether, during which time there was a noticeable, although not dramatic, lessening of his hostile attitude toward women. He would occasionally date a woman from his own social class, but such relationships remained on a superficial level. It no longer cost him any mental effort to refrain from exposing himself in public. Because that symptom had been the motivation for his entering therapy, its disappearance served, in his eyes, as justification to discontinue treatment. He did not feel motivated to use psychotherapy as a mechanism for enhancing his ability to establish intimacy. For this reason, I felt discouraged about his long-term prognosis. He was in his late 30s when he left treatment, and although he had symptomatic improvement, he had no close relationships with women, and it seemed that he was too old to make much progress in that area.

My pessimism turned out to have been unwarranted. At follow-up 20 years later, I learned that he had left his old job and was now running a successful business of his own and that he had married and was raising three children. In retrospect, it was perhaps useful to have pursued a psychodynamic psychotherapy where the aim was to reduce his animosity toward women. His main conflict centered on his heterosexual desires versus his hatred of women. If a behavioral technique had succeeded in reducing the tendency toward exhibitionism, he might have emerged symptom-free but still incapable of trusting a woman in an intimate relationship. I had focused on reducing his negative feelings toward women and on bolstering his sense of masculinity (which had been enfeebled by his early experiences at home), with the hope that this approach might take away the exhibitionistic urges. It is hard to know whether this approach contributed to his being able to establish a good relationship some years later, but it was gratifying to learn that he ultimately became less rigidly obsessive-compulsive and better able to lead a fulfilling life.

A 30-year-old woman became depressed after the breakup of a romantic relationship and sought treatment at that point. The only girl in a family of five children, she was burdened with the care of her elderly parents. Her brothers had abandoned responsibility toward their parents either because they felt this was a "daughter's proper role" or because none of them liked either parent very much. She was also the youngest of the five and the only one not married, all the more reason, according to the brothers, that their parents' care should be entrusted to her. Meanwhile, her position as a middle-level executive in a large accounting corporation left her little time for activities not related to work. Both parents were in poor health, and their needs took precedence over her social life, especially because of the unwritten rule that the brothers were not to be called on to help in managing their parents' affairs or even in making decisions involving their living arrangements.

The patient showed a fair degree of psychological mindedness and high motivation to solve the seemingly intractable problems of her family life, but she appeared to me, after I got to know her a little better, as one of those hapless persons in whom an unextractable "bad-luck magnet" has been placed. She had become the designated companion of her parents' old age, and to walk away from that obligation would be to abandon them altogether. Her brothers no longer even visited them. Thus, if she were to meet a suitable man and marry him, let alone have a family of her own, her parents would be left to fend for themselves. The idea of a nursing home was not acceptable, so that alternative was not available.

The little time the patient set aside for dating was spent with men who were grossly unsuitable. With some she had strong cultural and religious differences. Others had an unpromising work history, treated her shabbily, or had serious personality problems and were sexually avoidant. I made the interpretation on many occasions that she was drawn to these unsuitable men as a means of resolving the conflict between her needs and those of her parents. As long as she picked "losers," she could maintain the illusion that she was giving adequate thought to her own future but was simply cursed by a malevolent fate never to meet the right man. The situation did not improve after the death of her father, 2 years after she began treatment. The patient moved her mother into her small apartment. A hired companion looked after her mother during the day, and the patient looked after her during the evening. This change brought her relationships with men almost to a halt. She and her mother then moved to a different city, and her treatment was interrupted.

Treatment was resumed several years later, by which time she had married and had taken a position closer to home in order to work nearer her husband. She was in crisis when she called me, feeling depressed, anxious, and entrapped, because her husband had turned out to be controlling, hot-tempered, and at times physically abusive. He was secretive about money, doled out an allowance barely sufficient for household expenses, and complained of an "Everest" of debts, yet he spent lavishly on his own hobbies and pursuits. If she protested about his behavior or his stinginess, he would stalk out of the house, disappearing for hours or even overnight. When she mentioned such incidents to a friend who was an attorney, the friend urged her to divorce.

This course of action seemed impossible to the patient, partly for economic reasons and partly because she felt pessimistic about ever finding someone to marry. Her therapy was by now purely supportive and crisis oriented. I urged her to send out résumés in hopes of securing a higher-paying job, so that she might have the option of leaving the marriage. In a self-defeating way, she could never seem to follow through with this task. Eventually, she did go for two interviews, but she gave up after the second rejection. When she recounted another episode of cruelty on her husband's part, she would beseech me with questions of "Why does he do this?" My response was to ask her, "Why do you remain in a joyless and at times downright dangerous marriage?" She had no answer, although her fear of being alone played a role in her reluctance to leave a bad situation. Therapy was stalemated because she could not bring herself to implement the changes she knew were necessary.

Although this patient exemplifies depressive-masochistic personality, such a label cannot do justice to the complexity of intertwined forces that directed her behavior. Part of her problem was an outgrowth of her good character. Unlike her brothers, she did not abandon her parents in their declining years. Neither was she content simply to serve as their companion in their old age. She also wanted marriage and children, and hence her conflict arose. She could not leave her marriage, because she was too fearful of living alone until she met a more compatible partner. Earlier she had been too guilt-ridden to place her parents in a nursing home to facilitate her ambition to have a life of her own. This choice was also inspired by fear—fear of the parents' silent disapprobation. A neurobiologist might suspect that she had an overactive amygdala (see LeDoux 1996, pp. 157–165; LeDoux 2002, pp. 120–124), as a genetic legacy or as the by-product of repetitive frightening interchanges with family members while she was growing up. This difference in brain structure might be part of the reason she emerged as a finer person than her siblings, but she was also unfulfilled, unhappy, and unable to change. Despite her capacity for insight, her good character, and her motivation, she defeated every opportunity for self-fulfillment and thwarted almost all therapeutic efforts aimed at springing her "trap." Thus she showed an intermediate level of treatability. Had her parents died at younger ages, freeing her at an earlier age of the guilt she felt about not remaining by their side, she might have used her many positive qualities to better advantage vis-à-vis her own future, but this interpretation remains a speculation.

The following case example illustrates the interaction between personality and an underlying symptom disorder. The man depicted in the example showed the traits of narcissistic personality disorder along with those of what was formerly called "explosive-irritable" personality. The latter shares some of the features of Kraepelin's "irritable temperament" (1921), which he felt was associated with manic-depressive psychosis. This man's bipolar II variant of mood disorder served to intensify the expression of his personality tendencies. He was given to outbursts of rage that adversely affected all his interpersonal relationships, especially with his wife and with his subordinates in the workplace.

A 46-year-old man was referred for psychotherapy because of trouble on two fronts: severe marital conflict and a crisis in his business. Both troubles stemmed from a common source—his explosive temper and its impact on all the people whose lives intersected with his. A handsome man with a powerful athletic build, he was a formidable ladies' man and even more formidable as a competitor in business. The business he owned took him to many countries, and, like Mozart's Don Juan, he had liaisons with women in whichever country he visited. These affairs had led to the downfall of his two previous marriages but were not the main issue with his current wife. The problem was his temper. He had few complaints about his wife, but he hated his in-laws. If she dared to take their side on any issue, he would explode in anger, call her disloyal, and sometimes hit her. At other times, he took out his frustrations about work once he got home, and he might overturn the dinner table or smash down a door. He could be cordial, even complimentary, to his employees who performed well. Those whose performance displeased him, however, were subject to his rage and humiliating remarks.

He was given to mood swings, with mild hypomanic episodes that alternated with occasional but deeper depressions. This pattern was compatible with a diagnosis of bipolar II disorder. His symptoms were not very responsive to mood stabilizers. In other respects he showed the features of malignant narcissism (Kernberg 1992, p. 77). Ordinarily cheerful, with a breezy sense of humor (he referred to his medications as his "M&Ms," because they didn't seem to have much greater effect than those candies), he could suddenly descend into a profound sadness, crying with remorse if he had struck his wife the day before.

After he had been in treatment with me for half a year, his tendency to extremes of mood intensified. He was in the midst of selling his firm, which offered the possibility of a comfortable retirement if the sale was made or of more years of ungratifying work if it failed. On one occasion he came home after a frustrating day with the prospective buyers and lost control with his wife, hitting her in the face and giving her a black eye. He threatened to kill her, as he had threatened on other occasions, but this time she was quite frightened. I scheduled an emergency meeting with both of them. I insisted he live apart for a few days in a kind of cooling-off period, which he was reluctant to do. I asked his wife to leave, so I could talk with him alone in the hope of getting my point across. The dialogue went this way:

Patient: Why do you say I have to go somewhere else? I just lost my temper. I could never kill her. She's my only friend, even though I hate her at times.

Therapist: You know what? I don't know you could "never" kill her. You gave her a black eye. You scared her out of her wits. You smashed the kitchen door. You've been way out of control. And you don't have to go "somewhere else." You can sleep in your office for three or four nights, get hold of yourself, and then we'll see.

Patient: I can't do it. I feel lost without her. Even three days alone.... I promise I won't lay a hand on her....

Therapist: She's gotta know she's safe. That's the first thing. Three days without her—that's a small price to pay for making sure nothing bad happens. You're a 220-pound weight lifter. She's a 100-pound woman. You could accidentally kill her, not even meaning to. They find a married woman murdered—what do the cops know? Ninety percent of the time it's the husband; 5%, it's the ex-husband. The trial is window dressing. They'd know it was you. And you'd be looking at 20 years of bad food and no women. Do the 3 days. If you get lonely, call me.

Cajoling him in this way, I was able to persuade him to spend 4 nights in his office, by the end of which he had regained his composure and returned to his wife with much better self-control. This was a time of crisis, and I felt an exhortatory comment—a distinctly supportive intervention, laced with humor to make it more palatable—was needed. During the several years between that crisis and this writing, he and his wife have been on consistently better terms, and he has kept his promise not to get "physical" with her, no matter the situation. The outcome at work was not nearly as good. He remained a tyrannical boss, until he finally did retire, which reduced his explosive temper by eliminating the chief source of irritation.

There are many ways of making sense out of this patient's approach to life and many concepts derived from various theories of personality development that render his behavior understandable. His early years were marred by a mother who was forever belittling him for being merely a top student, not *the* top student. She urged him to be a lawyer and put down his preference for a business career. In addition, his mother much preferred his sister and looked down on her husband as "weak" because he earned only a modest living. The patient grew up forever trying, always in vain, to earn his mother's respect, and trying—with success—not to end up in "mediocrity" like his father. From a psychodynamic viewpoint, these experiences could be identified as the seeds of his narcissistic defenses. One could also see in his philandering—using his charm to seduce women whom he then emotionally wounded by dumping them and going on to another—an endless cycle of getting women to care about him, as he could never do with his mother, and of then exacting his revenge on these mother surrogates (as he unconsciously regarded them).

But I am also drawn to an explanation in the language of cognitive-behavioral schema theory, as set forth by Jeffrey Young et al. (2003). In their understanding of narcissistic personality, they draw attention to three prominent schemata: the lonely child, the self-aggrandizer, or the detached self-soother. As the "lonely child," the narcissistic person struggles against emotional deprivation and comes to utilize a coping style of overcompensation accompanied by feelings of entitlement, which leads such persons to "demand much and give little to the people closest to them" (Young et al. 2003, p. 374). These authors went on to say that narcissistic persons typically are competitive, grandiose, abusive, and status-seeking. Furthermore, as the patient in the vignette showed, they commonly lash out at others who fail to meet their needs; they bully others and behave like tyrants (Young et al. 2003, p. 377). Many narcissistic persons, as Young et al. pointed out, have difficulty relating to others as objects to love and cherish, because they did not feel loved and cherished. Instead, they relate to others as objects from whom to extract the necessary things of life, just as their parents may have used them to fulfill unrealized dreams of their own.

This man felt his mother's love was contingent on his being the valedictorian of his class and on his following her, not his, choice of profession. Because he did neither, her love remained bottled up. As for his mood disorder, I find that many men with bipolar illness, especially those who are particularly aggressive, show little psychological mindedness and little sensitivity to the feelings of others. The machismo that brought this man to the heights (thanks to his drive) nearly toppled him (thanks to his abrasiveness). I believe I fell into the pattern of talking to him like the cop on the corner as a way of parrying his belligerent style.

In general, when confronting personality-disorder patients of intermediate levels of treatability, therapists find themselves working harder than they do with the most accessible patients. It helps to have some of the actor's ability—or perhaps the salesperson's ability—to shift one's style to an approach that is more adaptive to the task at hand. Therapists who work with hysteric persons, for example, find themselves reacting with more than customary reserve and precision. With the obsessive patient, whose isolation of affect makes for arid sessions, we often become more dramatic in our way of speaking. I was able to reach the man in the previous vignette with a mixture of humor and tough talk. I happened to find this man very likeable, and I think he knew this. Because of our camaraderie, he was willing to "do the right thing," including live apart from his wife until he gained the inner strength to control any aggressive impulses toward her.

REFERENCES

Alden L: Short-term structured treatment for avoidant personality disorder. J Consult Clin Psychol 56:756–764, 1989

American Psychiatric Association: Diagnostic and Statistical Manual of Mental Disorders, 4th Edition, Text Revision. Washington, DC, American Psychiatric Association, 2000

Barber JP, Morse JQ, Krakauer ID, et al: Change in obsessive-compulsive and avoidant personality disorders following time-limited supportive-expressive therapy. Psychotherapy 34:133–143, 1997

Barley WD: Behavioral and cognitive therapy of criminal and delinquent behavior, in Unmasking the Psychopath: Antisocial Personality and Related Syndromes. Edited by Reid WH, Dorr D, Walker JI, et al. New York, WW Norton, 1986, pp 159–190

Beck A, Freeman A: Cognitive Therapy of Personality Disorders. New York, Guilford, 1990

Black DW: Bad Boys, Bad Men: Confronting Antisocial Personality Disorder. New York, Oxford University Press, 1999

Brenner C: The masochistic character: genesis and treatment. J Am Psychoanal Assoc 7:159–226, 1959

Brown EJ, Heimberg RG, Juston HR: Social phobia subtypes and avoidant personality disorder: effects of severity of social phobia, impairment, and outcome of cognitive-behavioral therapy. Behav Ther 26:467–486, 1995

Chodoff P, Lyons H: Hysteria, hysterical personality and "hysterical" conversion. Am J Psychiatry 114:734–740, 1958

Cooper AM: Narcissism, in Essential Papers on Narcissism. Edited by Morrison AP. New York, New York University Press, 1986, pp 112–143

Davanloo H: Intensive short-term psychotherapy with highly resistant patients, I: handling resistance. International Journal of Short-Term Psychotherapy 1:107–133, 1986

Easser R-R, Lesser S: Hysterical personality: a reevaluation. Psychoanal Q 34:390–405, 1965

Easser R-R, Lesser S. Transference resistance in hysterical character neurosis: technical considerations, in Essential Papers on Character Neurosis and Treatment. Edited by Lax RF. New York, New York University Press, 1989, pp 250–260

Eidelberg L: A schizoid patient. J Am Psychoanal Assoc 26:298–300, 1957

Emmelkamp PMG, Scholing A: Behavior treatment for simple and social phobias, in Handbook of Anxiety, Vol IV. Edited by Noyes R Jr, Rith M, Burrows GD. Amsterdam, Elsevier, 1990, pp 327–361

Fleming B: Cognitive therapy with histrionic personality disorder. International Cognitive Therapy Newsletter 4:4–12, 1988

Gabbard GO: Psychodynamic Psychiatry in Clinical Practice: The DSM-IV Edition. Washington, DC, American Psychiatric Press, 1994, pp 601–608

Goldberg A: Self psychology and the narcissistic personality disorders. Psychiatr Clin North Am 12:731–739, 1989

Grinberg L, Rodriguez-Perez JF: The borderline patient and acting out, in Technical Factors in the Treatment of the Severely Disturbed Patient. Edited by Giovacchini PL, Boyer LB. New York, Jason Aronson, 1982, pp 467–485

Guidano VF, Liotti G: Cognitive Processes and Emotional Disorders. New York, Guilford, 1983

Horowitz M, Marmar C, Krupnick J, et al: Personality Styles and Brief Psychotherapy. New York, Basic Books, 1984

Jacobson E: Transference problems in the psychoanalytic therapy of severely depressed patients, in Depression. Edited by Jacobson E. New York, International Universities Press, 1971, pp 284–301

Kernberg OF: Further contributions to the treatment of narcissistic personalities. Int J Psychoanal 55:215–240, 1974

Kernberg OF: An ego psychology object relations theory of the structure and treatment of pathologic narcissism: an overview. Psychiatr Clin North Am 12:723–729, 1989

Kernberg OF: Aggression in Personality Disorders and Perversions. New Haven, CT, Yale University Press, 1992

Kohut H, Wolf E: The disorders of the self and their treatment: an outline. Int J Psychoanal 59:413–425, 1978

Kraepelin E: Manic-Depressive Insanity and Paranoia. Edinburgh, E & S Livingstone, 1921

LeDoux J: The Emotional Brain: The Mysterious Underpinnings of Emotional Life. New York, Simon & Schuster, 1996

LeDoux J: Synaptic Self: How Our Brains Become Who We Are. New York, Viking, 2002

Leszcz M: Group therapy, in Treatment of Psychiatric Disorders. Edited by Karasu T. Washington, DC, American Psychiatric Press, 1989, pp 2667–2678

Liberman D: Interpretación correlativa entre relato y repetición: su aplicación en una paciente con personalidad esquizoido. Rev Psicoanal 14:55–62, 1957

Marks IM, Marks M: Exposure treatment of agoraphobia/panic, in Handbook of Anxiety, Vol IV. Edited by Noyes R Jr, Roth M, Burrows GD. Amsterdam, Elsevier, 1990, pp 293–310

McWilliams N: Psychoanalytic Diagnosis. New York, Guilford, 1994

Meissner WW: Psychotherapeutic schema based on the paranoid process. Int J Psychoanal Psychother 5:87–113, 1976

Meloy JR: Antisocial personality, in Synopsis of Treatments of Psychiatric Disorders, 2nd Edition. Edited by Gabbard GO, Atkinson SD. Washington, DC, American Psychiatric Press, 1996, pp 959–967

Millon T, Davis R: Personality Disorders in Modern Life. New York, Wiley, 2000

Modlin HC: Psychodynamics and management on paranoid states of women. Arch Gen Psychiatry 8:263–268, 1963

Overholzer JC: Facilitating autonomy in passive-dependent persons: an integrated model. Journal of Contemporary Psychotherapy 17:250–169, 1987

Rockland L: Supportive Therapy: A Psychodynamic Approach. New York, Basic Books, 1989

Salzman L: Paranoid state: theory and therapy. Arch Gen Psychiatry 2:679–693, 1960

Salzman L: The Obsessive Personality. New York, Jason Aronson, 1973

Sifneos PE: Psychoanalytically oriented short-term dynamic or anxiety-provoking psychotherapy for mild obsessional neuroses, in Essential Papers on Obsessive-Compulsive Disorder. Edited by Stein D, Stone MH. New York, New York University Press, 1997, pp 113–123

Stone MH: Schizoid and schizotypal personality disorders, in Synopsis of Treatments of Psychiatric Disorders, 2nd Edition. Edited by Gabbard GO, Atkinson SD. Washington DC, American Psychiatric Press, 1996, pp 953–957

Vanggaard T: Borderlands of Sanity. Copenhagen, Munksgaard, 1979

Winston A, Pollack J, McCullough L, et al: Brief psychotherapy of personality disorders. J Nerv Ment Dis 179:188–193, 1991

Winston A, Laikin M, Pollack J, et al: Short-term psychotherapy of personality disorders. Am J Psychiatry 151:190–194, 1994

Young JE, Klosko JS, Weishaar ME: Schema Therapy: A Practitioner's Guide. New York, Guilford, 2003

6

PERSONALITY DISORDERS OF LOW AMENABILITY TO PSYCHOTHERAPY

Borderline Personality Disorder

> If you understand others, you are astute;
> If you understand yourself, you are insightful.
>
> Lao Tzu, *The I Ching*

Many years ago I attempted to well-order the various personality disorders from most to least treatable with psychotherapy (Stone 1979). That analysis was written shortly before the publication of DSM-III (American Psychiatric Association 1980), and I made no allusion to personality disorder "clusters," but I did assign the highest degrees of treatability to the personality types that were about to be gathered into Cluster C, the anxious cluster. I included the obsessive-compulsive, dependent, and "phobic" (avoidant) types and also the *hysteric* type—that is, the milder form of the dramatic personality type that is currently conflated with its more seriously disturbed counterpart, the *histrionic* type. I also mentioned the *depressive-masochistic* type as among the more readily treatable, in line with the experience of Kernberg (1967) in his typology of patients who manifest borderline personality organization. I assumed that the lowest levels of treatability would be found among patients with schizoid, paranoid, and (worst of all) antisocial personality disorders. I assumed that patients with borderline or narcissistic personality (and also those with passive-aggressive personality) would be between the highest and lowest levels of treatability. In general, such a mapping is not too wide of the mark, even by current standards. My original list encompassed all of the important personality variants, but the remainder—hypomanic, explosive-irritable, sadistic, and psychopathic personalities—are among those that are less amenable to treatment.

In line with the epigraph from Lao Tzu at the beginning of this chapter, it often (though not always) turns out that borderline patients who have some self-reflective capacity ultimately do better than those who understand only others but not themselves. Borderline patients, especially those with low amenability to psychotherapy, are typically so much at the mercy of whatever strong emotions are affecting them at the moment that they cannot simultaneously think *about* and react *to* the situation that elicited these emotions. So they react without thinking. Insight does not come easily, nor does the self-control that insight ideally engenders.

In everyday clinical experience, any such well-ordering of the personality types can be only an approximation. The generalization holds up well for the extremes at the negative end—the sadistic and psychopathic types. But among patients with the anxious cluster disorders, one regularly finds patients with obsessive-compulsive, dependent, or avoidant personalities who are highly resistant to psychotherapy of any sort or who may become actively engaged in therapy yet show such inertia that no progress is made even after years of treatment.

Patients with borderline personality disorder (BPD), as defined in DSM-IV-TR (American Psychiatric Association 2000), span the spectrum of treatability, and much of the variation depends on their accompanying personality traits. Those with mainly depressive-masochistic or dependent traits tend to have better outcomes with psychotherapy than those with predominantly narcissistic or paranoid traits. Where the admixture of antisocial features is particularly strong, the accessibility to therapy and the long-term outcome are correspondingly poorer. In addition, treatability is affected by certain traits, independent of the DSM personality disorder they are associated with. Borderline patients, for example, often show inordinate anger, and this trait is one of the defining attributes of BPD. But some bor-

---

TABLE 6–1. Factors associated with low treatability in borderline personality disorder patients

---

1. Persistent anger, hostility, or irascibility, particularly if directed toward the therapist or toward the significant others in the patient's interpersonal life
2. Chaotic life (manifested by, for example, multiple, indiscriminate, brief sexual liaisons with strangers; irresponsibility about appointments or about showing up on time for work; hastily quitting one job after the other; disappearing for days with telling anyone)
3. Marked dismissiveness or contemptuousness toward the therapist
4. Erotomanic preoccupation with either the therapist or someone in the patient's external world (especially if accompanied by stalking)
5. Poor motivation for therapy
6. Marked mistrustfulness and paranoid trends
7. Deceitfulness and other antisocial features
8. Extreme manipulativeness (manifested by, for example, marked seductiveness, demandingness)
9. Chronic and persistent abuse of alcohol or other substances, with refusal or strong disinclination to enroll in the appropriate 12-step program

---

derline patients seem to confine their outbursts of anger (or outright rage) to family members, lovers, and others in their world outside therapy. This pattern is often easier to deal with in therapy than anger or hostility displayed directly to the therapist. When the therapist is the target, countertransference problems are much keener and more adroit interventions (and greater sangfroid on the part of the therapist) are required than when the anger is just something the therapist hears about in session. A list of attributes—personality traits, symptoms, and attitudes—that correlate with poor amenability to therapy in borderline patients is shown in Table 6–1, and illustrative clinical examples are provided later in this chapter.

The list shown in Table 6–1, which includes qualities that are the extreme opposite of those associated with optimal treatability, can be understood as the inverse of the treatability scale as shown in Table 1–1 in Chapter 1. But the two lists are not neatly paired. Among borderline patients, for example, some patients who are not particularly psychologically minded and who begin therapy with a limited capacity for mentalization respond well to certain therapeutic approaches and later begin to demonstrate great improvement in these attributes. The same could be said of certain spirituality factors, such as hopefulness and forgiveness, that might be all but absent at the outset but as treatment progresses may become present in good measure.

As noted earlier in Chapter 2, for borderline patients, more so than for patients with other personality disorders, any dramatic shift that takes place in accessibility to psychotherapy may depend on the psychological "fit" between therapist and patient. This scarcely definable quality, often referred to colloquially in such terms as *clicking* or having the right *chemistry*, must be akin to the largely unconscious processes that underlie the mother-child bond and sexual attraction. Some borderline patients may go from one therapist with whom they do not "click" to another and then another, during which time an observer might conclude that these patients had low levels of treatability. Some of these patients eventually find the right therapist, and the estimate of their amenability to therapy suddenly zooms upwards. Because of this phenomenon, it is important to reexamine the list of negative qualities in Table 6–1 in relation to the question of whether the patient nonetheless has certain qualities whose presence augurs poorly for accessibility to therapy, independent of the "chemistry" between therapist and patient.

I consider mistrustfulness, substance abuse, and erotomania to carry less ominous overtones for treatability and prognosis than do the other factors listed in Table 6–1. Some forms of substance abuse are harder to ameliorate than others, but 12-step programs such as Alcoholics Anonymous (AA) and other rehabilitative programs exist for most varieties. In evaluating borderline patients with substance abuse, the personality attributes outlined under the heading of spirituality in Table 1–1 are important. Patients who have enough humility, forbearance (or patience), and orientation toward others, for example, are likely to benefit greatly from AA or an analogous program. After the substance abuse problem is conquered, accessibility to psychotherapy may quickly shift from low to adequate.

I believe that some borderline patients who fail to "click" with a particular therapist—or even a series of several different therapists—may do so because of a mistrustfulness born not of a marked paranoid personality (which is much harder to fix) but rather of a fearfulness of most people or a need for a rare combination of personality qualities (based in an internalized image of the "ideal" parent the patient never had) found only in a handful of therapists. Erotomanic fixation on a therapist may represent the opposite side of the same coin—inordinate idealization of a therapist who becomes elevated in the patient's eye as the God-like ideal parent or lover who alone can rescue the patient. With borderline patients of this type, the task is to help the patient understand, through a slow, painstaking process, that the therapist is not, and does not need to be, this sort of Supreme Being in order to be of genuine help. It is sufficient for the therapist to be what Winnicott (1965), who coined the phrase *good enough mother* (p. 145), might have called the *good enough therapist*.

Deceitfulness, chaotic life, and profound hostility, in contrast, create nearly insuperable barriers to treatability. A patient who chronically attempts to deceive the therapist is, in effect, a patient in costume—someone hiding behind the facade of a false persona that is being held up in front of the therapist. Many patients (borderline and otherwise) boast about sexual exploits they never made and about money they never possessed or earned in order to impress others or to appear the equal of co-workers or friends whose success in these areas is much greater than theirs. As long as they reveal these face-saving fibs during their sessions, they are at least not trying to deceive the therapist. For those whose deceit carries over, repeatedly, into the sessions, the outlook is much less promising. There is no Liars Anonymous to which such patients can be referred. Perhaps the closest modality to such an organization would be a therapy group consisting of patients who lie a great deal. Chances are good that each such patient would quickly see through the prevarications of the others, and all of them might find it easier to accept the inevitable confrontations from peers than from the therapist. In any form of dyadic therapy, however, the therapist has much less leverage, especially if there is no access to family members or friends who could reveal what is really happening in the patient's life.

Borderline patients whom I consider *chaotic* are those whose impulsivity is so extreme and whose judgment is so impaired that their lives begin to resemble the once-popular film series *The Perils of Pauline*. The 20 chapters of the silent film classic, shown between 1914 and 1915, featured a heroine who managed to evade attempts on her life by pirates, Indians, gypsies, rats, sharks, villains who tied her to railroad tracks, and so forth. The analogy does not quite hold, however, because chaotic borderline patients place their *own* lives in jeopardy—for example, by placing themselves at risk of rape by getting into cars with strangers, engaging repeatedly in unprotected sex or various self-destructive or self-mutilative acts, running away, skipping sessions, becoming embroiled in destructive relationships with cruel partners, inadvertently overdosing on street drugs of unknown ingredients and strength, engaging in senseless quarrels with teachers or family members, and behaving irresponsibly at work. Some borderline patients of this type remain well motivated for therapy, but they often come late to sessions, show up on the wrong day, or forget to take care of their bill, such that the therapy lacks any smoothness and is in any case wholly absorbed in dealing with the latest crisis. Persons in continual crisis have no leisure to reflect on the underlying dynamics or the nature of their acting out, let alone on ways to restore some semblance of order and predictability in their lives.

Inordinate anger is one of the defining features of BPD and is common enough in the larger domain of patients with borderline personality organization (Kernberg 1967). Whether anger lowers accessibility to psychotherapy depends on a number of factors. Unremitting anger directed at the therapist represents a kind of extreme dismissiveness that is destructive of any efforts to achieve a working alliance and cooperative atmosphere in the sessions. This kind of anger usually bespeaks great mistrust of the therapist—the very opposite of the ideal situation described by Thomä and Kächele (1987), who wrote, "If a patient's trust outweighs his mistrust, stable unobjectionable transference…can be expected" (p. 61). These authors discussed at length the connection between the early mother-child relationship and the formation later in life of an adequate therapeutic alliance (pp. 61–71).

Many, although not all, borderline patients experienced difficulties in the early mother-child relationship, for a number of reasons. Some had adequate mothers but were born with an "overheated" nervous system that interfered with perceiving the mother as sufficiently attentive and nurturing. Others became attached to mothers who were truly inadequate, as assessed by objective standards such as those researched by Fonagy (2001). Still others may have had a good enough mother, but her efficacy was nullified by a father who committed incest or beat the mother for spending "too much time" with the infant. Therapists differ in their capacity to serve as "containers" of the anger their borderline patients direct at them. Here again, the chemistry between the two participants becomes important. An initially angry patient with a therapist who is comfortable with angry outbursts or with being disliked for long periods of time may be experienced as eminently treatable. The same patient coupled with a therapist who has no stomach for such negativity will be experienced as barely treatable or as altogether untreatable. Even borderline patients who confine their anger primarily to persons outside therapy—to parents, lovers, spouse—may seem scarcely treatable if the anger and hostility persist at high levels over time. Such patients may come faithfully for their sessions and may seem to show adequate motivation, yet may remain "stuck" in their fury over past injustices and in their undiminished hostility toward persons who, in retrospect, may not have been all that bad.

FACTORS ASSOCIATED WITH LOW TREATABILITY

MISTRUSTFULNESS

Borderline patients who exhibit mistrustfulness can be grouped into those who show *significant paranoid trends* and those who show a *wariness* that stems from an all too accurate history of abuse. Many patients with marked paranoid features also have a history of abuse, but an abusive childhood does not always conduce to paranoid ideation. Wariness or uneasiness in the presence of strangers is, however, a common accompaniment of early abuse.

The following two vignettes depict borderline patients whose mistrust-fulness was associated with paranoid features:

> **A borderline patient** with significant paranoid trends had come from a family where the parents had divorced when he was quite young. The family atmosphere had been one of pitched battle—a Hobbesian war of "all against all"—that did not cease even after the divorce. He and his younger sister continued to live with their mother, who alternated between screaming and cursing at her children over trivial matters and collapsing into states of depression, tearfulness, and helplessness. The salient features of the patient's personality, as he reached his late 20s, were narcissism (arrogance and contemptuousness) and a profound misanthropy. He disliked and distrusted everyone, with the exception of his boss at the bank where he was a middle-level executive. He sought treatment because of his loneliness and inability to form intimate ties with anyone. He had made a number of suicide gestures, out of despair over his isolation, and was poignantly aware of the paradox between his hatred of people and his wanting to be loved by someone. A man of unusual intelligence and energy, he was in his workplace envious of those above him (except for his boss) and short-tempered with his subordinates.
>
> Therapy seemed to be proceeding reasonably well in the beginning, but after a few months he learned by chance that I had been a fact witness in a murder case. He began to fear that I would somehow turn him in to the authorities because of the murderous thoughts he had expressed, although he had never even whispered that he had actual intent, nor had he ever threatened, let alone struck, anyone in his life. No amount of interpretation and reassurance restored his trust, and he quit treatment in the third month. Likeability was not the problem here. I had great respect for this man, liked him, and felt compassion for him for the truly wretched childhood he had experienced. Perhaps he was blind to these feelings.
>
> Another paradoxical situation that we never had a chance to talk of and resolve had to do with envy. He told me he had chosen to work with me because I had a "certain reputation" in the field of personality disorders. But this situation was a "catch-22." Having a good reputation meant I was "above" him (never mind that I was three times his age) and would therefore "look down on him," as he imagined his superiors at work did, apart from his boss. All through his early years he felt his schoolmates looked down on him, because he lived in a poor section of town after his parents divorced. His father was wealthy, and the patient had lived in a splendid home until age 5 years, which doubtless intensified his reaction to the straitened circumstances that followed. He acknowledged to me shortly before he left that had I been a "nobody" in the field, I probably couldn't have helped him, although he would have at least felt more at ease.

Another borderline patient with paranoid features and limited amenability to psychotherapy had begun treatment in the hope of straightening out a difficult relationship with her boyfriend. Her parents had divorced when she was quite young. Afterward she lived with her mother, who had bipolar disorder. Her mother was supported by a trust fund from her wealthy relatives. Her mother was a tempestuous woman who oscillated wildly between nearly smothering displays of affection and outbursts of rage when she would refuse to let her daughter back in the house.

The patient's boyfriend was given to abrupt shifts of a similar sort. Half the time he was clingingly dependent; the other half, pathologically jealous. He grew so distrustful that she might be "cheating" on him that he began stalking her. Although this behavior annoyed her greatly, the thought of losing him and being alone seemed far worse. She had no faith in her ability, as a bright, attractive woman in her early 20s, to find another man if the current relationship ran aground.

In her sessions with me she was very secretive and grew antagonistic if I raised the slightest question about how comfortable she could be with a man whose jealousy drove him to spy on her and check on her every movement. She showed little psychological mindedness, and I sensed that she and I were not connecting in any meaningful way (no seeds of a working alliance were sprouting). After a month or so, she revealed that she had come to see me unwillingly and only under pressure from her family, who were alarmed about the jealous boyfriend. She also said that she was already in treatment and had been for the past several years with a therapist who practiced past-life regression. I regarded this "therapy" as a fraudulent enterprise, the more so because the patient had not been reared in a religion, such as certain forms of Hinduism or Buddhism, where belief in reincarnation is emphasized. Given the strength of her attachment to the past-life regression therapist, who did not attempt to dissuade her from continuing to see the jealous boyfriend, I felt it would have been inappropriate for me to discourage her from remaining with that therapist. The various interpretive arrows I might have used—pointing out, for example, the eerie similarity between her mother and her boyfriend and that he represented a hidden aspect of her ambivalent relationship with her mother—I simply left in my quiver. She told me she wanted to continue with her original therapist, a decision in which I readily acquiesced, as it was the only reasonable alternative under these unusual circumstances. Some years later I learned that she had married the boyfriend, in what had become a somewhat shaky albeit viable arrangement. He was still jealous, but she was the major earner in the family, and what she sacrificed in personal freedom she made up for in power.

As for a borderline patient whose past led her to regard others with wariness, the following vignette is illustrative:

The young woman, who had been hospitalized throughout her late teens and early 20s, was initially unable to connect with any of several therapists who were assigned to her. Intensely despairing and self-punitive, she had made a number of suicide attempts during these years and had strong urges to end her life that hardly ever left her mind. While she was in treatment with a previous therapist, she often wrote down her thoughts and impressions. In one entry she wrote, "I don't know what to say or how to say it. I saw Dr. C__, and it was again a waste of time. I think I'm giving up. There's no good in me." A little later: "The session with Dr. C__ was dreadful. There's so much I want to say, but it wouldn't come out....I don't think he'd understand." Some weeks later: "I must kill myself. I cannot tell anyone; I cannot go for help. There's no one here to go to." Two months later she was assigned to a new psychiatrist. In her first entry after the change, she wrote: "A lot has happened since [my last note]. I have a new doctor who is really wonderful. I had almost given up hope. I like Dr. T__ so much. Can you imagine liking someone so much and then being afraid of him because you know he doesn't like you?" Such sentiments, reflections of a long-standing self-loathing, gradually dissipated while she worked with the new therapist. A year later she penned her last entry: "Oh my...I've gotten so much better...Things are so much better now."

These brief snippets cannot do justice either to the seriousness of the patient's original condition or to the profound and totally unanticipated change brought about by the therapist with whom she finally was able to "click." Having languished for years in a state that was so unreachable that most of the clinicians who had worked with her in any capacity had given up on her, she suddenly blossomed when her treatment was taken over by someone she felt understood and respected her. The change transformed her, literally overnight, from a patient with low—or seemingly no—amenability to therapy to a highly responsive and treatable participant in the therapeutic process. This patient took the "high road" from most unpromising beginnings and sustained the enormous gains she subsequently made over the ensuing 40 years.

The story of this former patient is at once frightening, sobering, and inspiring. It reminds us that the lives of many borderline patients hang in the balance, with death circumvented only by a chance encounter with a therapist who, for them, makes the difference between recovery and continued despair leading to suicide. It is inspiring to know that sometimes therapists can make a tremendous difference in the lives of patients. It is sobering to know that the alarmingly high suicide rate among borderline patients— from 3% to 9% in long-term risk (McGlashan 1986; Stone et al. 1987)— might be lowered if it were possible to better predict which patients are most likely to form a life-saving attachment and working alliance with which particular therapists.

SUBSTANCE ABUSE

Concomitant substance abuse dramatically lowers amenability to individual psychotherapy of whatever type, such that even if adequate psychological mindedness, likeability, motivation, and other therapy-promoting factors are present, their positive effects may be compromised or nullified owing to the brain changes, temporary or otherwise, induced by the substance(s) in question. In relation to alcoholism, Babor et al. (2003) discussed the role of AA and other mutual-help organizations in the promotion of abstinence. These authors regarded AA as a well-respected resource in the treatment of persons with alcoholism, although they mentioned that those who are most highly motivated to achieve abstinence might do as well with other forms of supportive therapy. Citing the work of Ogborne and Glaser (1981), they added that personality variables seem not to differentiate between persons with alcoholism who affiliate with and persevere in AA and those who do not.

Simultaneous abuse of alcohol and cocaine is common in borderline patients and is associated with a worse outcome than is noted among those who abuse only alcohol. Marijuana abuse is common also (singly or in combination with alcohol or other substances). Affiliation with and remaining in specialized treatment programs are the key to overcoming marijuana abuse (Gruber and Pope 2003). Such programs include AA, Narcotics Anonymous, and the newer Marijuana Anonymous. The psychological addiction to cocaine can be quite powerful and difficult to overcome, especially in patients with severe personality disorders (BPD, antisocial personality disorder) whose lives are often in considerable disarray for reasons other than the substance abuse. The various residential and other modalities in current use to combat cocaine addiction were outlined by Jin and McCance-Katz (2003).

My own clinical impression is at variance with the view of Ogborne and Glaser that personality variables do not make a difference in the propensity to remain with and benefit from AA. I have in mind those alcoholic patients who, in addition to their substance abuse, show dismissiveness, contemptuousness toward 12-step ideology, superciliousness, lack of perseverance, impulsivity, and denial about the nature of their condition. I find that this mixture of narcissistic and impulsive personality traits militates strongly against accepting, let alone remaining in, AA. For these patients, the usual end result is continuance of the alcoholism and a downward life course. In my long-term follow-up study (Stone 1990), BPD patients who refused AA had outcomes that were exceedingly bleak and a suicide rate far in excess of that for borderline patients with any other combination of factors. The number of cases was small, but of the seven BPD patients who refused AA, three committed suicide within the 10- to 25-year follow-up period.

In addition, many authors have emphasized the link between alcoholism and *violence*. This aspect of uncorrected alcoholism was reviewed by Klassen and O'Connor (1994). As Volavka (2002) pointed out, BPD is "partly defined by impulsive and aggressive behaviors" (p. 189) and will at times overlap with antisocial personality. Persons exhibiting this combination of traits are notorious for their disinclination (or outright refusal) to remain with AA or with any other rehabilitative program designed to curb substance abuse. Goldman and Fishbein (2000) and Linnoila et al. (1983) have commented on the low brain levels of serotonin associated with alcoholism and their correlation with suicidal, aggressive, and impulsive behaviors. There is consensus that alcoholism predisposes individuals to impulsivity and can exaggerate a preexisting personality trait of impulsivity. Still *other* personality traits, mentioned earlier in this section, interact with the underlying substance abuse disorder to steer affected persons either toward help or away from help—the latter direction favored by those with a haughty disregard for social norms, a denial of illness, and a continuing preference for thrill-seeking and a life of irresponsibility.

The two clinical examples that follow derive from my experience with two alcoholic borderline patients, one who only pretended to abide by the rules of AA and another who (begrudgingly, at first) accepted AA:

> **A 51-year-old woman** was referred for therapy because her life "lacked direction." She had made a few suicide gestures with overdoses of aspirin or antihistamines in the preceding few years, after the death of her mother. She had finished college but had rarely worked, except for brief odd jobs over the next 25 years. During this time she continued to live at home, supported by her father, who was a well-to-do retired merchant. At our first session, I was struck by her appearance. Her hair was completely gray and reached down to her shoulder blades. She appeared much older than her stated age and was morbidly thin, weighing perhaps 90 pounds. She acknowledged having been anorectic in her teens, but there was no evidence that the eating disorder had ever ceased. She wore "bobby-soxer" clothes: socks and sneakers, a miniskirt, and an inappropriately revealing halter top that might have been appropriate for a 20-year-old at a dance, but not a 51-year-old at a psychiatric consultation.
>
> Her speech was rapid, disjointed, and somewhat slurred, and it proved difficult to obtain a coherent picture of the flow of events in her life. She had never married. She had one brief affair in her 20s with a man she still considered her lover, although she had not seen him in almost 30 years. Mainly she took care of her elderly father, who in turn took care of her, as she often had injuries resulting from automobile accidents, falling down stairs, or collapsing at dinner, and so on. She could not handle money properly, and her father doled out to her just enough to get her where she was going and back. Her self-image was that of a model or an actress. It did not seem incongruous to her that she was way past the age for the former and without any training for the latter. She had a pleasant, engaging manner.
>
> Her motivation for therapy seemed strong, almost as if her twice-

weekly sessions were the high points of her week. I wondered whether her speech reflected excessive use of alcohol, but she hotly denied this possibility. A month later, however, her father phoned to tell me that he had found a half bottle of vodka in her carrying case. He shared with me his suspicion that she may have been drinking much more than he was aware. When I confronted her about her use of alcohol—and about the seriousness of an alcohol problem—she admitted that she had been drinking, but "only that one time." Only a week later, a doorman in my office building told me he had noticed her swallowing something from a brown bag while she was in the lobby.

At that point I told her that she must begin going to AA meetings, and she promised she would go. She did begin attending with some regularity, but the secret drinking continued. Around the time of the Christmas holidays, someone left four bottles of liquor in a gift box in the lobby as a present for the concierge. The box mysteriously disappeared at a time when the patient was waiting in the lobby, where she had come 5 hours before her appointment, ostensibly to get away from her father for the day. She then wandered into the basement of the building and was seen drinking from one of the bottles. Faced with such irresponsible and destructive behavior, I felt there was no choice but to have her hospitalized in an alcohol rehabilitation unit, which was effected later that day.

A man in his mid-20s was encouraged to begin treatment for having failed to get his life in order after graduating from college. He lived alone in an apartment, supported by his parents, and had done no real work since graduation. The girl he had been seeing over the last few years had broken off their relationship, seemingly because of the aimlessness of his life, coupled with the fact that he had begun to abuse alcohol heavily and to move in a crowd of young persons who did likewise. He had also become neglectful of his hygiene.

A crisis point was reached when he played a hurtful prank on a family member and also fell asleep while smoking, causing a small fire in his bedroom. These acts necessitated hospitalization for several weeks. Among other therapeutic interventions, the staff insisted he join AA as a condition of his release. When I resumed working with him, he was still going to AA meetings, but he found them distasteful and protested strongly that AA was a waste of time. The following conversation between us took place about this time:

Patient: Why do you insist I keep going? There's all this God crap…all this talk about a "higher power." My family's not religious, and I'm not religious. It really grates on me.

Therapist: I don't see AA as a religious organization to begin with. It's true, it was started by Bill Wilson and his friend—both alcoholic men who were staunchly Christian—but that was in 1930-something. And even they weren't trying to convert people to being Episcopalians. All AA means by a "higher power," as I understand it, is that as social animals, we're all answerable to the whole human community. None of us can survive without all the other people we depend on. So that's the "higher power." The 30 or so people you join when you go to the meetings and the sponsor they give you—who you can call in the middle of the night, if you feel tempted to take a drink—they all care about you and want to help you quit drinking, so that's a "higher power" right there. I can't do all that by myself, but if I can help you to see that you can be a total atheist, if you want, and still take advantage of the higher power of the AA group, then I become part of that higher power, too. Think of "God" as a symbol for the *whole human race*, if you're more comfortable with that—one slice of which is the AA group that's trying to help you. Main thing is, for God's sake, *keep going to it!* End of sermon.

Fortunately, my "sermon" worked with this patient. Within a few weeks he began to complain less about AA. He got along well with his sponsor, who was there for him when he felt the need for reassurance and support, no matter what hour. Gradually, he gave up all his drinking buddies and began to form solid friendships with other AA members who had already achieved long periods of abstinence. As he progressed through the 12 steps, he began to speak about spirituality and about the need to bond with other abstinent people who, collectively, helped him resist temptation during stressful times. In place of his original contempt, there was now genuine enthusiasm for the organization that had, as was obvious in hindsight, saved this man. After a year and a half, he had risen to a well-paying managerial post in the company he had begun working for, at first in a very humble position.

As I noted earlier in relation to mistrustfulness, substance abuse may be associated with varying degrees of amenability to psychotherapy. In the case of alcoholism, the presence of a *mitigating* factor—a personality configuration disposed to accept the need for the help that AA or related organizations can provide—can make the difference between a patient who can be "reached" therapeutically (and who can make significant improvement, as in the latter case) and a patient who is likely to defeat any therapeutic effort.

EROTOMANIA OR OBSESSIVE LOVE

One of the most prominent features of borderline patients is their longing for attachment. The evolutionary psychiatrists McGuire and Troisi (1998) in fact view BPD as a "failed attempt at attachment," in reference to the often extraordinary lengths certain borderline patients will go to in order to secure and hold on to an intimate partner. Many of the defining items for a DSM-IV-TR diagnosis of BPD, such as stormy relationships, manipulative suicidal acts, and pathological reactions to rejection, may be understood as misguided and exaggerated efforts to establish a close and lasting attachment. The chronic feelings of emptiness and the tendency to boredom also fit into this picture, for they reflect the emotional state common to many borderline patients who for the time being *lack* this desired attachment.

It is not surprising that clinicians working with borderline patients encounter examples of *obsessive love* or even of *erotomania*, as described by de Clérambault (1923/1942). Obsessive love consists of intense preoccupation with the love object (to the point where the brain seems emptied of other content), coupled with an obstinate refusal to relinquish the loved person in the face of that person's flagging interest or outright rejection. The term *lovesickness* has also been used to designate a condition of craving for unconditional affection as an antidote for loneliness or other types of insecurity (Tennov 1979). Pathological jealousy often forms the other side of the coin of obsessive love (White and Mullen 1989). Erotomania also includes intense preoccupation with the love object, but it has the unusual feature that the erotomanic person is convinced of being loved secretly by someone, usually of much higher social status, who is "not at liberty" to reveal his love openly. I say "his" because the usual pattern is that of a woman in humble circumstances who imagines herself to be loved by the nobleman from the castle (or the equivalent). This condition is a species of *unattainable* love.

Among borderline patients one occasionally finds another type of unattainable love, in which the therapist supposedly loves the patient but is hindered in his expression of that love because he is already married. In another variant, more like obsessive love, the patient is passionately in love with the therapist but is tormented by the conviction that the therapist is totally consumed by a similar passion for his wife and could therefore have no positive feelings left over for anyone else, least of all the patient, who, through self-denigration, sees herself as worthless and not even likeable. The clinical example that follows concerns a borderline patient with obsessive love:

> **A woman in her mid-20s** had met a man of similar age at the tennis court of a private club. They dated for a while, but his enthusiasm for her was much less than hers for him. The relationship had not quite progressed to include sex, but after about 2 months he told her that he didn't think they were right for one another and that they would be better off seeking other partners. She felt devastated. She had already begun, while at work or alone in her apartment, to write her name on scraps of paper, adding his last name to her first name, as if trying to get the feel of what it would be like to be his wife.
>
> She convinced herself that the breakup was merely temporary. They encountered each other on many occasions, as they both went to their club on a regular basis. Sometimes she would violate her own code, according to which the man must initiate the date, and ask him out. He would always politely decline. None of these rejections diminished her preoccupation with him or challenged her conviction that he was destined by God to be her "intended" and that he would sooner or later acknowledge this destiny and return to her. She became depressed over the "tardiness" of this acknowl-

edgment and made a small number of suicide gestures and wrist-cuttings, two of which necessitated brief hospitalizations. By now 4 months had gone by since the breakup. She began to telephone him at his office and at home 20 or 30 times a day and also drove to the place where he lived and stared at his house with binoculars.

It was difficult to get an accurate picture of what was happening at this point because she related stories about her boyfriend (not a "former" boyfriend) that seemed fantastical or that seemed to be projections from her own life onto him. She spoke, for example, of his having been sexually abused by his father and of his father's having taken nude pictures of him. But the doctor who referred her for therapy felt convinced, from material she related to him, that she had been molested by her own father during her adolescence. The previous therapist had begun treating her when she was 18 years old, and her father had died when she was almost 20 years old. The incestuous activities apparently included both sex and taking pictures of her when she was naked. She began, around the time I started treating her, to put messages on her boyfriend's phone and send letters to him that she knew of *his* sexual trouble and that she was eager to help him. In response, he instituted a lawsuit, claiming she was harassing him. She signed a paper, accepted by both his attorney and hers, that if she refrained from all contact for 6 months the case would be dropped. She was able to comply, and the suit was eventually dropped.

In the meantime she had nightmares in which a man she could not recognize would touch her breasts. Her associations led to memories of her father touching her breasts. She tried to downplay the significance of the memory, saying, "He probably meant nothing by it; it's no big deal!" and adding, "I shouldn't talk about these things, since he's dead." But she reported dreams that hinted at the incest memories. One such dream occurred on the day the Pope was visiting New York: "I'm playing tennis with someone, and the guy hits the ball. Suddenly it went 'pop' and all the air went out of it and it exploded; I worried about the Pope because there were bomb threats." She made the connection between *Pope, pop,* and the *Holy Father* but denied that these words related in any way to her own father. The subject was off limits.

She then began to experience dissociative states in which she would "lose" minutes or hours, emerging bewildered and with no recollection of what had occurred during these "blanks." A curious development now took place—the traumatic events involving her father were converted exclusively into worries that her boyfriend was being victimized in various ways and that it was her mission to rescue him. A whole segment of her past was now projected onto him. She insisted he had once asked her to marry him and had then revealed "horrifying secrets" about himself. She had almost given up hope that her love could cure him, or at least motivate him to seek treatment for his "multiple personality." He had never done any of the things imputed to him, and these beliefs were emanations of her own mind, but even the gentlest interpretations that the troubles she was assigning to him were really *her* troubles met with denial and anger. In the midst of this minipsychotic episode she wrote me a politely worded letter breaking off her treatment and expressing her dismay that I had doubts about the accuracy of her story. In her mind, it was beyond dispute that in time her love would restore her boyfriend's equilibrium and help him overcome the effects of his sexual abuse.

The interruption of therapy with this woman occurred after 4 months. Apart from the week she spent at the hospital, she was able to work throughout this period. But her accessibility to therapy remained diminished, owing to the impregnable wall she built around her love for her former boyfriend and around the belief that what had happened in *her* adolescence had really happened in his adolescence and that these tragic circumstances had plunged him into depression, which her love would ultimately cure. Motivation, perseverance, and spirituality were all present, but her psychological mindedness and capacity for mentalization were distorted by her tendency to dissociate and project whenever the sensitive areas of her mental life were touched on. Delusional ideas then surfaced, including the belief that it was her boyfriend, not herself, who had become "amnestic" for the sexually traumatic events of the past. Denial of her own illness led her to refuse medication, which further hampered her recovery. As for her personality in general, most of her traits belonged to the borderline, histrionic, narcissistic, and, to the extent that she resorted for a time to stalking her former boyfriend, antisocial categories of Cluster B, in that order. Some schizotypal traits were also present. In terms of the continuum of borderline conditions developed by Grinker et al. (1968), her clinical picture represented Type I, the "border with psychosis."

This patient's case raises the controversial issue of whether her initial revelations about incest to the former therapist were veridical or fantasized. If they were real, should the therapist attempt to bring the memories more to the surface, to help the patient deal more effectively with what is "down there" and ultimately overcome the deleterious effects of the traumatic experiences? Or should one assume that the unconscious past, relegated to the procedural rather than to the declarative memory system, cannot be exhumed by analysis (or by other approaches), in which case the focus should be on the here and now and on the transference as it is lived out in the course of therapy? The latter school of thought treats the memories of traumatic experiences that patients might reveal as so much *ignis fatuus* (fool's gold), not to be relied on as the foundation for their true life story.

The contrasting psychoanalytic theories—some of which emphasize the earlier view that recovery of memory is important to the efficacy of therapy, and others disputing this view—are discussed in an excellent review by Rangell (2004, pp. 285–293). Representing the object relations school and focusing on contemporary neuroscience, Fonagy (1999) argued against the faith many have placed in the therapeutic effectiveness of recovering memories, especially traumatic memories. Fonagy drew attention to two important memory systems: one system that subserves declarative memory and relies on the hippocampus and the temporal lobes, and the other system that subserves procedural memory (habit memory), relies on the amygdala and the basal ganglia, and is involved both in learned repetitive activities such as driving a car and in fearful emotion.

These memory systems are not as independent as Fonagy contends, even though for didactic purposes, they can be separated *conceptually*. A useful summary of the neuroanatomy of memory, with especially helpful diagrams, can be found in Rita Carter's *Mapping the Mind* (Carter 1998, pp. 158–179). The summary includes not only *procedural memories*, which are stored in cerebellum and putamen (with deeply ingrained habits stored in the caudate nucleus), and *episodic memories*, which are encoded in the hippocampus for a time, then stored in the frontal cortex, but also *fear memories* (including phobias and flashbacks), which are stored in the amygdala but may be delivered to the frontal cortex, and *semantic memories*, involving facts without emotional overtones, which are encoded in cortical areas of the temporal lobe and retrieved from the frontal lobes. As for *traumatic memories*, of the sort that were at issue with the patient in the previous vignette, John Morton (1998) made the point that an impossible element in someone's story of abuse does not negate the possibility that abuse nevertheless occurred, just as the report of some verifiable fragments does not guarantee the validity of the rest of a patient's recollections. Memories, including those of traumatic experiences, are reworked over time, and new information may be added as one matures and gets older, such that a patient's recollection may represent the "accurate" memory of a more recent, somewhat altered memory of an original event that is no longer retrievable in its pristine state.

This view does not imply that the memory is totally false. Morton (1998) outlined a number of situations in which a person may be unable to recall an earlier trauma. When a memory is much at variance with a person's habitual self-image, a conscious effort must be made to recall the memory. A woman who had been sexually molested at an early age by her father, for example, and who experienced pleasurable sensations at the time may, as an adult, recall only the shame and the anger at the father, because the pleasure does not fit with her self-image as a respectable woman. I agree with Rangell (2004), who wrote: "There can be general agreement...that the pursuit of memories, as of knowledge, is a valid process, even though the results may never be absolute or complete" (p. 293).

To return to the patient in the vignette, was it necessary to recapture what really happened to her in the past in order for her to get better? I believe there had been incestuous molestation, the precise details of which remained obscure. From the time before her father died to the time afterward, she seemed to have shifted from a willingness to discuss the matter, at least in broad outline, to a position where she adopted the old adage *de mortuis nihil nisi bonum* ("of the dead we say nothing except what was good"). The bad things her father had done to her were taboo and, in her case, not only taboo but (because of her proneness to psychosis) largely exported to her boyfriend. He became in her mind the repository of the father-child incest and the victim in urgent need of love and psychiatric help.

DECEITFULNESS

As Clarkin et al. (1999) stated in their comments on dishonesty, "The process of therapy is particularly vulnerable to dishonesty, as the problem may exist for a long time before the therapist is aware of it" (p. 196). The authors mentioned several underlying motives that may be operative, such as 1) the wish to avoid taking responsibility for certain actions, 2) the wish to avoid the therapist's disapproval, 3) the desire to exert control over the therapist, and 4) interest in duping the therapist in order to prove a kind of superiority. They asserted that *consistent* dishonesty, deceptiveness, and manipulation may be part of a pervasive defense against an underlying paranoid transference in which the patient fears being mistreated or disliked by the therapist. They mentioned as an example a paranoid patient who refused for some time to give his real name.

These remarks are very useful and cover much of the territory pertaining to patients who exhibit deceitfulness. Now and again, however, one encounters a characterologically deceitful patient—someone who is nearly always dishonest, even in the most trivial situations. The primary motive of such patients seems to be merely to con others, therapists included. Here one can speculate about hidden contemptuousness, but most apparent on the surface are the desire to demonstrate superiority over other people and the delight in doing so. One cannot show that a paranoid transference is always at work in deceitful patients or that all deceitful patients fear their therapists' reactions.

Perhaps because psychopaths and chronic liars were mercifully rare among the patients of the psychoanalytic pioneers, the analytic literature is not rich in material relating to such persons. Melitta Schmideberg's paper on the psychopath (1947) and Helene Deutsch's article on the imposter (1955) are important exceptions to this generality. More recently, Kernberg (1992) distinguished among various forms of narcissistic personality and mentioned that the antisocial personality (as outlined in DSM, for example) presents severe superego pathology. He wrote, "These patients' antisocial behavior includes lying, stealing, forgery, swindling, and prostitution—all of a predominantly passive-parasitic type," and added that the behavior of those who committed violent acts can be categorized as the "aggressive" type (p. 74).

Within the domain of borderline patients, chronic lying does not emerge as a major stumbling block. Linehan (1993), for example, stated, "It is difficult to answer contentions by some theorists that borderline individuals frequently lie. With one exception, that has not been my experience" (p. 17). In my private practice over the past 40 years, I have not been as fortunate as Dr. Linehan. Lying was a notable feature in 9 of 76 borderline patients (12%), although 8 of these patients also had antisocial personality.[1] During the early months of my work with her, the patient who was not simultaneously antisocial often lied to her friends, in hopes of gaining some advantage. She would, for example, tell one friend a negative and fictive story about another person in their circle as a way of ingratiating herself with the listener. But she readily told me about these manipulations and felt quite remorseful.

The only deceitfulness she showed toward me occurred during my absences. She had a morbid preoccupation with my wife, whom she had occasionally encountered in the hallway leading to my office, because of her conviction that my absorption with my wife was all-consuming and effaced from my psyche any awareness that my patient even existed. In this regard, her dread reduplicated her experience of her parents, whom she saw as so devoted to one another—and so indifferent to their children—that she had "disappeared" from their mental map, especially when they went on vacation. Whenever I was about to go abroad for a psychiatric meeting, she would try to learn whether my wife would accompany me. Rather than tell her, I would try to learn what fantasies lay behind her question. But when I was actually gone, she would call my home number. If no one answered, she assumed the worst and grew quite anxious. If my wife answered, she would hang up, content in the knowledge that I was traveling alone. She did not tell me about this behavior until much later in the therapy. In general, her amenability to psychotherapy was of a fairly high level, in marked contrast to the patient of the following example, whose level of mendacity was much greater and whose lying extended into the therapy:

---

[1]These patients were treated in private practice and were not part of the previously mentioned long-term follow-up study.

A woman in her early 30s was referred for therapy because of anxiety concerning her complicated life situation. She and her three brothers were raised in affluent circumstances; their father was a prosperous manufacturer as well as an accomplished artist. Her mother, with whom she was never close, died when the patient was 20 years old. Her brothers all held responsible positions in their father's company. She was given a post there also, but she had little enthusiasm for the work and soon quit. Clearly her father's favorite during her early years, she grew up with a sense of entitlement and became progressively more self-indulgent and indifferent to social convention. As a child she frequently had tantrums if she didn't get her way. In her 20s she was noticeably moody, sometimes depressed and tearful. Her tearfulness had a manipulative quality, as she seemed to cry mostly to have an effect on people—to make them feel sorry for her or to extract something she demanded. On several occasions these behaviors escalated into suicide gestures or wrist-cutting.

When I began treating her, she was living alone with her 4-year-old son. The paternity of the boy was in question, because she had been promiscuous around the time she became pregnant. She claimed that the father was a married man she had been seeing, and she subsequently threatened to inform his wife of his adultery unless he gave her a generous monthly sum for child support. This arrangement "worked," because whenever he insisted on DNA testing to confirm his paternity, she again threatened to inform his wife. The payments were made in cash through an intermediary. Because the sums were unverifiable, she found it tempting to lie to her father, as though the amounts were very little. He suspected the deceit, but to make sure his grandson, of whom he was very fond, would not go wanting, he gave in to her demands as well, effectively doubling her income. She would often "plead poverty" to me during her sessions, urging me to intervene with her father and to persuade him to be still more generous with her. Instead, I insisted she find at least part-time employment so she could be less dependent on her former lover and her father.

Finding a job was to be step 1 in discontinuing the blackmail. I had little confidence in the efficacy of such a plan, knowing that in a person of her character structure the satisfaction of earning an honest dollar through work would not compete with the satisfaction of obtaining much more through deception. For several months she made some halfhearted attempts to find jobs at various charity organizations where the hours were not too strict. Even so, she showed up late and did so little work that she was fired from one such post after another. To explain why she was late, she told her bosses stories that strained credulity, as did the stories she told me about why she was let go.

By now she had alienated the other members of her family, especially because she tried to cadge money from her brothers for some "emergency" whenever her father was out of town. Her father was now at his wit's end about what to do in the face of her lying and manipulations. He knew she had been extorting money from the father—if he was the father—of her son, but there seemed no easy way to stop the extortion unless he gave her an even larger allowance. If her father refused her money, she would threaten suicide, and he was reluctant to take the risk that she would carry out that threat. At this point, I felt it was necessary to confront her about her behavior in a family meeting that included her father, her brothers, and their wives.

She was willing to have the meeting, partly because, I believe, she felt I was "on her side." She had always come faithfully and on time to her twice-weekly sessions, she was likeable because she had considerable charm, and she showed what seemed to be a measure of genuine regret that she had made such a mess of her life. I was not optimistic about the meeting, but I was not totally pessimistic about working out some arrangement that would end the extortion and lessen her dependency. I had spoken with her father privately to reassure him that her threats of suicide were more a bluff than real and that she had little chance of getting better unless he could call her bluff and cease support unless she abided by the rules that would be established at the meeting.

The meeting took place, and all seemed to go well. Limits were set. Promises were made. A "fail-safe" scenario was outlined. Everyone seemed pleased. But later that evening I heard from one of her brothers that when his wife had briefly left the meeting, his sister had stolen from his wife's purse an expensive watch and several hundred dollars. That behavior proved to be the last straw. The fail-safe scenario was then implemented—her father and brothers ceased to support her financially, and she and her son went to live with a distant relative in another city. In the end, her antisocial traits reduced her amenability to psychotherapy from low to negligible.

CHAOTIC LIFE

Borderline patients whose lives seem in perpetual chaos often exemplify *all* the items of the current DSM definition for BPD (Stone 1990), but the idea of chaos accords most closely with the extremes of two of these items, *impulsivity* and *stormy relationships*.

A chaotic life and the endless string of crises that make up such a life obviously interfere with the flow of psychotherapy, reducing amenability drastically in two main ways. First, crises call for urgent actions that usually take precedence over the themes and topics that were the focus of the therapy beforehand. Second, even in the brief respites between crises, chaotic patients often skip appointments, show up late, disappear for a few days, or have minor crises, such as losing a wallet on the way to a session or losing a prescription. The flow of psychotherapy—which ideally involves sustained work on a particular problem over weeks and months until the problem is resolved—becomes disjointed. Both the therapist and the patient find it difficult to pick up the thread from the preceding session or even to recall what the thread was.

Some borderline patients who present with this picture are able in time to strike a better balance—less chaos and more regularity—in their lives. Their treatability may then ascend to a higher level. For others, however, chaotic tendencies are seemingly insurmountable, and therapy is unsuccessful, as in the following example:

A woman in her mid-30s sought treatment for depression and outbursts of anger. She had a 2-year-old son, and she was particularly upset over her tendency to flare up suddenly and "explode" about minor annoyances. Like any 2-year-old, her son made messes or sometimes tossed food on the floor. She would become enraged, just as her mother used to react to her and her four siblings. The patient said, "I want to be a changed person; I don't want to be like my mom." Her life seemed out of control in general; every chore and task overwhelmed her. She saw her life reduplicating that of her mother, which added to her desperation.

Her parents both grew up in a farm region; her mother was only 15 years old and her father only 16 years old when the patient was born. Her parents fought violently, until her father initiated a divorce when the patient was 9 years old. She and her four siblings then lived in poverty. At age 9 years and for several years following, she was molested by a man in his 50s who owned the restaurant where she helped out. Although she was an A student, her mother would rebuke her, saying she was a "pig" or a "nobody." She and her sisters were, like their mother, quite beautiful, and all became models at about age 18 years. The modeling was done with no encouragement from their mother, who would taunt each of them, saying: "You can't be a model. You're just white trash! Who do you think you are?!"

The patient's modeling career took her to many different countries, lasted until she was 30 years old, and lifted her into much better economic circumstances, but her impulsivity and jealousy got in the way of her finding any contentment. If a boyfriend so much as looked at another woman, she would attack him physically and break off the relationship. She used marijuana and cocaine addictively and often drank to excess.

In her mid-20s she met a wealthy, divorced 50-year-old man, who arranged for her to have an apartment and an allowance in return for companionship and sexual favors. The father of her son was a man her age whom she had known from high school. They had been together on and off for a number of years, during which time he was often physically abusive toward her. He was a drug addict who was chronically out of work and who contributed nothing to the support of his son. The patient had sole custody of her son. Now that she had a child to care for, her 50-year-old friend also paid for a live-in housekeeper. This arrangement was a mixed blessing, because it relieved her of many responsibilities that would have been hard for her to fulfill, yet she had a great deal of time on her hands and was easily bored.

A psychiatrist she had seen earlier had prescribed fluoxetine, which had relieved her depression to some extent. I urged her to stay away from cocaine and other drugs, but she could abstain only for short periods. In the beginning, she came twice a week for sessions, always on time, and sometimes accompanied by her friend, who was quite concerned about her well-being. In her sessions, she was extremely emotional, often sobbing when recounting the dreadfulness of her upbringing. She had once aspired to be an actress, but she felt now that her "days were over." Yet when, in her 20s, she had taken acting classes, she had usually failed to show up for auditions, sabotaging her chances of any success in that profession. After about 2 months, she began to miss appointments, often because she was "strung out" on cocaine she took at parties with her friends. One could communicate with her only by cell phone, but the phone was usually turned off or not answered because she wasn't in the mood to talk with the caller. At times I could get in touch with her only through her friend, who would urge her to keep her next appointment. After 3 months, she drifted away from treatment and remained unreachable.

This patient showed mainly the traits of the dramatic cluster of personality disorders, chiefly, borderline and histrionic. Jealousy was no longer an issue during the time she was in treatment, and it is not clear to which DSM personality disorder this trait belongs. One of the descriptors of paranoid personality disorder, for example, is suspicions about the fidelity of one's partner. But not all jealous persons are paranoid *in general*, and jealousy can accompany any of the named disorders as a separate but prominent trait. When jealousy is present to a marked degree, it can present major obstacles to treatability. This issue will be discussed in Chapter 8, "Personality Traits at the Edge of Treatability."

CHRONIC INTENSE ANGER

Clinicians often focus on inordinate anger and self-damaging acts as the prototypical features of BPD. Either of these traits can create roadblocks in the path of psychotherapy, at least in the beginning, but various therapeutic approaches have shown impressive results in reducing the tendency for self-mutilation and suicide gestures, even within the first year of therapy (Bateman and Fonagy 1999; Clarkin et al. 2001; Linehan et al. 1991). In many borderline patients, *anger* out of proportion to the stimuli that engendered the emotion and *chronic hostility* are enduring personality traits that do not quickly melt away in therapy of any kind. To the extent that these attributes are readily apparent in the therapeutic *mise-en-scène*, they pose major countertransference problems. These traits alienate the key people in the patient's life outside therapy, weakening the patient's stability and increasing the likelihood of an interruption in treatment.

In recent years there has been a proliferation of "anger management" groups designed to minimize the tendency of such patients to hamper their lives because of anger or to pass beyond verbal expressions of anger into outright violence. Group therapy for anger management is a mainstay in treatment in forensic settings. In the forensic hospital, for example, patients are taught to appeal to a staff member for help rather than touching or hitting another patient who might have offended them. This strategy is often effective in the intramural setting, but it is of unknown effectiveness in extramural life, because methodical follow-up of the behavior of released forensic patients is, in the United States at least, next to impossible.

Guidelines for dealing with anger in forensic settings, including the use of skills training techniques and cognitive therapy, were outlined by Quinsey et al. (1998, p. 204). Beneficial results with dialectical behavior therapy in dealing with anger-related problems in borderline patients were mentioned by Linehan (1993, p. 23). As for group therapy with borderline patients, Leszcz (1992) suggested that "continuous rages with persistent angry devaluation of the group or therapist serve no useful function for the patient, the group, or therapist, and the attacking patient should not be allowed to ride roughshod over the group" (p. 460).

Beck and Freeman (1990), in their book on cognitive therapy, provided general advice about dealing with anger in borderline patients, and their advice would apply with equal relevance to other therapeutic approaches. They described, for example, a therapist who was able to avoid explosive confrontations in an angry borderline patient by being "alert for non-verbal indications of anger and resentment, such as clenched fists...or a defiant attitude" (p. 194). The therapist went on to encourage the patient to describe in greater detail the sources of the anger. Sometimes the patient's anger exploded anyway. In those situations, the therapist acted as a container for the outbursts of emotion, and in situations where the therapist felt in the wrong, open acknowledgment of the mistake served further to defuse the patient's anger and to restore calm in the therapeutic atmosphere. As Beck and Freeman mentioned, these interventions helped to overturn the patient's preconceptions about authority figures. In the language of cognitive theory, the patient was able gradually to replace older inappropriate schemata with more adaptive schemata for reacting to the various figures in her interpersonal world.

The following two vignettes, which illustrate chronic anger and hostility in borderline patients, were chosen to show how this trait can interfere grossly with accessibility to psychotherapy. The ultimate outcome of such patients, however, is not always as bleak as their stories suggest. Some make satisfactory adjustments many years later, but others continue to lead unhappy, unfulfilling lives.

This example concerns a woman I began treating when she was 35 years old. I have presented her story in greater detail elsewhere (Stone 1993,

p. 250). Her most noticeable traits at the time I treated her were anger, argumentativeness, scornfulness, irritability, and vanity. She had been raised in a family where psychoanalysis enjoyed a high social regard, and she insisted on working only with analysts (I was her fifth), even though she had very limited psychological mindedness. Her low psychological mindedness was but one of the obstacles in accessibility to therapy. Another obstacle was her qualified motivation—she was motivated to be in psychoanalytic therapy, but she had little motivation to make meaningful changes in her life.

She grew up in a family of considerable wealth, where there was not a whisper of abuse of any kind. To the contrary, both parents were thoughtful, considerate, and indulgent persons who bent over backwards (without success) to help her overcome her childhood shyness. They supported her with a generous trust fund, which unfortunately ended up providing secondary gain that was too tempting. She grew scornful of the entry-level jobs she could have obtained, and she would not enroll in courses that could have qualified her for positions more in keeping with her grandiose self-image.

I became convinced that her anger arose primarily from biological rather than environmental forces and that she had a predisposition to bipolar illness, of which her extreme pressure of speech was the most prominent index. On days when I tried to interject a word or two, she would pounce on me, saying: "You're interrupting me!" If in the next session I remained mostly silent, she would tell me, "This is a wasted session! You didn't do anything! You're supposed to make an interpretation about what I've said!" If in the session that followed, I hazarded an interpretive remark such as "You know, when I interrupt, you get angry with me that I didn't let you finish your thought. If I let you talk on, you get angry with me that I've wasted your time and haven't earned my fee. So it seems anything I try to do strikes you as wrong! What do you think about that?" she would come back with, "That's just some stupid comment you got from a book!"

Her interest in dating men, which she did only rarely and never seriously, was only in having them compliment her on her attractiveness. Once the right words were spoken, she allowed no further contact. Perhaps this pattern was the moving force behind the only dream she mentioned in almost a year of therapy. This dream stands out in my memory as the most grotesquely picturesque I have heard in 40 years of practice and the most dramatic depiction of a patient's contempt for a therapist. She reported, "You're gay, though you have a crush on me. I tell you I'm quitting therapy for good, and you make a pass at me. You pull a gold chain off my neck. Also, you kept my mail. In one envelope there was a picture of me, which you jealously hold on to, in order to masturbate with."

She had not a single association to the dream, not even when I inquired about the various elements in it, one by one, or when I commented to her that she seemed to see me in very degraded terms and asked whether that interpretation sparked any thoughts in her mind. By this time, she had shown signs both of deep depression with suicidal ideation and of swings to hypomania. When I suggested she might benefit from lithium, she was enraged at the idea that I felt she was needed medication and was therefore "crazy," and she stormed out of the office, never to return.

I try to do extended follow-up of all my patients, even when, as in this case, the therapy was a total flop. When I (hesitantly) phoned her 10 years later, she was delighted that I called and told me she had gone into therapy with a female therapist, whom she found very helpful, and was now working in an executive position in a media-related industry. Three years after that, she was most cordial and happy to see me when she noticed me sitting two rows behind her in the theater. Time and a sixth therapist—in what proportions I can only guess—combined to mellow her personality so that in her late 40s she was no longer the angry person she had been when I first knew her.

The second of these vignettes concerns a borderline patient for whom hostility toward the therapist was a major obstacle to treatment.

The patient was a single, 40-year-old woman when I began treating her. She had been in a psychoanalytic therapy for the preceding 8 years in four-times-a-week analysis on the couch. Depression, angry outbursts, and irritability were her major problems. Because of her irritability and waspish sarcasm, she had alienated most of her friends, and she led an isolated existence. During the lengthy analysis she had been hospitalized on three occasions for suicide gestures. In the aftermath of the last hospital stay she had parted from the previous analyst, who referred her to me.

Her early life had been especially traumatic. She had an ongoing incestuous relationship with her father, who in other respects was very kind to her. Her mother, whom she described as ill-tempered and cruel, would, under one pretext or another, periodically do genital examinations on her during her adolescence. Her mother, as well as an uncle and grandfather, had all received a diagnosis of manic depression.

The marked mood lability and irritability of the patient could be ascribed to a combination of her own bipolar condition and the traumatic experiences. These qualities lent a turbulent and disjointed atmosphere to the sessions. Although she was bright and insightful, there were rarely 3 days in a row when she was calm enough to do expressive or exploratory therapy. I didn't regard her as an appropriate patient for the couch, and I did not think she needed (or could afford) four sessions a week. We met instead twice a week.

During her frequent crises and suicide threats, I felt that supportive interventions were often indicated. Some of the interventions consisted of suggesting to her more diplomatic ways of relating to others so that she did not lose her few remaining friends. Having lost her job, she now received disability payments from social services, plus an allowance from her family. I urged her to resume work, in order to escape from dependence on external support. Whenever I switched to a supportive or behavioral mode to cope with the crisis of the moment, she would rail at me, "What the hell kind of therapy is this? Is there a name for this? This isn't analysis!" Sometimes she would then abruptly leave my office, vehemently slamming the door on her way out. She smoked a great deal, but I do not permit smoking in my office, and she took offense at this restriction. On rainy days she would bring her wet umbrella to her chair instead of leaving it in the umbrella rack by the door, which was only one of her many annoying habits.

In the 2 and a half years I worked with her, she did manage toward the end to find a job, which was less rewarding than her previous editorial job but which sustained her. She still led an isolated life, having by now exhausted the patience of all but one or two friends. When she failed to come for two appointments in a row, I called a relative, who informed me that she had had a stroke and had been hospitalized. Probably her three-pack-a-day cigarette habit had contributed to this illness. She never fully recovered, and 2 months later she died from a second stroke while still in the hospital.

In this patient, chronic anger was not merely a behavior that occurred in interactions with *others* and that was dutifully reported to a therapist she liked. Instead, her anger and hostility intruded directly into the sessions, making her not very likeable. The anger, coupled with her dismissiveness of suggestions about how to deal more effectively with people, limited the level of gains she could make in therapy. The same traits severely limited both her capacity to build a satisfying and supportive social life and her ability to enhance this capacity through therapy.

GENERAL FACTORS THAT INTERFERE WITH TREATABILITY

PATIENTS WHO ARE HARD TO LIKE

As the previous clinical examples illustrate, chronic anger or hostility need not always detract from a patient's likeability. Amenability to psychotherapy is usually fairly well preserved when therapists deal with patients they like, even though some of these patients may have so many negative factors operating in their lives that treatment founders or fails. When patients inspire intense dislike in the therapist, that factor by itself constitutes a major interference with treatability, particularly when this dislike is a reflection of a terrible imbalance in a patient's personality—where "bad" traits (offensive, socially repugnant, and personally threatening qualities) grossly outweigh "good" traits.

In this situation, the therapist is faced with the following problem: if the therapist is candid and honest in pointing out traits that offend other people, even if the remarks are couched in the most diplomatic language, the patient may take umbrage and feel (or say), "You don't like me; you just think I'm a bad person." If a patient begins to think that the therapist finds hardly any of his or her traits acceptable, the patient tends to become silent, to hide his or her true self behind a facade, or to quit therapy altogether.

Fortunately, therapists in private office or clinic settings do not often face this problem, but it does emerge in forensic work. In offenders who have committed grievous bodily harm or murder, respect and likeability may come only at the price of their acknowledging their actions and expressing genuine remorse, which many forensic patients are not willing to do. It is true that many violent offenders have had tragic early lives full of abuse and neglect, and this background may elicit the therapist's sympathy and open the door to treatability. But if their subsequent lives have been filled with brutal acts of vengeance against others—the result of development along a path from victimization in childhood to later belligerency and finally to what Lonnie Athens (1992) called "virulence"—this sympathy fades, and treatability vanishes. Likeability is hard to preserve in these circumstances. These patients also have low scores in the corresponding dimension of *agreeableness* in the Five-Factor Model of personality (Widiger and Frances 2002). I will have more to say about patients of this sort, some of whom I encountered in private office or clinic settings, in the chapters that follow.

SEVERELY TRAUMATIZED PATIENTS

Patients who have endured repeated traumatic experiences during their early years, especially before age 10 years, often show severe difficulties not only in the retrieval of these memories but in making seemingly obvious connections between what they are communicating at the moment during a session and what they said a half hour earlier or in a session a few days before. It is as though, when dealing with emotionally painful areas, they have been stripped of what Edelman (2004) called "secondary consciousness," which is peculiar to the human species and includes syntactic language, the ability to think about the distant past or guess about the future, and the phenomenon of *self*-consciousness. In these patients, certain painful memories become fragmented and their elements disconnected, such that the original agent of the painful experience becomes lost to declarative memory. This phenomenon was examined by Breuer and Freud in their *Studies on Hysteria* (1893–1895/1955). In Breuer's chapter "Unconscious Ideas and Ideas Inadmissible to Consciousness—Splitting of the Mind" (pp. 222–239), Breuer mentioned Freud's observation that "splitting of the mind can also be caused by 'defence,' by the deliberate deflection of consciousness from distressing ideas" (p. 235). Probably some of the "hysterics" of Freud's day would be reclassified "borderline" today.

Many patients with BPD have experienced severe trauma that is more likely to be sexual than physical, and many antisocial patients also have histories of trauma, although it is more likely to be physical than sexual. Males and females tend to process such experiences differently, with men becoming more aggressive and women becoming more self-punitive and depressed (Stone 2002). The disconnection between the memory systems may be so great in formerly traumatized borderline patients that it may give rise not only to dissociative disorders, but to phenocopies of *schizoaffective disorder*. As one borderline patient said of herself, "I am a person without chronology," which suggests the kind of *dyschronia* that may result from disruption of communication between the frontal lobes and the limbic system. Other severely traumatized borderline patients are prone to circumscribed delusions, such as a patient who was thought to be schizoaffective and whom I evaluated in Australia. She had been the victim of incest by her father and, worse still, of traumatic injury to her genitals that resulted when her fanatically religious mother scrubbed her vulva with steel wool before going to church, to make sure she was "pure" enough to enter that holy place. This patient developed the delusion that the woman who had violated her was not her real mother—her "real" mother was, in her mind, a "kindly lady dressed in white, living somewhere in the outback."

Certain borderline patients with significant trauma histories react as though they have an impairment in working memory (i.e., short-term memory that may be stored temporarily in multiple sites in the brain) (Bear et al. 1996, p. 518). Such a patient may, for example, unearth a long unavailable memory that her mother screamed at her for falling when she was learning to roller-skate and then hit her with a stick for being "careless." In the next session, the patient may report a dream in which an older woman, glimpsed in the shadows and not readily identifiable, is beating the patient with a whip. Asked what comes to mind by way of association, the patient would say, "Nothing" or "I have no idea." The patient, who may be very intelligent, suddenly appears dull. This phenomenon may be better understood as a kind of "pseudo-imbecility" (Schoenberger-Mahler 1942) that forestalls angry feelings toward an abuser, lest the abuser inflict even worse punishment.

Even as such patients begin to trust a therapist, it remains difficult for them to speak aloud the words that signify the connection between the traumatic memory and the ambivalently regarded parent. This phenomenon in and of itself does not result in low amenability to psychotherapy, because many borderline patients of this type have counterbalancing positive factors, such as high levels of motivation, perseverance, empathy, and likeability. Rather, this effect of trauma may slow down the process of therapy and may require the therapist to be especially adroit in helping the patient to feel entitled, emboldened, and (above all) safe enough to make the necessary emotional connection. I stress *safety*, in line with the remarks of Winston et al. (2004), in their essay on supportive therapy: "Creating a sense of safety can help the patient begin to develop a more integrated sense of self and others in the context of reduced anxiety" (p. 123).

REFERENCES

American Psychiatric Association: Diagnostic and Statistical Manual of Mental Disorders, 3rd Edition. Washington, DC, American Psychiatric Association, 1980

American Psychiatric Association: Diagnostic and Statistical Manual of Mental Disorders, 4th Edition, Text Revision. Washington, DC, American Psychiatric Association, 2000

Athens LH: The Creation of Dangerous Violent Criminals. Urbana, IL, University of Chicago Press, 1992

Babor TF, Kranzler HR, Hernandez-Avila CA, et al: Substance abuse: alcohol use disorders, in Psychiatry, 2nd Edition, Vol 2. Edited by Tasman A, Kay J, Lieberman JA. New York, Wiley, 2003, pp 936–972

Bateman A, Fonagy P: Effectiveness of partial hospitalization in the treatment of borderline personality disorder: a randomized controlled trial. Am J Psychiatry 156:1563–1569, 1999

Bear MF, Connors BW, Paradiso MA: Neuroscience: Exploring the Brain. Baltimore, MD, Williams & Wilkins, 1996

Beck AT, Freeman A: Cognitive Therapy of Personality Disorders. New York, Guilford, 1990

Breuer J, Freud S: Studies on hysteria (1893–1895), in The Standard Edition of the Complete Psychological Works of Sigmund Freud, Vol 2. Translated and edited by Strachey J. London, Hogarth Press, 1955, pp 1–319

Carter R (ed): Mapping the Mind. Los Angeles, University of California Press, 1998

Clarkin JF, Yeomans FE, Kernberg OF: Psychotherapy for Borderline Personality. New York, Wiley, 1999

Clarkin JF, Foelsch PA, Levy KN, et al: The development of a psychodynamic treatment for patients with borderline personality disorders: a preliminary study of behavioral change. J Personal Disord 15:487–495, 2001

de Clérambault G: Les psychoses passionelles (1923), in Oeuvre Psychiatrique, Vol 1. Edited by Fret et J. Paris, Presses Universitaires de France, 1942, pp 323–451

Deutsch H: The imposter: contribution to ego psychology of a type of psychopath. Psychoanal Q 24:483–505, 1955

Edelman G: Wider Than the Sky: The Phenomenal Gift of Consciousness. New Haven, CT, Yale University Press, 2004

Fonagy P: Memory and therapeutic action. Int J Psychoanal 80:215–225, 1999

Fonagy P: Attachment Theory and Psychoanalysis. New York, Other Press, 2001

Goldman D, Fishbein DH: Genetic bases for impulsive and antisocial behaviors: can their course be altered? in The Science, Treatment and Prevention of Antisocial Behaviors: Application to the Criminal Justice System. Edited by Fishbein DH. Kingston, NJ, Civic Research Institute, 2000, pp 9-1–9-18

Grinker RR Sr, Werble B, Drye RC: The Borderline Syndrome: A Behavioral Study of Ego Function. New York, Basic Books, 1968

Gruber AJ, Pope HG Jr: Substance abuse: cannabis-related disorders, in Psychiatry, 2nd Edition, Vol 2. Edited by Tasman A, Kay J, Lieberman JA. New York, Wiley, 2003, pp 995–1009

Jin CY, McCance-Katz EF: Substance abuse: cocaine use disorders, in Psychiatry, 2nd Edition, Vol 2. Edited by Tasman A, Kay J, Lieberman JA. New York, Wiley, 2003, pp 1010–1036

Kernberg OF: Borderline personality organization. J Am Psychoanal Assoc 15:641–685, 1967

Kernberg OF: Aggression in Personality Disorders and Perversions. New Haven, CT, Yale University Press, 1992

Klassen D, O'Connor WA: Demographic and case history variables in risk assessment, in Violence and Mental Disorder: Developments in Risk Assessment. Edited by Monahan J, Steadman HJ. Chicago, IL, University of Chicago Press, 1994, pp 229–257

Leszcz M: Group psychotherapy of the borderline patient, in Handbook of Borderline Disorders. Edited by Silver D, Rosenbluth M. Madison, CT, International Universities Press, 1992, pp 435–469

Linehan MM: Cognitive-Behavioral Treatment of Borderline Personality Disorder. New York, Guilford, 1993

Linehan MM, Armstrong HE, Suarez A, et al: Cognitive-behavioral treatment of chronically parasuicidal borderline patients. Arch Gen Psychiatry 48:1060–1064, 1991

Linnoila M, Virkkunen M, Scheinin M, et al: Low cerebrospinal fluid 5-hydroxy-indoleacetic acid concentration differentiates impulsive from nonimpulsive violent behavior. Life Sci 33:2609–2614, 1983

McGlashan TH: The Chestnut Lodge follow-up study, III: long-term outcome of borderline personalities. Arch Gen Psychiatry 43:20–30, 1986

McGuire M, Troisi A: Darwinian Psychiatry. New York, Oxford University Press, 1998

Morton J: Making memories, in Mapping the Mind, by Carter R. Los Angeles, University of California Press, 1998, p 170

Ogborne AC, Glaser FB: Characteristics of affiliates of Alcoholics Anonymous: a review of the literature. J Stud Alcohol 42:661–675, 1981

Quinsey VL, Harris GT, Rice ME, et al: Violent Offenders: Appraising and Managing Risk. Washington, DC, American Psychological Association, 1998

Rangell L: My Life in Theory. New York, Other Press, 2004

Schmideberg M: The treatment of psychopaths and borderline patients. Am J Psychother 1:45–70, 1947

Schoenberger-Mahler M: Pseudo-imbecility: the magic cap of invisibility. Psychoanal Q 11:149–164, 1942

Stone MH: Psychodiagnosis and psychoanalytic psychotherapy. J Am Acad Psychoanal 7:79–100, 1979

Stone MH: The Fate of Borderlines. New York, Guilford, 1990

Stone MH: Abnormalities of Personality. New York, WW Norton, 1993

Stone MH: Violence in adolescents, in Proceedings of the 5th Congress of the International Society of Adolescent Psychiatry. Edited by Gutton P, Godenne G. Paris, Les Editions GREUPP, 2002, pp 175–192

Stone MH, Hurt S, Stone DK: The PI-500: long-term follow-up of borderline inpatients meeting DSM-III criteria. J Personal Disord 1:291–298, 1987

Tennov D: Love and Limerence: The Experience of Being in Love. New York, Stein and Day, 1979

Thomä H, Kächele H: Psychoanalytic Practice, Vol 1: Principles. Translated by Wilson M, Roseveare D. Berlin, Springer-Verlag, 1987

Volavka J: Neurobiology of Violence, 2nd Edition. Washington, DC, American Psychiatric Publishing, 2002

White GJ, Mullen PE: Jealousy: Theory, Research, and Clinical Strategies. New York, Guilford, 1989

Widiger TA, Frances AJ: Toward a dimensional model for the personality disorders, in Personality Disorders and the Five-Factor Model of Personality, 2nd Edition. Edited by Costa PT Jr, Widiger TA. Washington, DC, American Psychological Association, 2002, pp 23–44

Winnicott DW: The Maturational Processes and the Facilitating Environment: Studies in the Theory of Emotional Development. New York, International Universities Press, 1965

Winston A, Rosenthal RN, Pinsker H: Introduction to Supportive Psychotherapy. Washington, DC, American Psychiatric Publishing, 2004

PERSONALITY DISORDERS OF LOW AMENABILITY TO PSYCHOTHERAPY

Other Personality Disorders

Poor amenability to psychotherapy cuts across *all* categories of personality disorder, a list that extends beyond those enumerated in Axis II of DSM-IV-TR (American Psychiatric Association 2000) and includes the Kraepelinian temperaments (Kraepelin 1921) (hypomanic, irritable, depressive), as well as passive-aggressive, sadistic, masochistic ("self-defeating"), and psychopathic personality (Cooke and Michie 1997; Hare et al. 1990). Although some of these constellations—psychopathic, sadistic, and hypomanic—are associated with low treatability in general, at least some patients with a primary personality disorder diagnosis that is considered more reachable by therapy (the inhibited types, for example) prove difficult to treat by any psychotherapeutic approach.

As a concept and as a measure, amenability to psychotherapy is different from *impairment,* a term used by Winston et al. (2004) in relation to personality disorders. These authors wrote about a continuum of impairment, specifically "impairment of psychic structures or ego-functions...such as cognitive abilities, reality testing, thought process, the capacity to organize behavior, affective regulation, and the capacity to make relational contact with other people" (p. 6). In this schema, the most impaired persons would best be served by a supportive approach; the least impaired, by an "expressive" approach. The latter type of approach includes mainly psychoanalytically oriented techniques, but Winston and his colleagues emphasized that supportive psychotherapy itself relies on psychodynamic principles. Supportive psychotherapy makes much more liberal use of interventions such as *suggestion, advice, explicit direction, limit-setting, education, modeling,* and *ventilation,* as outlined in the recent article by Aviram et al. (2004). Kernberg (1984) took a contrasting view, advocating expressive psychotherapy for patients with nonpsychotic, nonorganic psychopathology and supportive psychotherapy for patients with ego weakness (as in the psychoses), poor motivation, or poor psychological mindedness even with adequate ego strength (p. 168). Although both Kernberg and Winston et al. would favor supportive psychotherapy for the most impaired patients, such as those with schizophrenic conditions, Kernberg would continue to rely on expressive therapy for patients who were further toward the "impaired" end of the continuum, including most borderline patients, except for the most fragile or least motivated patients in that group.

In this chapter I focus on patients who are least impaired (that is, who are nonpsychotic) but who still prove scarcely reachable by psychotherapy, for reasons adumbrated by Kernberg, such as poor motivation and poor psychological mindedness, and for other reasons as well. Many patients with the personality disorders generally associated with more dysfunction also prove difficult to reach, even with supportive or cognitive-behavioral techniques. It is worth mentioning that supportive psychotherapy does *not* always connote a psychodynamically oriented approach, as it does in the treatment philosophy of Winston et al. and of Rockland (1989). Many clinicians use the term "supportive therapy" to refer only to the set of interventions listed earlier (suggestion, advice, etc.) and do not include exploratory techniques in this category.

The following clinical examples highlight factors that interfere with treatability by any approach in patients with a variety of personality disorders.

ECCENTRIC CLUSTER PERSONALITY DISORDERS

A 50-year-old man sought treatment in the hope of improving his ability to get along with women. He had a clerical job with the local government, a post he had held for several years after discharge from a psychiatric hospital where he had been admitted for a combination of bipolar disorder and paranoid personality. Apart from being morbidly obese, he was in reasonably good health. His mood disorder had been stabilized with valproate and small doses of fluphenazine. He had few friends and led a lonely life, but occasionally he would meet women in public settings and ask them for a dinner date. But he would quickly find fault with each woman or with the people encountered in the course of the evening, including waiters and salespersons. He was sure all of these people were taking advantage of him in some way. He reported that the women "just want to be with me for the free meal" or that a waiter tried to cheat him out of 15 cents in adding up the bill.

He was deeply prejudiced against many of the ethnic groups to which some of his co-workers belonged, and he assumed they harbored similar degrees of ill will against him. These sentiments were echoes of his upbringing in a family where prejudice against outsiders was rivaled only by the scorn and contempt in which his parents had once held him because he was the more fragile of their two sons. At least one of the roots of his paranoid distrust of others and his angry insistence on "justice" was a belated attempt to get even with his parents, who had died long ago.

Yet this man had redeeming features that made his level of treatability merely low rather than negligible. There was something likeable about this outwardly gruff and unprepossessing man. He had candor and a sense of humor, a rare quality in patients with more entrenched forms of paranoid personality, and his motivation was unusually good for someone so mistrustful in general. He actually took to heart, for example, my suggestion that, in restaurants, he muster his courage and willpower and give the waiter a large-denomination bill, without even looking at the tab, and, when his change was brought, leave a generous tip. That way, there would be no unpleasant scenes and the woman he was with would have a good feeling about him. He trusted me enough to put this plan into action. In time he came to realize that retaining a friendship by being polite and generous was worth much more than the dime or quarter he might save through haggling over prices. This change did not happen overnight, because he needed to overturn habits of many years.

Similar lessons relating to his behavior at work were put into practice. He sometimes worked as a receptionist, greeting employees as they entered the building in the morning. Some were in a rush and barely said hello. He took umbrage, as though they were slighting him, and occasionally made rude remarks that got him in trouble with his supervisor. It was important to persuade him not to feel personally slighted if an employee in a hurry failed to notice him. Many repetitions of this suggestion were necessary, but he eventually succeeded in learning this lesson. The therapeutic interventions in this man's treatment were clearly supportive in nature, consisting of suggestion, education, and exhortation.

In assessing a paranoid patient's level of treatability, the therapist factor becomes particularly important. Meissner (1986b, 1996) wrote extensively about how paranoid patients, who tend to project the uncomfortable aspects of their inner conflicts onto others, including the therapist, can convert the therapist into the "enemy." Paranoid patients behave in certain respects like persons with myopia or astigmatism who are trying to read an eye chart. The big "E" can be read, but from there on down, the finer the letters, the worse the mistakes. The eye doctor does not take these mistakes personally; the mistakes are merely taken as cues for the eyeglass prescription.

The patient in the previous vignette, unlike more seriously "astigmatic" paranoid persons, was at least willing to acknowledge his tendency to misread others. As long as the therapist does not overreact to the typical mistakes of paranoid patients, which often make them seem "difficult, resistant, provocative and contentious" (Meissner 1996, p. 949), countertransference need not become too great an interference. The patient in the vignette came to appreciate his new "prescription," although he stumbled at first, as one tends to do with a new pair of glasses that make the world look different. Had his argumentativeness and anger overwhelmed my flexibility and tolerance, I would have failed to help him and would have unfairly considered him untreatable.

With the most seriously paranoid patients, in contrast, therapeutic failure is almost inescapable. My impression is that when paranoid personality is associated with schizophrenia or heightened risk for schizophrenia (as suggested by a strong family history of either that condition or schizotypal personality disorder), amenability to psychotherapy is poorer than when the underlying condition is in the affective spectrum, as in the patient in the previous vignette. In cases of paranoid personality where genetic factors do not seem important, amenability depends on the intensity of various environmental factors. Paranoid persons who were reared in a setting organized around religious fanaticism, for example, may be hostile to the very idea of "therapy," because they feel their ideas alone are valid, and they may remain quite immune to change by any means. It is not surprising that Kurt Schneider (1923/1950) chose the term "fanatic" personality—with chief traits of combativeness, aggressiveness, and litigiousness—for what is now called paranoid personality.

The following case example concerns a patient whose personality configuration was primarily schizotypal. But, as one finds in many patients with this personality disorder, a few elements of the other Cluster A disorders were also discernible. His tendency to choose solitary activities and his meager interest (when he was first in treatment) in sexual experiences are schizoid traits; his tendency to read hidden and negative meanings into benign events is a paranoid trait.

A man in his early 20s was referred for treatment because of despair over not being able to find his way in life. He often had suicidal ideas, and he made occasional suicide threats, although he had not committed any self-damaging acts. His father was a well-to-do businessman, much older than the patient (almost 80 years old), who hoped his son could assume a position of responsibility in his company. But his son was ill at ease meeting people and felt he didn't fit in at all in the business world. He lived in a separate wing of his parents' house and interacted as little as possible with his sister and brother, both of whom were conventional persons who functioned with considerable success in their respective professions. Their mother, however, had been twice hospitalized for a schizophrenic illness.

The patient's one passion in life was computer baseball, which he played on the Internet with acquaintances from distant cities. Although free of delusory ideation, he did experience ideas of reference when he was in social situations. He imagined that people commented on his stoop-shouldered habitus and gawky appearance, which he believed suggested that he wasn't "manly." He had dated a few girls briefly when he was in high school, but by the time I began treating him he had not dated in 6 years. His father was unsympathetic about his son's plight and lost no opportunity to humiliate him about his "laziness."

Diagnostically, he showed many of the characteristics of schizotypal personality. Further evidence came in the form of his strange mystical and philosophical concerns. He speculated about whether what people assumed was reality might be the manifestation of a gigantic dream that had been conjured up by a demiurge of supernatural powers and that enveloped us all. This concern was not so much a delusion as it was an *overvalued idea*, a phenomenon discussed by Hoch and Polatin (1949) and later Kernberg (1967). He was willing to concede that his dream theory might not be correct. When I got to know the painful details of his everyday life, I suggested as an interpretation that his idea of everyone's being locked up in a bad dream was inspired by the wretchedness of his life and that if the demiurge decided to release us from the "dream," better days might follow. In a role reversal typical of patients with borderline organization, he then, treating me as his father treated him, mocked my comment as unimaginative and pedestrian.

When he felt intensely suicidal, as he did from time to time, he was grateful for my availability. I met several times with his parents, in hopes of persuading his father to adopt a more understanding and less punitive attitude. This effort met with little success. His father remained fixed in his harsh ways, although the patient at least appreciated my attempt to intervene. After about 6 months, he began canceling sessions, and then he stopped his therapy altogether.

His low amenability to psychotherapy rested on both internal and external factors—the meagerness of his motivation and psychological mindedness, coupled with parental uncooperativeness. At follow-up 20 years later, his story had a happier-than-expected ending. His father died a few years after he stopped therapy, leaving him with his mother, a kinder and more tolerant person. The patient channeled his mystical preoccupations into religiosity and joined a strict, all-embracing religious cult. In the process, he met a similarly minded woman whom he eventually married. In the late 1990s, they moved to the country in which their religious group is based, and they have been living there happily ever since.

DRAMATIC CLUSTER PERSONALITY DISORDERS

Among patients with personality disorders of the dramatic cluster, those with *antisocial personality disorder* usually prove to be the most challenging in psychotherapy. Unlike histrionic and narcissistic patients (or borderline patients, as discussed in Chapter 6), for whom the level of treatability depends considerably on the skill and personality of the therapist, psychotherapy with *antisocial* patients is often a frustrating venture irrespective of the therapist's personality or the specific therapeutic approach. Here, low amenability to psychotherapy is primarily a function of the condition itself. In general the prognosis is better when the patient's antisocial features are less ominous (less violent and less accompanied by callousness) and occupy less of the patient's life—that is, when the patient's life is not wholly given over to antisocial behaviors and deceitfulness.

If psychotherapy is to be useful at all, a cognitive-behavioral approach will almost surely be needed, rather than a psychoanalytically oriented approach. A good example of the former approach, used with a mildly antisocial patient, can be found in the chapter on antisocial personality disorder in Beck and Freeman's book (1990, pp. 147–175). For more seriously disturbed adolescents with antisocial personality disorder, cognitive-behavioral techniques may be combined with special forms of parental training and family-based methods (Southam-Gerow and Kendall 1997). Berlin (2000) outlined behavior therapy techniques for antisocial persons whose main problem lies in the area of sexual offending.

Many authors who wrote on the subject of therapy for antisocial persons acknowledged the guarded prognosis associated with all but the mildest cases. Dolan and Coid (1993), for example, in their book on psychopathic and antisocial disorders cautioned that "engaging personality-disordered patients in outpatient therapy is a difficult task and often only achievable when clients are on probation or under court orders of treatment" (p. 127). Other authors suggested that the outlook is better for self-referred male voluntary patients with impulsive character who undergo outpatient group therapy (Lion and Bach-y-Rita 1970). The key word here is "voluntary," which implies that the patient has sufficient motivation, awareness of his antisocial proclivities, and a desire to change. These attributes are lacking in the more "hard-core" antisocial persons, who often remain resistant to positive change from psychotherapy and may be slow to improve.

Donald Black (1999), in his monograph on antisocial personality, gave the example of a patient who showed considerable progress, although much of it was unrelated to therapy. This man, called Russ by Dr. Black, had been alcoholic when he was younger (he was age 49 years at follow-up) and had once been jailed for a month on a charge of assault and battery. Black wrote that "change for Russ seemed to come from within, perhaps at a fortuitous time when he was poised for progress," adding that "[t]he blend of personal motivation and circumstance is essential to any discussion of antisocial personality disorder treatment since there are no proven methods for overcoming the disorder" (p. 127). Russ gave up alcohol at age 34 years, having become "sick and tired of being sick and tired." In agreement with the majority of clinicians who devote themselves to this area, Black wrote that uncovering unconscious mental processes, as in psychoanalytic psychotherapy, is a futile exercise with antisocial patients. The chances for reaching this population are better with cognitive therapy focused on inaccurate beliefs and cognitive distortions. When Russ was interviewed at follow-up, he revealed to Dr. Black that at the time of the assault, he believed the victim thought of himself as a "tough guy," and Russ felt that he "needed a lesson." This view is similar to that often expressed by antisocial men who rape women—that the woman was "asking for it" (by walking in the wrong part of town, wearing revealing attire, and so forth). Cognitive therapy or cognitive-behaviorally oriented group therapy for antisocial patients may eventually succeed in driving home the lesson that their views on such matters are self-serving and wrong.

As for prognosis in antisocial personality, an important point—one that is not often voiced—should be emphasized: the fewer in number and shorter in duration the humanizing influences in the formative years of persons who go on to develop antisocial personality disorder, the worse the chances that any therapeutic modality, whether outpatient or institutional, will succeed in their socialization. Work in forensic settings quickly reveals that persons who were treated cruelly early in life—those who were brutalized repeatedly from their earliest years, outrageously neglected, shunted from one foster home to another with rarely a stay of more than 6 months at any one place, sexually violated before puberty, and humiliated at every turn—grow up with no template either for feeling "human" in themselves or for feeling compassion for other people. A kind of induced paranoid personality develops alongside the antisociality, and it becomes impossible for such persons to believe in the goodness and consistently caring attitude of anyone, including the therapists who try to reach them. Here I am describing basically untreatable patients—who are discussed in more depth in Chapter 8—rather than those with low amenability to psychotherapy, but the topic of untreatability is hard to avoid in any discussion of antisocial personality disorder, let alone of psychopathy strictly defined. Some of the more favorable cases described by Lion (1978/2001) were labeled "psychopaths," but these patients would probably now be classified as young offenders with antisocial personality disorder, as they indulged in property crimes, not violent crimes.

No discussion of therapy with antisocial persons would be complete without attention to the powerful countertransference feelings regularly elicited in their therapists. Strasburger (1986/2001) outlined six main stumbling blocks for therapists who treat antisocial patients: fear of assault or harm, helplessness and guilt, loss of professional identity, denial of danger, rejection of the patient, and the rageful wish to destroy (p. 297). But Strasburger's warning signs pertain to the more severe and violent regions of the antisocial domain, not to the group of milder rule-breakers who are hard, but not impossible, to treat. Predatory or impulsively violent patients inspire fear and hatred; patients whose worst offenses are shoplifting, driving while intoxicated (as long as they haven't committed vehicular homicide), or embezzling inspire less drastic countertransference reactions such as contempt, envy (at getting away with things), or annoyance (at skipping appointments). The example that follows concerns a patient with antisocial personality whose amenability to psychotherapy was low, but still present:

> **A 23-year-old man** was referred for therapy because his behavior was getting out of control in relation to a woman with whom he had become involved. Their relationship was sometimes "on" and sometimes "off," but when they were temporarily not seeing one another, he was consumed with jealousy of the men she might be with in the meantime. While in this state of mind, he stalked the place where she lived and threatened her. On a few occasions, when they got back together, he hit her. She pressed charges because of the stalking, and he had to hire an attorney and meet with the police.
>
> There were striking parallels between his current life and his life as it unfolded during his childhood. As a child, he frequently had tantrums and was later considered hyperactive to the point of receiving a diagnosis of attention-deficit/hyperactivity disorder. His mother was by all accounts a beautiful woman who came from a disturbed family. She was heavily involved with drugs and died, perhaps because of an overdose, when the patient was 9 years old. Her behavior was erratic, and she alternated between being loving and "cuddly" with her son and being physically abusive. She was not faithful to his father, and the patient would see other men emerge from her bedroom in the last few years before she died.
>
> Although he was a bright student at school, his behavior was disruptive and, at times, combative, and for extended periods he was truant. Expelled in the middle of high school, he was sent to a camp specializing in the re-

habilitation of behavior disordered adolescents. His behavior improved, and he no longer got into fights, but he began to use drugs, and later he began to deal in drugs, which became his major livelihood. Although he had short-term liaisons with many women, he developed a meaningful attachment to the woman with whom he had the tempestuous relationship. Unlike the other women he dated, this woman was considerably older than he was; she was the same age as his mother when she died.

In the beginning of his therapy his motivation was high because he was in trouble with the law. By promising to stay away from his girlfriend, he was able to avoid incarceration, and after a short time she dropped the charges, so that he ended up with no record. It seemed prudent in our sessions to focus on the danger he might put himself in if he continued to pursue that relationship, rather than on its psychodynamic roots. That the woman represented a transference object—one might even say a revivification—of his dead mother was clear enough, but he was not comfortable dealing with this topic. After a few months he formed a new relationship with a woman his own age. She was a model, as was the other woman, but she had a calmer disposition, and she did not behave in ways that incited jealousy.

Having gotten used to making substantial sums of money through drug dealing, the patient had little incentive to try his luck in the conventional workplace. Besides, he had dropped out of college after a few semesters and had not acquired the skills that would have led to an equally remunerative job on this side of the law. His aspirations for the future consisted mainly of acquiring enough cash from the drug dealing to start a legitimate business, such as owning a bar and restaurant. He looked forward to marriage and children. In this way he differed from a more typical antisocial person, for whom the nurturing of long-range plans and conventional goals such as supporting a family is anathema. He saw himself as half an "outlaw," like his mother's side of the family, and half an ordinary person, like those on his father's side. As he began to settle in with the new girlfriend, and as his law troubles were behind him, his motivation flagged. He would skip every other session, reassuring me that he felt "cured," and after about 4 months he stopped coming to therapy. The low amenability to psychotherapy in his case had primarily to do with his wavering motivation and limited psychological mindedness. In other respects, he was bright and assertive. He was cautious in his business dealings and quite successful with women. One could picture him making his way in life rather successfully, provided he avoided the pitfalls of jealousy and made the transition into legitimate business in the near future.

Besides antisocial patients, patients with *narcissistic personality disorder* often have low amenability to psychotherapy. Clarkin et al. (2004) wrote that patients with narcissistic personality disorder are "more difficult to engage in treatment and have a poorer prognosis" (p. 60). Similar impressions led Swenson (1989) to speculate that patients in these categories would be less reachable by a transference-oriented approach, as compared with a cognitive-behavioral approach, such as Linehan's dialectical behavior therapy (1993).

Narcissistic personalities come in many shades and gradations, some of which were described by Ben Bursten (1973/1986) under the following headings: the *craving*, the *paranoid*, the *manipulative*, and the *phallic-narcissistic*. By the craving type, Bursten had in mind overly dependent persons who were demanding and pouty. One of his patients spoke of himself as feeling more than just neediness: "It's craving. I'm like a little bird with a wide-open beak" (p. 384). The paranoid narcissistic person is argumentative and litigious and subject to jealous rages. Bursten's manipulative type is equivalent to the current category that includes sociopathic or antisocial personality. Finally, Bursten's phallic-narcissistic type, described originally by Wilhelm Reich (1933), primarily designated men who parade their masculinity and tend to be reckless and exhibitionistic. In their attitude toward women, these men show polar opposite reactions of disparagement and idealization, depending on the occasion. Add aggressiveness to this constellation of traits, and the phallic-narcissist becomes the malignant narcissist, as limned by Kernberg (1992, p. 77), with the salient characteristics of narcissism, antisocial behavior, ego-syntonic sadism or characterologically anchored aggression, and a paranoid orientation, albeit with a capacity for loyalty that would not be found in the thoroughgoing antisocial person. Many of the narcissistic patients in Bursten's classification showed poor amenability to psychotherapy and also could be considered to have *borderline personality organization*, as described by Kernberg (1967), although only a few might simultaneously qualify for a DSM-IV-TR diagnosis of borderline personality disorder (BPD) (American Psychiatric Association 2000).

There are higher-functioning persons with marked narcissistic features, such as those sketched by Meissner (1986a), in whom stable characterological traits, minimal regressive tendency, and a stability of functioning are all present. Among the recommendations for treatment of these better-functioning narcissistic patients are those of the Kohutian Self Psychology school (Goldberg 1989) and the Kleinian school, as represented by Riccardo Steiner (1989). Steiner emphasized the manner in which greed, envy, omnipotent denial of dependence, and megalomanic idealization of the self dominate the mind-set of the narcissistic patient. These attitudes and emotions can be found both in the poorer-functioning and the better-functioning persons with narcissistic personality disorder. But even patients in the latter group often prove challenging and difficult to treat psychotherapeutically, regardless of the approach. Less difficult, but still challenging, is another group of narcissistic patients who often show low amenability to therapy—those who are quite high-functioning in their occupations but whose interpersonal relationships are strained because of their self-centeredness. These patients may be socially affable, polite, and neither demanding nor aggressive or manipulative, but they may be remarkably negligent in meeting the needs of those in their intimate life, such as their spouse, children, and friends. They seem tuned in only to their own station, preoccupied with their own interests, and not closely connected to anyone else. The following vignette describes this type of patient:

A 51-year-old man was referred for therapy because of a vexatious marital problem. An attorney at a large law firm, he had been married for 25 years to a woman who had become seriously depressed. Her depression occurred within the context of a deteriorating marriage, with her husband having shown less and less interest in her over the preceding 10 or 12 years. She had made several suicide threats in the recent past and told him she would definitely kill herself if he ever left her. The patient dealt with this problem, one could say, by not dealing with it. He buried himself in his work and had long ago given up on urging her to go into treatment, which she had anyway refused to do. Their sexual relations had ceased shortly after the birth of their second child some 20 years earlier. For the past 10 years the patient had been having an affair with a wealthy 40-year-old divorcée, whom he would be with every Tuesday or Wednesday. Several times a year he would travel abroad with her on the pretext of conducting law work at the London or Hong Kong office. This woman was mild-mannered, aristocratic, and undemanding, and thus quite the opposite of his wife, whom he described as whining and shrewish. But marriage seemed out of the question, because of his wife's suicide threat.

The complexity of his life did not end with this clandestine affair, however, for he had also been carrying on a still more secretive affair with one of his firm's paralegals, a woman in her late 20s, to whom he was drawn because of her beauty and passionate nature. The trouble was that she was also volatile, intensely jealous, and stormy, and she demanded more time from him than the few hours they spent together in his office after the business day once or twice a week.

Although the patient complained that his life had somehow descended to the level of a bad movie, it soon struck me that his complex situation supplied the drama that energized his otherwise humdrum life. He frequently used the image of the Gordian knot in describing the ties that bound him to these women—an image I found worrisome, because the Gordian knot of classical mythology was impossible to undo. I took his use of this phrase as his way of announcing to me that my task was hopeless: he was coming for help, which intellectually he knew he needed, for a problem he didn't want solved.

He had been the pampered first-born child of indulgent parents who fostered in him the belief that it was not necessary to make choices between desirable alternatives. As a child, for example, he didn't have to choose between the toy truck or the stuffed giraffe, because he could have both. It offered him little relief when I pointed out that his wife's suicide threat was essentially a form of blackmail for which he was not responsible. Even if he imagined a life without her, there still remained the choice between the tranquility he might enjoy with the divorcée and the passion he might enjoy with the glamorous woman from the workplace. None of the three possible combinations (wife + divorcée; wife + paralegal; divorcée + paralegal) had greater appeal than the other two, and the idea of making a new life with just one of the other women seemed equally unattractive, since he would have to sacrifice passion in the one instance and tranquility in the other. There was the added difficulty that if he broke off the relationship with the paralegal, she might make a scene at the office that would threaten his job.

Like a chess match destined to end in a draw, therapy gradually wound down and stopped. The patient seemed satisfied that he had made an "honest effort" to resolve his problem. This effort was as far as his motivation would carry him. It was clear to both of us that he could not keep the young woman "on hold" forever and that eventually she would insist on marriage and children of her own, for which he had no interest. It was equally clear that the only reasonable choice was to marry the divorcée and give up the passionate encounters, which would have been hard to maintain past a certain age in any case. He was not prepared to make this choice.

Time, however, has a way of providing solutions where therapy fails. When I followed up the case 10 years later, I learned that the young woman had lost patience with her lover's indecisiveness and had moved to a different city. The divorcée was at an age when she was no longer content to be caught up in a secret affair. The attorney revealed the long-standing affair to his wife, who, as promised, did commit suicide. After waiting a "decent interval" and after becoming estranged from his (now grown) children, he married the divorcée. His contentment was marred only by a twinge of remorse over his wife's suicide and a twinge of regret over the loss of the younger woman.

In patients with histrionic personality disorder, amenability to psychotherapy is often lower than what could be expected from patients who would have been identified as having "hysteric character" in the older psychoanalytic literature. Hysteric character was described by Reich (1933) as representing the "simplest type of character armoring" whose most outstanding qualities are "an obvious sexual behavior in combination with a specific kind of bodily agility with a definitely sexual nuance" (p. 189). Reich mentioned that the connection between female hysteria and sexuality "has been known for a very long time" and is evidenced by "disguised or undisguised coquetry in gait, gaze and speech." Men may at times show this configuration, but in them one may notice a "softness and over-politeness, feminine facial expression and feminine behavior" (p. 189). Accompanying these traits is a certain apprehensiveness or fearfulness—in effect, a backing away from the desired accomplishment of sexual intimacy because of conflictual feelings about actually fulfilling these desires.

It was accepted in the psychoanalytic community during the early years that hysterical character was the outgrowth of fixation at the "genital phase" of infantile development, as adumbrated, for example, in a paper by Karl Abraham (1926). Patients with this diagnosis were optimistically considered to be ideal candidates for psychoanalytic therapy, because they were poised nearest to the developmental goal of full "genitality"—that is, the capacity for mature sexual intimacy. More recently it became clear that no simple isomorphism exists between the Freudian developmental stages and various psychiatric conditions; for example, some "oral" depressive persons functioned better than certain highly disturbed hysteric persons (Easser and Lesser 1965; Stone 1980).

The concept of hysterical character was felt to be marred because of gender bias and was replaced in DSM-III (1980) by histrionic personality disorder (Millon and Davis 2000, p. 244), but the new set of criteria described a sicker personality constellation than the old hysterical character. Women with histrionic personality disorder were found, in comparison to a control group, to show less sexual assertiveness, more fearfulness about sex, and greater marital dissatisfaction (Apt and Hurlbert 1994). Persons with hysterical character, in contrast, generally show emotional lability and warmth, a controlled and socially adaptive quality, and a capacity for appropriate social interactions, except for those that involve sexuality (Kernberg 1984, p. 80).

There is an overlap between DSM histrionic personality disorder and "infantile personality," which is outlined in Kernberg's schema for personality disorders. The characteristics of infantile personality include childlike dependency, as well as crude and inappropriate use of sexual behavior, a tendency to make manipulative suicidal threats or suicide gestures when under stress (especially in response to the threat of loss of a close relationship), and, in general, a greater proneness to displays of hostility and anger, in response to disappointment, than one sees in persons with hysterical character. The concepts of histrionic personality disorder and BPD merge in many particulars. Although patients in either of these categories span the range of treatability from low to high, many patients with histrionic personality disorder prove extremely frustrating to work with in therapy, because of the childlike quality that Kernberg alluded to and because of the lack of seriousness about their condition that often accompanies their immature attitude toward the demands of the adult world. The following vignette concerns such a patient:

> **A 26-year-old woman** was referred for therapy because she was in the throes of a dilemma concerning which of two men she should marry. She

had a position in an import-export company and traveled extensively around the world in connection with her work. One of the men was a soldier she had met while in California; the other, a businessman from Stuttgart who did business with her company. Because she was based in New York, she was thousands of miles from both men, and she knew neither of them very well. She retained idealized images of them that were undiminished by the flaws and faults that would be revealed during extended intimacy.

The only daughter of a prosperous Midwestern family, she had grown up the clear favorite of her father, whereas her mother doted on her two brothers. During her adolescence these preferences grew more polarized, such that her mother became intensely jealous of her daughter and equally resentful of her husband for his spending so much time with her. Although there was no hint of gross sexual misuse on the father's part, his kisses and hugs even throughout her adolescence were ardent enough to raise suspicions in her mother about how far he might be tempted to go in that direction.

As I got to know the patient in the opening sessions, she struck me as both dramatic and shallow emotionally, given to enthusiasms that could shift from moment to moment, and more interested in a "quick fix" for her romantic conflict than in any serious exploration of why she so often ended up in unworkable situations with men. This superficiality extended to her attitude toward therapy. She spoke, albeit in a breezy way, of being very committed to working on her problems, yet she often canceled appointments on the spur of the moment for unimportant reasons.

This pattern, coupled with her need to be away for a week or two every month for her work, gave a disjointed quality to the therapy. Besides showing this deficiency of motivation, she also displayed a lack of psychological mindedness that was, in its way, as dramatic as her self-presentation. In the first dream she reported, for example, she saw herself on the lawn of the home where she grew up, being embraced by an amorous tiger while her mother looked on with a furious expression. She had no associations to the dream, even though she had been speaking in the preceding sessions about her mother's jealousy, her father's physique—which she much admired—and his habit of treating his daughter as his "little wife."

This dream was followed some weeks later by another dream in which she was riding in a subway and holding on to one of the straps for the standing passengers, but the "straps" consisted of so many penises suspended from the top of the subway car. Here again she had no associations, apart from being amused by the graphic imagery. Yet this was one of those dreams where even the manifest content points clearly to the hidden meanings—in this case, to the patient's lifelong need to hang on (literally) to men for her emotional support. I made an interpretation to the effect that she had always hung on to her father (as in the dream of the tiger) in a way that interfered with her choosing a mate of her own, because a prospective mate could never measure up to the "tiger." I went on to suggest that imagining herself in love with two men at once was a convenient illusion that covered up her still greater attachment to her father. Nothing need interfere with that attachment, so long as she kept picking either unsuitable men close to home or suitable men at the far corners of the globe whom she could never really get to know. The implication was that her struggle to decide between the California man and the Stuttgart man was not so much a genuine conflict as it was a mechanism to ensure that she would choose neither and would therefore not leave her father.

What ensued was an acting out in which she absented herself from therapy for several weeks on a business trip to New Zealand. While she was there, she had an affair with a client of the firm—a man much older than she was—by whom she became pregnant. When she returned to the United States, she realized the inappropriateness of the situation, concluded that the man was not the "love of her life," and terminated the pregnancy. After about 6 months she drifted away from treatment.

When I contacted her again 20 years later in a follow-up effort, she told me that 2 years after she stopped coming to therapy she met another man, whom she eventually married. Their relationship was stormy at first, but eventually it grew calmer. She had a daughter who was then in her teens. She had returned to work after a lapse of some years when she was busy raising her daughter and was now a more settled and less impulsive person. Her father was still her "hero," but now that she had a husband of her own, her father was no longer the center of her emotional life.

ANXIOUS CLUSTER PERSONALITY DISORDERS

The *anxious cluster* (Cluster C) designation is probably more appropriate for the dependent and avoidant types (or even for the passive-aggressive type, which is no longer included in DSM) than it is for the obsessive-compulsive type. The disorders of Cluster C are also characterized by an inhibited manner of dealing with other people, in contrast to the more impulsive manner of patients with Cluster B disorders. But just as narcissistic persons are by no means regularly impulsive, some obsessive-compulsive persons are neither particularly anxious nor inhibited. Politicians and high-level executives with pronounced narcissistic traits are as a rule measured and cautiously calculating in their interactions. Similarly, accountants, bankers, engineers, and academic professors of a decidedly obsessive-compulsive bent often show the triad of *orderliness, obstinacy*, and *parsimony* of which the first generation of psychoanalysts spoke (Freud 1929/1961, p. 96), but not all are notably anxious or inhibited in their dealing with the external world. At least such persons would not describe themselves as anxious, whereas in dependent and avoidant persons, anxiety is usually readily discernible.

The subgroup of Cluster C patients who have major impediments to psychotherapy present a paradoxical situation. The intense anxiety and suffering of certain dependent and avoidant patients may render them eager to seek and to remain in therapy. But their anxiety may be so crippling that it places a low ceiling on their potential for benefit. In contrast, certain obsessive-compulsive patients may show so little outward anxiety and so little awareness of emotion as to create, for the opposite reason, a nearly insuperable barrier to therapy. It is for this highly resistant, rigidly compulsive sort of patient that Davanloo (1986) devised his confrontational, not to say pugnacious, style of therapy, which was designed to blast his patients out of their complacency and into feeling *something*, if only annoyance at Dr. Davanloo.

Millon (1999) in his discussion of difficult-to-treat obsessive-compulsive patients gave the example of a man with concomitant paranoid features. Lest any doubt remain as to whether this man would score low in treatability, Millon provided a lengthy menu of his unflattering traits: "rigid, perfectionistic, grim, humorless, controlled, inflexible, dyspeptic, peevish, cranky, legalistic and self-righteous" (p. 706). Millon's patient experienced anxiety, as well as a fear of ridicule, but even so, "therapeutic procedures could not confront more than he could tolerate" (p. 707). Millon pursued a path that relied on brief, focused, primarily cognitive techniques, rather than on insight-based interpretations, and was able at least to help the man become less preoccupied with rules, regulations, and the inevitably hopeless quest for faultlessness. Anxiety was even less of a factor with the obsessive-compulsive patient in the following vignette, whose amenability to therapy was diminished for other reasons:

A 38-year-old middle-level executive at a prestigious brokerage house had been struggling to decide whether to marry the woman he had been dating on and off for the past 4 years. He entered therapy in the hope that it would help him resolve the issue. His girlfriend, who was a year older than him, worked in a similar post in a different firm. She felt he was "commitment shy," as he told me, whereas he was concerned that she might not remain faithful to him if they were to marry. That worry had arisen because, during a 5-month period when they had been apart, she had become involved with a married man.

The patient had grown up as the eldest of three children. His parents had both held good jobs, but they managed their money poorly and had financial difficulties. His personality was quite the opposite of everyone else's in the family. He was a highly responsible, cautious, and diligent "workaholic" who was as meticulous about his attire and his grooming as he was about his profit-and-loss sheets. A man of considerable reserve and taciturnity, he gave few clues to his feelings, volunteered little information in general, and insisted on being asked questions to get the wheels of dialogue moving. When he did speak, he often used trendy clichés. If he overlooked a detail at work, for example, he would comment: "If you look away for a second, the curveball goes right past you." He earned a high salary, a good portion of which he set aside in order to bail out the other members of his family, who were as profligate as he was prudent.

It soon became apparent that part of his attraction to his girlfriend was also a factor in his reluctance to "tie the knot." She supplied the emotions that were lacking in his life, but she was stormy and volatile, given to making scenes in restaurants and running off without him. I mentioned that men with constricted emotionality often gravitate to flamboyant women, which reminded him of his previous girlfriends, whose flamboyance was indeed the "red thread" that ran through their personality profiles. A vicious circle was at work in his relationships with women in that his icy reserve and judgmental nature were guaranteed to exaggerate the very moodiness and irascibility that he so disliked in the women he dated.

His hesitancy in making a commitment was highlighted in the first dream he reported. He saw himself falling through the air, holding on to a parachute that was not working. He waited too long, and it wouldn't open. He wondered, "What will my last thought be as I strike the ground and die?" In his associations to the dream he spoke of having let too many years go by without having "gotten his house in order" either financially or socially. For his girlfriend, time on the biological clock was beginning to run out, and he did want to have several children. But if he left her and searched for a suitable younger woman, he would be older still by several years, and it might be increasingly hard to find a woman in her 20s who would be willing to marry a man in his 40s. He tried to resolve the dilemma by drawing up lists of his girlfriend's good points and bad points, but given the bewildering complexity of people, compared with stocks and bonds, this exercise did not prove useful.

Because his psychological mindedness was not well developed, and because he was more interested in factual "answers" than in exploration of his own conflicts, therapy was conducted along primarily cognitive lines. His jealousy was reactivated after one of his absences, when he had a dream in which his girlfriend had taken up with another man. In the dream, the man had "moved in with her; she and I couldn't meet with any ease, because this man was now living with her. She said she was sleeping with him, which made me go berserk."

He voiced his ambivalence in the following way: "Right now, I'm 85% against marrying her and 15% for it; yet she's 85% perfect, and if she got into therapy and took care of that other 15%, I would marry her." I was intrigued by his use of the phrase "85% perfect." That very number had often been used by other patients I had worked with as a rationale *for* marrying: in their opinion, "85%" was about as compatible as any two people could get. Why didn't 85% suffice for this patient? I suggested that he was using his girlfriend's shortcomings as a shroud to cover his own imperfections and his own private reasons for avoiding marriage that had little to do with her. This suggestion spurred him to reflect on his fears about married life that stemmed from the picture he had built up over the years of his parents' marriage. They quarreled often over money and also seemed to favor the two younger children, who were still unable to fend for themselves. All of the burden fell on the patient, whose conscience would not let him simply walk away from them. Unless he could get a "100%" guarantee that he would not end up with similar burdens if he married and had children of his own, then bachelorhood seemed the safer course. In his risk-averse state of mind, 85% was still too dicey.

He also had a great deal of unprocessed anger at his parents, especially his mother. It appeared that he was drawn to unstable women partly because of positive feelings toward his mother, herself an unstable and mercurial woman. But he was not much in touch with those feelings. By choosing unstable women, however, he gave himself ample justification for avoiding marriage, without ever having to confront his own conflicts. So in that sense they were "perfect" after all.

His anger came through in the following dream: "I was out to dinner with my family. My brother wandered off, and my parents went in search of him, leaving me standing by the receptionist's table. When they came by me a little later, I grew furious and threw glasses and plates at my mother, and then stormed out of the restaurant." The dream encapsulated his feelings about the family during his early years. His mother in particular took pity on the two younger children, leaving the patient feeling misunderstood and neglected. He saw himself as "stuck" with all the responsibilities by virtue of his being the only capable one. In his current life, he calculated that if he dipped into his capital enough to stave off his parents' threatened bankruptcy and then dipped further in order to rescue his siblings, he himself would be in a precarious financial position. I asked him in what Bible was it written that where four family members are drowning, the fifth must also drown in the impossible task of rescuing them? He understood the advice hidden in the question: if he could help them to become self-sufficient without endangering himself, no more could be asked of him. If their prodigality continued, no one could say that he had failed them.

He then drew up a logical plan of action that enabled his parents to avoid bankruptcy and advanced them a small loan that was well within his means. To his siblings he gave no money; instead, he offered them help in finding job opportunities. He was finally able to accept the "logic" we worked out together: that it was better to have his siblings hate him and find work than to love him for the money he let them squander while they did nothing. Having lasted about 6 months, his treatment stopped at this point.

Patients with *avoidant personality disorder*—even those with milder expressions of the condition—present major challenges to psychotherapy. The similarities between avoidant personality disorder and schizoid personality disorder were emphasized by Millon (1999), who drew attention to the ways in which both types may "appear withdrawn, emotionally flat, and lacking in communicative and social skills" (p. 309). Persons with avoidant personality disorder are usually at pains to fend off depression or intense anxiety in social situations, especially in intimate situations. Thus agoraphobia and avoidant personality disorder secondary to the severe anxiety symptom disorders (especially social anxiety) may be understood as the opposite ends of a spectrum. For these patients, retreating to the safety of home becomes a defense against the anxiety that would be generated in social or intimate situations. The anxiety would be reawakened immediately if the avoidant person were thrust into a social encounter where it seemed to him or her that rejection or humiliation was nearly certain. In contrast, persons with schizoid personality disorder show an emotional blandness, along with an inability to experience profound feelings of any sort. They tend to choose occupations (such as that of the night watchman) and hobbies (such as video games) that do not push them into interaction with others (see Millon 1999, p. 283).

Avoidant persons are experienced by others as timorous, anxious, hesitant, lacking in self-confidence, and awkward socially; the term "mousy" is often applied, a reflection of the fearfulness and vulnerability of that small creature. "Self-fulfilling prophecies" are attached to many of the attitudes of persons with personality disorders. A bedeviling conviction of many avoidant persons is that others must regard them as inept, undesirable, and socially and, often, physically unattractive. But in a person who has avoided customary social scenes for a number of years, refused to accept dates, and shunned friends (believing "they really don't like me"), social skills fail to develop. Likewise, the self-acceptance that comes from a history of being liked or admired by the majority of one's acquaintances—and of being rejected or disliked only by a few—does not develop.

Avoidant persons become hardened in their beliefs because they cut themselves off from the feedback of the external world, which would normally serve to fine-tune perceptions of self and others along ever more realistic lines. These beliefs are generally quite distorted and may include "I'm ugly," "I'm fat" (in an underweight patient), "I have nothing to say," and "people think I'm dull." Tragically, after years of lack of interaction with others, some of their initial depreciatory views of themselves become true. If, for example, avoidant persons have kept themselves "out of the loop" for many years, they end up with very little to say to other people, because, for example, they haven't traveled, haven't taken interesting jobs, haven't married or raised families, and haven't joined any organizations. The wells of conversation soon run dry, and others may indeed think of them as dull, even though they had the capacity—before they shut themselves off from the outside world—to be as interesting and broad in their experience as other people. Avoidant persons are also prone to develop strange views—not just about their weight or attractiveness—that may come to resemble those of schizotypal patients.

Whatever form of psychotherapy is applied in the treatment of avoidant persons, at some point the supportive intervention of *exhortation*—specifically, urging the patient to face the feared social situations—will be necessary. This point was recognized years ago by Alexander and French (1946), who echoed the still earlier observation of Freud that interpretive work alone yields few results with "phobic" patients, as patients with avoidant personality were then known. The following clinical example is based on my work with an avoidant patient who had markedly diminished amenability to psychotherapy, which was attributable at first to the severity of her social anxiety. The situation was aggravated by the years she spent shut up in her private "safe house," cut off from both the dangers she feared and the experiences that might have taught her that these "dangers" were not so perilous after all.

A 20-year-old woman was admitted to a psychiatric hospital in the mid-1960s and was treated on a unit specializing in the long-term psychotherapy of severe personality disorders. She had been morbidly shy most of her life, a condition that declared itself first in the form of "school phobia" when she was 6 years old. Apart from a maternal aunt who had experienced postpartum depression, her extended family had no history of mental illness. She had a few friends during her school years, including one confidante (a girl in the same class), but she never dated during her high school years. She was accepted to a nearby college, but she became so anxious at the prospect of leaving home that she put off attending for a year.

By the time she was scheduled to start her freshman year she was nearly housebound. She was able to complete one semester, but she dropped out halfway through the second semester. Although she never accepted a date, she did form a brief friendship with a student in one of her classes who was about to return to his home in Europe. They had long talks over coffee but never got so far as to hold hands. For the first time in her life, she entertained fantasies of sex and marriage, but she imagined that he found her unattractive. She felt that his imminent return to Europe was the result of a desire to distance himself from her, rather than part of his original plan to spend only 1 year in the United States. She took his leaving as a rejection, as well as a confirmation of her self-image as a "boring, homely girl." She found it increasingly difficult to concentrate on her studies, and left college.

When she returned home, she rarely ventured out of her room and had little contact with others. The psychiatrist she had begun to see recommended hospitalization in the hope of effecting a speedier resolution of her agoraphobia and social phobia. Therapy was successful enough that when she left the hospital 4 months later, she was able to take transportation to and from her therapy sessions. In time she was able to work for a firm that published children's books, where she could use her artistic talents. She interacted scarcely at all with the other employees or even with her former friends.

The patient now spent considerable time thinking about the causes of her symptoms. She began to jot down notes and to elaborate her own theories about the root causes of mental illness. In her view, everything led back to some form of child abuse at the hands of the parents. She showed no awareness that people are born with various temperaments or biological predispositions that interact with parental influences in creating a path to either mental health or mental illness. There was no evidence that she had ever been subjected to any verbal, physical, or sexual abuse in her preadult years. Even her agoraphobia, for example, she ascribed to having probably been kept for long periods in a small crib by her "unthinking parents," such that now, 20–30 years later, she felt ill at ease in the vast outdoors.

At the time of follow-up, nearly 40 years later, the patient continued to show avoidant characteristics. She led an isolated life and had few outside contacts apart from occasional visits with family members. In recent years, she has seen a psychopharmacologist every month or so, who prescribed small amounts of risperidone (to reduce the cognitive distortions). With this regimen, she became less embittered toward her now-deceased parents. She continued to believe that her avoidant pattern stemmed from improper handling when she was a baby, but she was willing to forgive her parents on the grounds that they were probably mishandled in similar ways by their parents, and so on back through the generations.

REFERENCES

Abraham K: Character formation on the genital level of libido development. Int J Psychoanal 7:214–222, 1926

Alexander FG, French TM: Psychoanalytic Therapy: Principles and Applications. Lincoln, University of Nebraska Press, 1946

American Psychiatric Association: Diagnostic and Statistical Manual of Mental Disorders, 3rd Edition. Washington, DC, American Psychiatric Association, 1980

American Psychiatric Association: Diagnostic and Statistical Manual of Mental Disorders, 4th Edition, Text Revision. Washington, DC, American Psychiatric Association, 2000

Apt C, Hurlbert D: The sexual attitudes, behavior, and relationships of women with histrionic personality disorder. J Sex Marital Ther 20:125–133, 1994

Aviram RB, Hellerstein DJ, Gerson J, et al: Adapting supportive psychotherapy for individuals with borderline personality disorder who self-injure or attempt suicide. J Psychiatr Pract 10:145–155, 2004

Beck AT, Freeman A: Cognitive Therapy of Personality Disorders. New York, Guilford, 1990

Berlin FS: The etiology and treatment of sexual offending, in The Science, Treatment and Prevention of Antisocial Behaviors: Application to the Criminal Justice System. Edited by Fishbein DH. Kingston, NJ, Civic Research Institute, 2000, pp 21-1–21-15

Black DW: Bad Boys, Bad Men: Confronting Antisocial Personality Disorder. New York, Oxford University Press, 1999

Bursten B: Some narcissistic personality types (1973), in Essential Papers on Narcissism. Edited by Morrison AP. New York, New York University Press, 1986, pp 377–402

Clarkin JF, Levy KN, Lenzenweger MF, et al: The Personality Disorders Institute/Borderline Personality Disorder Research Foundation randomized control trial for borderline personality disorder: rationale, methods, and patient characteristics. J Personal Disord 18:52–72, 2004

Cooke DJ, Michie C: An item response theory evaluation of Hare's Psychopathy Checklist. Psychol Assess 9:2–13, 1997

Davanloo H: Intensive short-term psychotherapy with highly resistant patients, I: handling resistance. International Journal of Short-Term Psychotherapy 1:107–133, 1986

Dolan B, Coid J: Psychopathic and Antisocial Personality Disorders: Treatment and Research Issues. London, UK, Gaskell, 1993

Easser R-R, Lesser S: Hysterical personality: a reevaluation. Psychoanal Q 34:390–405, 1965

Freud S: Civilization and its discontents (1929), in The Standard Edition of the Complete Psychological Works of Sigmund Freud, Vol 21. Translated and edited by Strachey J. London, Hogarth Press, 1961, pp 59–145

Goldberg A: Self psychology and the narcissistic personality disorders. Psychiatr Clin North Am 12:731–739, 1989

Hare RD, Harpur TJ, Hakstian AR, et al: The revised Psychopathy Checklist: reliability and factor structure. Psychol Assess 2:338–341, 1990

Hoch PH, Polatin P: Pseudoneurotic forms of schizophrenia. Psychiatr Q 23:248–276, 1949

Kernberg OF: Borderline personality organization. J Am Psychoanal Assoc 15:641–685, 1967

Kernberg OF: Severe Personality Disorders: Psychotherapeutic Strategies. New Haven, CT, Yale University Press, 1984

Kernberg OF: Aggression in Personality Disorders and Perversions. New Haven, CT, Yale University Press, 1992

Kraepelin E: Manic-Depressive Insanity and Paranoia. Edinburgh, Livingstone, 1921

Linehan MM: Cognitive-Behavioral Treatment of Borderline Personality Disorder. New York, Guilford, 1993

Lion JR: Outpatient treatment of psychopaths (1978), in The Mark of Cain: Psychoanalytic Insight and the Psychopath. Edited by Meloy JR. Hillsdale, NJ, Analytic Press, 2001, pp 265–281

Lion JR, Bach-y-Rita G. Group psychotherapy with violent outpatients. Int J Group Psychother 20:185–191, 1970

Meissner WW: Narcissistic personalities and borderline conditions: a differential diagnosis, in Essential Papers on Narcissism. Edited by Morrison AP. New York, New York University Press, 1986a, pp 403–437

Meissner WW: Psychotherapy and the Paranoid Process. Northvale, NJ, Jason Aronson, 1986b

Meissner WW: Paranoid personality disorder, in Synopsis of Treatments of Psychiatric Disorders, 2nd Edition. Edited by Gabbard GO, Atkinson SD. Washington, DC, American Psychiatric Press, 1996, pp 947–951

Millon T: Personality-Guided Therapy. New York, Wiley, 1999

Millon T, Davis R: Personality Disorders in Modern Life. New York, Wiley, 2000

Reich W: Character Analysis. New York, Noonday Press, 1933

Rockland LH: Supportive Therapy: A Psychodynamic Approach. New York, Basic Books, 1989

Schneider K: Psychopathic Personalities (1923). London, Cassell, 1950

Southam-Gerow MA, Kendall PC: Parent-focused and cognitive-behavioral treatments of antisocial youth, in Handbook of Antisocial Behavior. Edited by Stoff DM, Breiling J, Maser HD. New York, Wiley, 1997, pp 384–394

Steiner R: On narcissism: the Kleinian approach. Psychiatr Clin North Am 12:741–770, 1989

Stone MH: Traditional psychoanalytic characterology re-examined in the light of constitutional and cognitive differences between the sexes. J Am Acad Psychoanal 8:381–401, 1980

Strasburger LH: The treatment of antisocial syndromes: the therapist's feelings (1986), in The Mark of Cain: Psychoanalytic Insight and the Psychopath. Edited by Meloy JR. Hillsdale, NJ, Analytic Press, 2001, pp 297–313

Swenson C: Kernberg and Linehan: two approaches to the borderline patient. J Personal Disord 3:26–35, 1989

Winston A, Rosenthal RN, Pinsker H: Introduction to Supportive Psychotherapy. Washington, DC, American Psychiatric Publishing, 2004

CHAPTER 8

PERSONALITY TRAITS AT THE EDGE OF TREATABILITY

Even patients whose array of personality traits does not meet the established diagnostic criteria for a specific disorder almost invariably manifest a few unwelcome traits that have affected their lives adversely and that contribute to their motivation to seek help. Some of these traits are the very ones that have led family members or others to urge treatment for the person in question.

The criteria for DSM-IV-TR (American Psychiatric Association 2000) Axis II disorders contain collectively only about 100 different traits, and these traits do not constitute a comprehensive list of the pathological, aberrant, or otherwise bothersome qualities that have relevance to psychiatry and psychotherapy. A comprehensive list would be very long—about 500 negative traits and about 100 positive traits would be needed to cover the field adequately (Stone 1993, pp. 100–106). A few additional traits that are mild, neutral, or ambiguous—such as absent-minded or proud—could be included in this list. "Proud," for example, can denote either an excessive quality of haughtiness or arrogance or a justifiable awareness of one's positive accomplishments.

Some persons exhibit an extraordinarily intense degree of a pathological trait that is a criterion for a DSM personality disorder, yet they do not have enough of the other traits of the disorder to warrant an Axis II diagnosis. Examples are jealousy (paranoid personality disorder criterion A7, elaborated in DSM-IV-TR as "has recurrent suspicions, without justification, regarding fidelity of spouse or sexual partner") and stinginess/cheapness (obsessive-compulsive personality disorder criterion 7, "adopts a miserly spending style toward both self and others"). As it happens, not all jealous persons are paranoid in general, and not all paranoid persons are jealous.

Sometimes the pathological trait operates as a kind of monomania, as described by Esquirol (1838): "a chronic disorder of the brain, without fever, characterized by a partial lesion of the intelligence or the emotions or the will. The intellectual disorder usually is concentrated on a single object or on a series of narrowly circumscribed objects….but apart from this, the [monomanic] patient feels, thinks, and acts like everybody else" (p. 1, my translation). Esquirol went on to sketch a variety of monomanic conditions, one of which was erotomania. He drew a careful distinction between that condition, which he viewed as a chronic brain disorder characterized by excessive love for either a known person or an imaginary person, and nymphomania or satyriasis. The latter were for Esquirol maladies that originated, instead, in the reproductive organs, whose abnormal irritability then exerted its reaction on the brain (p. 32). In the current era, examples of monomanic (that is, single-trait) preoccupation could be found in the actions of certain high-level executives who face charges of having enriched themselves through corporate malfeasance. Some of these men appear to have led conventional lives; to have been devoted and caring husbands and fathers, sympathetic neighbors, and generous supporters of charities; and to have been sought after as friends and as participants in community affairs. Their personality profile not only fails to meet the criteria for a recognized disorder, but is tarnished only by one flaw, albeit a flaw of monomanic (and monumental) proportions: greed. Some of the others appear to have a number of narcissistic traits, such as a grandiose sense of self-importance, preoccupation with unlimited success, and a sense of entitlement, but whether they show a full-blown narcissistic personality disorder could only be determined by someone who had examined them personally.

The majority of these "singularities"—traits so markedly exaggerated as practically to define the person who manifests them—may be understood as threads of personality that converge toward a nodal point of narcissism. They may exist, as mentioned earlier, in men and women whose personalities are otherwise unexceptionable, or they may be the one outstanding trait in those with a definite personality disorder whose combined traits

---

TABLE 8–1.   Personality traits whose presence, if intense, creates severe problems for psychotherapy, even in the absence of a definable personality disorder

---

Abrasive	Lazy
Bigoted	Maudlin
Bitter	"Plastic," lacking in firm values
Bullying; "macho"	Procrastinating
Caddish	Prudish
Despotic	Quarrelsome, argumentative
Envious	Rude, tactless
Form-conscious (excessively)	Sanctimonious
Garrulous	Scatterbrained, "flaky"
Greedy	Sensation-seeking
Humiliating, shrewish	Spiteful, scheming
Hypocritical	Unappreciative
Impractical	Unforgiving
Indiscreet	Unreliable, undependable, untrustworthy
Insubordinate	Unsympathetic
Irritating	Vengeful, vindictive
Jealous	Vicious

---

may spread over several Axis II categories. Most of the traits that others experience as objectionable—enough to urge the person to seek treatment or enough to wish that the person would seek treatment, even if the likelihood of improvement seems remote—fall under the rubric of narcissism, as they seem to be manifestations of extreme self-centeredness (see Ronningstam 2005). Some of these traits, most of which have no counterpart in the criterion items of Axis II, are listed in Table 8–1. Even traits that are unrelated to the concept of narcissism may prove to be stumbling blocks to psychotherapy if they are present in an intense form, whether they are encountered in patients with personality disorders or in persons who are in other respects rather normal.

About half the traits pertain to the domain of narcissism (e.g., abrasive, bigoted, bitter, bullying, caddish, despotic, greedy). The importance of narcissism is not surprising, because it is seen as approximately synonymous with the concept of pride, the deadliest of the Seven Deadly Sins and the one from which all the others (envy, gluttony, greed, anger, sloth, and lust) are said to arise. The relevance to modern psychology of the Greek, Jewish, and Christian theologies concerning this catalog of sins has been discussed by Solomon Schimmel (1997). It is important to note that this catalog, based on religion, overlaps rather neatly with a list of personality traits whose presence pushes therapists to the very edge of their therapeutic ability and, all too often, beyond that ability. The following sections direct attention to a few of the more common traits in this group.

BIGOTRY

Bigotry belongs to the domain of (false) pride, and hence narcissism, insofar as bigoted persons operate under the all but unshakable assumption that the group to which they belong is manifestly superior to the groups certain others belong to. Most therapists have probably never had the experience of a patient's asking for help to overcome his or her prejudices. Any efficacy that psychotherapy has in the treatment of bigotry usually results from group techniques.

When bigotry is combined with psychopathy, treatment is unavailing. One has only to consider the tragic case of James Byrd, Jr., a black man in Jasper, Texas, who was abducted in 1998 by three white men, John-William King, Lawrence Brewer, and Shawn Berry, chained to the rear of a pickup truck, and dragged while still conscious for about 3 miles along a road, until his limbs and head were torn off as the drivers passed a culvert (Temple-Raston 2002). King and Brewer, released from prison not long before the murder, were "Aryan Pride" racists who harbored murderous hatred for blacks, Jews, Asians, inter alia, and their subsequent death penalties had no sobering effect on these sentiments. The people of the town of Jasper, in contrast, underwent painful self-reflection and made a sincere effort to conquer their racial prejudices, thanks to the moral suasion of spiritual leaders from the black and white communities.

Group therapy can exert a positive influence on prejudiced persons who are less "far gone" than King and Brewer. The adolescent psychiatrist, Anita Streeck-Fischer (1998a, 1998b), for example, has had success with a number of "skinheads," teenage boys in what was East Germany who torched the houses of Turkish immigrants and committed other race-based offenses. Many of these boys came from poor and broken families and could be understood as attempting to compensate for their feelings of hopelessness and inferiority by beating up foreigners. Streeck-Fischer's sensitive handling of these adolescents, using predominantly group psychotherapy with some individual psychotherapy, helped many of them make the transition from bigotry to acceptance. Even in their less dramatic forms, however, bigotry and prejudice have a tenacity and durability that often resist the powers of psychotherapy.

BITTERNESS

The trait of bitterness can accompany any of the named personality disorders, although it crops up most frequently in those with paranoid, irritable, or depressive personalities (Stone 1993, p. 437). Bitterness involves chronic disgruntlement with how one's life has unfolded, coupled with the feeling of having been cheated out of something that one had a right to—be that the love of a parent, more generous financial support, recognition for an accomplishment somebody else got the credit for, and so on. Bitterness is thus closely linked with envy and is perhaps a subtype of envy, as not all envious persons show bitterness as a readily discernible trait. In large families, bitterness may develop in reaction to parental abuse in some, but not other, children, and the differences depend on genetic predisposition, gender, differential treatment by the parents, and innate abilities.

The patient I described under the heading of bitterness in my 1993 book lamented the death of her father when she was an adolescent and was embittered about the behavior of her mother, who treated her like Cinderella. She was made to do the cooking and the cleaning and later to go to a nearby college so she could continue to serve as her mother's "maid." After a failed marriage, the patient made a number of serious suicide attempts and was hospitalized on several occasions. She derived little satisfaction from the responsible job she held, because it was more important to her to "be in a relationship," even though she turned people away with her sharp tongue and fault finding. During our sessions, I encouraged her to focus on certain solitary pleasures over which she had control. She was a competent musician and could aspire to join others eventually in a chamber music group, where she could develop friendships with people who had similar interests. Participation in such a group might be a stepping-stone to a new and better relationship than the one she had had with her ex-husband. I emphasized the need to lay down the sword, as it were, and to get past blaming her aging mother for all the shortcomings in her life. None of these suggestions were taken very far. After about 2 and a half years of twice-weekly sessions, she showed up one evening after a brief absence on my part. She was very suicidal. Not trusting her to go to a hospital on her own, I drove her to a psychiatric emergency room, whereupon she reproached me by saying, "Who told you to save my f——g life?!" I would have regarded her treatment—and with it, my effort to overcome her bitterness—as a failure, but when I phoned her, with some trepidation, 10 years later, she surprised me with the news that after several months in different hospitals and after losing her old job, she had finally developed a more accepting and spiritual attitude about her life. She made peace with her mother, acquired a circle of friends, and found a position that was more satisfying than her old job. She expressed her gratitude to me for having kept her alive—against her will at the time. This help had enabled her to advance, unexpectedly and some years later, to a place where she was, for the first time in her life, content to be alive.

In my recent follow-up work with borderline patients whom I have been tracing over intervals of 30–40 years (an extension of the follow-up of P.I.-500 patients I had traced at 10- to 25-year intervals [Stone 1990]), I have noticed that bitterness is emerging as a kind of rate-limiting factor in long-term outcome. It may also be that risk genes for mood disorder predispose individuals to bitterness, especially where the balance in the mood disorder tilts toward depression. Persons with depressive temperament, for example, often show the traits of pessimism and gloominess. I was struck by the contrast between the life trajectories of several borderline patients who experienced comparatively little in the way of adverse childhood events (let alone physical or sexual traumata) yet who remained markedly bitter many years later and those of other patients who had experienced severe and prolonged traumata yet who were currently living successful lives without a trace of bitterness. Those who remained bitter did, however, have both a depressive temperament and a family history of close relatives with depression. The severely traumatized patient in the case example at the end of Chapter 4, who did not have a family history of depression, was without bitterness at follow-up despite all she had been through. Misdiagnosed with schizophrenia in her teens, she was treated with nearly 100 electroconvulsive therapy treatments in a hospital where she was kept for 3 years and was then transferred to another hospital, where she was able to make a good alliance with her second therapist. No longer acutely suicidal, she began a long uphill ascent, to become, 40 years later, one of the best-functioning persons in her original group.

One of the reasons bitterness is so resistant to psychotherapy is that chronically embittered people alienate others through their querulousness, get sidetracked because of grudges they can't seem to get past, and in other ways mar their chances for the success in love or work that might have ended the bitterness. Bitterness, in other words, sets up a vicious circle.

ENVY

Many consider envy the most corrosive of the Seven Deadly Sins and in general one of the most treatment-resistant and troublesome of the negative personality traits. As Fairlie (1995) wrote, "There is no gratification for Envy, nothing it can ever enjoy" (p. 61), whereas each of the other deadly sins has its own potential gratification—gluttony can be gratified by good food; greed, by wealth. As for the source of envy, a number of psychoanalyst writers have drawn attention to events in the earliest stages of development. Anna Freud (1968), for example, described how young children, as their awareness of persons and events in their environment increases, "cease sooner or later to live in emotional partnership with the mother alone and enter into the larger family group," yet "jealousy and envy of older brothers and sisters may be very strong" (p. 466). The older children themselves are vulnerable, because "the arrival of the next baby, who takes the toddler's place with the mother, is bitterly resented. He feels intense jealousy [envy would be the more appropriate word here] and hatred for the newcomer who has dispossessed him and wishes for the newcomer's death and disappearance" (p. 467). Riccardo Steiner (1989), in his discussion of Melanie Klein's (1957) writings on primary envy, emphasized that for Klein, this primitive form of envy was an essential constitutional aspect of the earliest relationship to the maternal breast—an envy that could be mitigated by the adequacy of the mother's nurturing availability. Gratitude, in that sense, becomes the "cure" for envy.

This point makes sense from the standpoint of infant development: the good enough mother reduces the infant's tendency to envy through her nurturing. From a clinical standpoint, however, adult patients who are intensely envious seem all but impervious to gratitude, no matter what they are given. Envy is seen also as a primitive defense mechanism, along with devaluation, idealization, and omnipotent control—all aimed at protecting the grandiose self (Kernberg 1989). This explanation relates to the envy associated with narcissistic personality and underlying pathological narcissism in patients whose abnormal early development gave rise to this condition. In comments pertaining to a more normative aspect of envy, Melanie Klein (1957, p. 181) also spoke of creative capacities as being the object of the "greatest envy," harking back to the mother's capacity for bearing children. Artistic creativity in men, for example, has been linked to the desire to be able to procreate as women do (Chasseguet-Smirgel 1985, p. 145).

Patients in whom envy is the most salient personality trait are seldom able to overcome it simply by getting at its roots through psychoanalytic psychotherapy or any other psychotherapeutic approach. To recognize that "my mother was pretty neglectful" or "my older brother was a better athlete" or "my sister earns double what I make" provides only cold comfort—this recognition is step 1 in a two-step process. It seems more effective to help such patients accomplish step 2—ascending to the level of, or outperforming, those whom they chiefly envy. Although Professor Schimmel's treatise on sin was written in part from a theological and philosophical perspective, he is also a psychologist and psychotherapist, and he came to a quite similar conclusion in his recommendations for addressing envy. "One of the wisest ways of dealing with envy," he wrote, "is, where possible, to transform it into emulation. Instead of harboring resentment at the achievements of others we should undertake actions that will bring us closer to attaining those things" (Schimmel 1997, p. 81). Schimmel mentioned the view of Helmut Schoeck (1970), according to whom envy is a "necessary fuel for social and economic progress" (Schimmel 1997, p. 82), because it spurs people to work toward the elevation of their status. In the most envious of patients, however, this trait has an aura of malignancy and corrosiveness, as the following case example shows:

> **A woman in her mid-20s** had come to the United States with her family when she was quite young. Her parents were successful professionals, and she had grown up in an affluent community. Although her parents were easygoing, serene people and not in the least competitive, she got caught up in the intensely competitive atmosphere that had come to dominate her age-mates from other families in the community. Her life was shaped by issues such as which girl had the most porcelain-like complexion, which families drove cars even fancier than the ones her parents owned, which high school seniors were accepted into Ivy League colleges, and which boy was most likely to be a millionaire by age 30 years. Her envy of persons who occupied niches higher than hers on these scales was matched only by her contempt of those who placed lower. This contempt extended even to herself, because she was less gifted than some of the other children in this narrow social circle, and she ended up in a less prestigious college than they did.
>
> The man who became her "first love" was not nearly so taken with her as she was with him. He was critical and dismissive. At times he made hurtful remarks that would have sent an ordinary woman packing, but she clung to him tenaciously all the same. Dependency and masochistic surrender were not her only qualities, however. When he rejected her definitively, she began to pester him with frequent calls and letters. She was eaten up with envy that he could prefer some other woman and was seriously depressed for months after the breakup. All the men she dated afterward she compared invidiously with her former boyfriend. He remained the North Star by which she guided her life. Her pain at the rejection could be assuaged for a time if I recited to her the catalog of his various cruelties, but then she would pine for him with undiminished fervor all over again. A few years later she met a man of excellent character (quite in contrast to that of the men she had been dating in the meantime) who brought out the best in her. They married after a brief courtship, which was a turbulent time for her, because she often felt she was settling for someone who did not measure up to her first boyfriend. Her envy gradually lessened, as she began to realize that a virtuous man of modest means is better than a rich but contemptuous man who treated her shabbily.

HUMILIATION

Another branch on the malign tree of narcissism is humiliation, here referring to a personality trait where the focus is on crushing the spirit of another person through caustic and humiliating remarks. Such remarks are all the more potent if delivered in front of other people. Humiliation can take many forms, including sarcasm, gratuitous insults, disdainful or contemptuous put-downs, unwarranted criticism, ridicule, and verbal taunts.

Persons whose chief characteristic is to humiliate others seldom complain of their own offensive nature, much less seek psychotherapeutic help in order to correct it. Fewer than 1 in 100 patients whom I have seen in private practice exhibited this trait. Several dozen others, however, had been severely affected by a close relative—a parent or a spouse—who regularly humiliated them and other members of their family. My impression about those who habitually humiliate others is that, far from being self-reflective, they rely on externalizing defenses and are aggressive in their interactions with others. This characteristic explains both their rarity as "identified patients" and their all too great frequency as the key agents in their relatives' (or, from the workplace, their subordinates') seeking psychotherapy. The following example concerns an elderly woman whose chief narcissistic traits were haughtiness and disdainfulness. Her chief targets were her husband and her daughter:

> **The woman's** husband was the director of a large organization, a person regarded by the outside world as intelligent, scholarly, and successful, but by his wife, as a feckless stumblebum. When he was on his way to work, she would upbraid him by saying, for example, "How can you go to work in a brown jacket and gray pants and a blue tie?! Take it all off! *I'll* choose what you'll wear!" As he reached retirement and developed Parkinson's disease, his gait was affected, which brought on his wife's regular tirade of "Why do you walk so *slow*? I wish you were dead." Her daughter had been overweight more often than not since adolescence, and her mother bought her clothes that were uncomfortably small, rather than acknowledge that she needed a larger size, and scolded her about being "such a pig." When her daughter was older, no meeting took place between the mother and daughter without the mother's making an acid remark about her daughter's weight, even though this behavior put at risk the older woman's access to her grandchildren. The daughter's therapist met with the mother on a number of occasions and urged her to refrain from making hurtful remarks to her daughter, but this intervention had no effect.

QUARRELSOMENESS

The trait of quarrelsomeness (or querulousness) may be a dominant feature in patients with a variety of personality configurations, such as paranoid, narcissistic, obsessive-compulsive, or passive-aggressive personality. The underlying motives may differ according to the predominant configuration and may include the need to externalize and blame others, as in the paranoid person; the need to get one's own way or to prove one's superiority, as in the narcissist; the tendency to find fault, as in the obsessive-compulsive person with a perfectionistic or a miserly streak; and the need in the passive-aggressive person to "defeat" other persons through captiousness, poutiness, and a groaning reluctance to do the smallest favor. At least a modest narcissistic "core" may exist in all of these variants, because quarrelsomeness bespeaks a degree of self-centeredness and a lack of cooperativeness.

Markedly quarrelsome persons are generally averse to seeking help, because this trait, like most traits, is ego-syntonic. Those who do end up in therapy often quit prematurely and are inordinately difficult to treat. The countertransference reactions of impatience, irritation, and the wish to counterattack (to prove a point or win the argument) can be formidable, and there is no guarantee that conquering such feelings will conduce to a successful outcome of the therapy. In general, however, it is the relatives of quarrelsome persons who seek therapy, not the quarrelsome persons themselves, as in the following example:

> **The husband of one patient** combined passive-aggressive and obsessive-compulsive traits to an extraordinary degree. Of the latter, he showed two-thirds of Freud's triad—*obstinacy* and *parsimony*—or, as his wife experienced them, *stubbornness* and *stinginess*. Although a well-to-do physician, he hid his assets in devious ways and pled poverty, giving his wife a tiny household allowance that was insufficient to put food on their table unless she dipped into her much less ample earnings. At the same time, he lavished expensive gifts on the college-age children from his first marriage. He also treated them to expensive vacations but took his wife nowhere except to visit his mother, even though the two women detested one another. If the patient complained about any of these injustices, he would become quarrelsome to the point of abusiveness, at times striking her. He would then storm out of the house and disappear until the wee hours or the next morning, giving no indication of where he was. She did manage to have him join her in couples therapy, but this venture failed, as the therapist who undertook this thankless task soon gave up on the husband and ended the sessions. There are many men—and some women—who mask their insecurity by attempting to achieve total control over their mates through subjugation. The main difference between the partners in this marriage was that the husband mocked the very idea of therapy, whereas the wife was highly motivated to work on her problems. Unfortunately, although her suffering was enormous, she was too entrenched in her masochism to leave a bad situation.

In an earlier work, I gave an example of a paranoid querulant, a man whose quarrelsomeness had driven his family to distraction (Stone 1980, p. 461). He came for a consultation at the insistence of his father. Our interchange was remarkable in that anytime I made a comment or suggested an interpretation, he immediately shouted, "I disagree!" When, toward the end of our meeting, I told him that I had another observation to share with him but was hesitant to voice it because of his consistent disagreement, he again said with some vehemence: "I disagree!" This man was beyond treatability not only because of this trait but also because of his lack of self-reflection, candor, and motivation.

Narcissistic personality disorder is especially difficult to treat when it is combined with fame, wealth, political power, or other forms of unusual success. Some persons in this rarefied category equate success with wisdom and come to believe that they "know better" than others—all others—no matter the subject. Those who are in addition quarrelsome present even greater barriers to psychotherapy because of their conviction that they are right about whatever issue is under discussion and that their spouse, child, business partner, or therapist has regrettably missed the point, as the following case example illustrates:

> **Some years ago I treated** the wife of an opera star and then worked with the couple in the hope of resolving the tensions in their marriage. The singer's mother was an elderly woman whose prescription for dealing with loneliness was to bind her only child to herself by disparaging all the women in his life, including his current wife. The main arena of battle between the two women was the 4-month-old son of the singer and his wife. Everything the wife did was wrong in the eyes of her mother-in-law, who constantly intruded on the couple, alienating the wife with her criticism. Invariably, the singer sided with his mother to "keep peace in the family," but this led to acrimonious arguments with his wife. Then the singer would berate his wife with the comment, "It's all your fault." If, during the couple's session, I tried to point out that his mother seemed quite jealous of any attention he might bestow on his wife, he would berate me by saying, "You don't understand the situation. My wife should have compassion for my mother, and she doesn't." In my view, the worst that could be said of the wife was that in personality, she was of a depressive-masochistic mould, prone all her life to seek and then to endure humiliation. Yet at the same time she was a sympathetic and emotionally "tuned-in" person with unusually good instincts for grasping the psychological dynamics of the important people in her life. The family (including the singer's mother) all returned to France, their native country, shortly after I began seeing them. I referred them to a colleague in Paris, from whom I learned, a year later, that the quarrels had continued, the singer was still unable to see his wife's side of the conflict, and they were on the brink of divorce.

SENSATION-SEEKING

I am using sensation-seeking here as an umbrella concept covering a variety of personality traits that often coexist. Persons for whom the antidote to boredom is strong sensation tend to lack perseverance and to scurry from one "thrilling" experience to another. Millon and Davis (2000), citing Cloninger's model, refer to "novelty-seeking" (p. 19), which may have the neurobiological underpinnings of low basal dopaminergic activity in the central nervous system (Cloninger 1986). Sensation-seeking is found with regularity in persons with antisocial personality, and it is a common feature of psychopathy (Harpur et al. 2002). There is also a strong correlation between sensation-seeking and impulsivity (Harpur et al. 2002). But even in persons with substantial degrees of sensation-seeking who are not distinctly antisocial or psychopathic, a common attribute is irresponsibility. This trait often proves to be a major stumbling block in therapy. Patients with this attribute may come faithfully for appointments when they are in a crisis, but then, when their situation temporarily settles down, they may skip appointments because they feel they don't need to come anymore. This fragmentation interferes with the tasks the therapist set out to accomplish, and a patient who seemed treatable at the outset becomes someone who is not very treatable or at best "half-treatable." The following vignettes illustrate this point:

> **A 29-year-old woman** was referred for treatment by another psychiatrist. She had already been married and divorced three times and was again living at home with her parents. They were at their wits' end about what to do with her, because, as they discovered, she would often sneak out of the house in the wee hours and go to bars, where she would take up with some of the disreputable "regulars," men who were happy enough to buy her a few drinks in return for her sexual favors.
>
> She had been wild and impulsive since her adolescence, and she seemed to have a temperament that was very different from that of her parents, who were studious, methodical people who ran a highly successful business. She could be considered self-destructive because of her promiscuity, although she did not engage in self-mutilative or parasuicidal acts. In personality she was markedly histrionic and had some borderline features, especially an intolerance for being alone. Her life lacked all structure, as was clear from the initial consultation. I felt it best to refer her to a colleague who was skilled at creating a stabilizing environment for such a patient.
>
> For several months, all went better than expected. Her parents set her up in an apartment and paid for a live-in companion. My colleague helped her to enroll in a local college, and for a time she attended classes with commendable regularity. This part of her story seemed to indicate that she was at least "half-treatable." Three months later she became fed up with this discipline and virtuous living and decamped for Florida, where she became involved with a group of gangsters. At a certain point she jilted one of these men in favor of a rival, but not before she cast aspersions on the sexual prowess of the first lover. The man shot her to death, the details of which I learned from the New York City tabloids. I have since revised my assess-

ment about her suicidality, because her provocative behavior is probably best characterized as "suicide with the help of a friend."

A woman in her mid-20s was brought for consultation by her parents because of a multiplicity of problems, including alcoholism, anorexia, agoraphobia, depression, benzodiazepine abuse, episodes of running away from home, and promiscuity. In personality she met criteria for borderline personality disorder, histrionic personality disorder, and dependent personality disorder. She was well-motivated for therapy, although she had little psychological mindedness. All the women in her family for three generations were depressed, some abused alcohol as well, and two had been hospitalized for depression. There was no history of physical, sexual, or verbal abuse; to the contrary, she was a pampered child, indulged particularly by her father.

Since her teen years, she had shown a "wild" side, which took the forms of truancy and promiscuity. She sometimes disappeared for weeks at a time with a boyfriend to a different part of the country, which necessitated her parents' hiring private investigators to track her down and return her home. Then, for periods of time she would become agoraphobic. When she did venture out, she would go to bars, get inebriated, and dance on the tabletops, attracting rough men who would take her home in their cars after having sex. Sometimes, she would get into fierce arguments with them, be left on the side of the road in the middle of the night, and have to walk long distances to get home.

I managed to get her into Alcoholics Anonymous (AA)—with great difficulty, because she was very picky about choosing meetings that contained the "right kind of people." She gave up alcohol, only to ratchet up her abuse of diazepam to alarmingly high levels. She had no hobbies and no ability to amuse herself, apart from drowning out her thoughts and easing her boredom by listening to raucous music at high volume. When her parents left for a brief vacation, she became suicidal. Hospitalization was then indicated both for her suicidality and to taper the diazepam gradually, which she was unable to do while at home. The hospital stay proved to be a turning point. Although several months were required to taper the benzodiazepines completely, afterward she was able to live with another former patient, at first in a sheltered setting and later in a place of her own. She has never been rehospitalized, and at follow-up 25 years later she was asymptomatic and successfully running a business of her own. The sensation-seeking of her earlier years melted down into a manageable predilection for vigorous exercise; she no longer abused substances, and she surrounded herself with friends who were stable and behaved conventionally. Psychiatry played an important role in her recovery, but not the psychotherapy so much as the limit-setting and group encouragement that the hospital and AA provided.

SPITEFULNESS

Despite the old adage that "living well is the best revenge," relatively few people have the opportunity (or the means) to improve their lives so dramatically or to rise to such high position as to be able to have the last laugh, from a position of superiority, on someone who has mocked, betrayed, insulted, or otherwise hurt them. More commonly, people seek retaliation for real or imagined hurts in more direct ways that will not only redress, but outdo, the original hurt. The "payback" often far exceeds the insult. We reserve the word *spiteful* for retaliatory or vengeful acts and attitudes that are unjustified. The dictionary speaks of a "malicious, petty desire to harm." Etymologically, the word comes from the Latin *despectare*, which means "to look down on."

The impulse to get back at those who have hurt or insulted us is deeply embedded in the psyche, presumably for reasons that are as compelling from an evolutionary standpoint as those explaining why jealousy exists in relation to the threat of loss of a sexual partner. Recently, Harmon-Jones and his colleagues at the University of Wisconsin Department of Psychology (Harmon-Jones 2004; Harmon-Jones and Sigelman 2001; Harmon-Jones et al. 2004) demonstrated that trait anger, a "negative, but approach-related emotion," is associated with increased left prefrontal and decreased right prefrontal cortical activity. These investigators understood their results as suggesting that asymmetrical prefrontal activity is associated with motivational direction, rather than with the positive or negative valence of an emotion, as had been assumed previously. These neurophysiological correlates of insult-related anger shed light on the biological underpinnings of emotions such as spitefulness.

Spitefulness that is discernible as a prominent characteristic is both highly pathological and particularly difficult to remedy. The challenge to treatability probably stems from the pleasurable aspect of spitefulness. Revenge-related fantasies and urges have even been described, as with hunger and lust, as "delicious" and hence not readily given up (Carey 2004). Spiteful persons often behave as though they are compensating for distinct feelings of inferiority, whether or not they consciously acknowledge such feelings.

It is not at all necessary to insult or hurt the spiteful person literally to awaken the emotion. Persons of great accomplishment routinely elicit spitefulness in various strangers, who feel annoyed—or "put down"—by the mere example of a great person's fame and skill. One need only go to Web sites where anonymous messages can be posted to verify this tendency. After Lance Armstrong won his sixth Tour de France bicycle race, earning him a place among the greatest athletes of all time, hundreds of people posted their anonymous messages, some laudatory, but others pathetically invidious. One person wrote, "This guy is so wrapped up in himself, he's blind to everything outside him…Fall off your bike already. What a role model this jerk is." Another wrote, "Look in the mirror Lance. If you weren't worth millions, Cheryl Crow [his fiancée] wouldn't look cross-eyed at you." A third called the victor a "steroid-taking cheater." Celebrity stalkers are almost invariably spiritually small persons committed to making life miserable for—in effect, to tearing down—those who are beautiful, famous, talented, or otherwise gifted.

In clinical work, therapists see spiteful patients from time to time whose vengefulness has its origin in cruel or otherwise markedly unfair treatment by parents during the formative years. Because it is seldom possible to exact revenge on the parent(s) directly, spitefulness may emerge as a prominent trait, with the emotion now directed at those who either symbolize the original sources of hurt or betrayal or just happen to be "in the way" of a patient who is not easily able to deal with the challenges and annoyances of everyday life. The following vignette presents an example of spitefulness of the latter sort:

A 36-year-old woman was referred because of marital strife. She and her husband had two young children, a 6-year-old boy and a 4-year-old girl. Her husband had a 12-year-old daughter by his first wife. The patient was a woman of a markedly irascible nature, and although she was highly critical toward her husband, she was particularly venomous toward her stepdaughter, whom she permitted to visit only on Fridays after school. She could be counted on to insult and berate her stepdaughter during every visit, which required some inventiveness, because the girl was a sweet, pretty, straight-A student who offered little rationale for such negativity. One week, shortly after I began treating this patient, the stepdaughter, because of a school commitment, asked to visit on a Thursday rather than on the customary Friday. The patient experienced this change as a "willful disruption" of the schedule and reacted with gratuitous violence. While the stepdaughter was quietly playing a game with the two younger children, the stepmother stormed into the room and yanked a large swatch of hair from her stepdaughter's head, causing great pain and leaving a noticeable bald spot in the back of the girl's head. The girl vowed never to return to her father's new home. This incident severed their relationship almost completely, and because the divorce had been acrimonious, the father had no opportunity to see his daughter at the home of his first wife.

I met then with both the patient and her husband in the hope of dealing with the crisis that the hair-pulling incident had precipitated. I explained to the wife that, having alienated her stepdaughter and having made it next to impossible for her husband to see his older daughter, she was now risking divorce—not a desirable situation for her, because she would have to cope with two small children all on her own. I added that she seemed to have been acting out of spite, given that the girl had done nothing offensive to her, and I suggested that her anger might be meant for someone else, for whom the girl was the "fall guy." I had been thinking of the woman's own father, who had molested her sexually when she was a teenager. Over the years she had stored up a great deal of anger about these experiences. Her reaction to my suggestion was swift and violent. She screamed invective at me (denying that she was "angry"), ran out of the office, slammed the door, and disappeared for several months. On her eventual return, her husband sued for divorce.

I have thought about this patient many times in the 20 years since the final session I just described. There is no question that I registered strong antipathy (or negative countertransference) toward her when I heard what she had done to her stepdaughter. This antipathy may have shown through in my less than sympathetic remarks about her spiteful behavior and unjustified anger. Another therapist might have handled the meeting better, and the outcome might have been less drastic. But to convert a chronically hostile and vituperative person of this age into a calm, good-natured, and (in this case) remorseful person whose marriage could be preserved is a task that is at best difficult, lengthy, and without any guarantee of success. One cannot state categorically that such patients are untreatable, but at the same time, one can say—categorically—that they belong to a most difficult domain of personality disorders, where successful psychotherapy is the exception rather than the rule.

DISCUSSION

Thus far the clinical vignettes have focused on traits that are actively offensive to others. Some of the personality attributes listed in Table 8–1 are close cousins of those traits. Spitefulness, for example, is related to vengefulness and also to viciousness, the latter being reserved for patterns of behavior that are more repugnant than those associated with spitefulness. Persons who predictably and repeatedly behave in vicious ways toward others are usually considered sadistic as well, because of their enjoyment in making others suffer. Sadistic personality is discussed in Chapter 9, which deals with untreatable personality disorders.

Elsewhere, I gave detailed descriptions of persons who were indiscreet, callous, or vengeful (Stone 1993, Chapter 20), along with brief allusions to other barely treatable or untreatable character types, including the despotic boss, the tyrannical father, and the explosively violent person who is nevertheless capable of some remorse, such as the prizefighter Jake LaMotta (1970). Also mentioned were certain narcissistic and intrusive parents whose efforts at self-magnification through forcing a talented child to achieve fame in the movies earned them the soubriquet "Hollywood mother." Maria Tatuloff, the mother of Natalie Wood (Lambert 2004), is an example.

People with the character types I have been sketching here seldom seek treatment, and they do not regard themselves as needing help. Therapists hear about these persons only indirectly, through the news media or in the accounts of an actual patient, who describes a relative or employer. Their amenability to treatment is reduced almost to the vanishing point, because they do not think of themselves as disturbed. They might be identified as personality disordered in an epidemiological survey, but they do not achieve "caseness" because they never present themselves to clinics or practitioners. Those whose chief characteristics are despotic, spiteful, vengeful, mean-spirited—in a word, hateful—create an even higher barrier against amelioration by therapy. Such persons inspire dislike in most people, including potential therapists. Should they somehow end up in a therapist's office, they tend to inspire strong countertransference feelings that interfere with—or defeat altogether—the development of a useful therapeutic alliance. They are in any case at the mercy of unpredictable particularities of the therapist's personality—qualities that permit some therapists to do good work with them, where another therapist, failing to find the "islands of humanity" in such patients, would soon give up. As the negativity in patients becomes more chronic and severe, this human factor in potential therapists advances to the forefront.

With patients who have very few likeable traits—or in language of the Five-Factor Model, very few "agreeable," as opposed to "antagonistic," traits (Costa and Widiger 2002)—therapists find themselves in the uncomfortable position of having to point out, again and again, that something a patient said or did was unpleasant, offensive, wounding, or tactless. In response, the patient tends to conclude that the therapist "doesn't like me" and quits treatment. If the therapist genuinely dislikes the patient and cannot get past this feeling, it may not be possible to do good work, and it would not be fair to the patient to continue. If the therapist likes or respects the patient, it may be possible to get around the impasse, if the therapist can bring enough art to the task of therapy. The therapist might save the day by saying, in effect, "Because I sometimes tell you that when you get angry or insecure, you deal with your discomfort by lashing out, it doesn't mean I don't like you, although it's true that people—me included—wouldn't like to be on the receiving end when you get upset. But I sense that underneath that tough outer shell is a good person trying to break through. I'm here to help that happen." Of course, a therapist can make such a remark only if it is sincere and genuine. In such situations, it is important to remember that likeability by itself is no guarantee of a patient's amenability to therapy; for example, many psychopaths of the "charmer" type are disarmingly likeable but remain untreatable and unchangingly dangerous.

Besides the difficult patients whose personalities display primarily narcissistic and antagonistic qualities, other patients have a markedly low amenability to therapy because of their passivity, clinging dependency, or other similar traits that quickly become irritating. These patients seem to lack all courage, become mired in self-pity, or, because of their feelings of utter helplessness, call their therapist too often and at inconvenient hours. The therapist who treats such patients soon comes to feel that the hole in their boat is much bigger than the little scoop that is being used in the hope of keeping them afloat. Some aspects of a patient exemplifying these qualities were described in Chapter 1, in the case example of the divorced woman who lived with her elderly mother. Here are some additional details concerning her dependency and her tendency to alienate others because of her self-pity and clinginess:

> **In the specifics** of her personality disorder she showed many of the signature or prototypical traits for both dependent and avoidant personality disorders, as demonstrated recently in the large-scale study by Shedler and Westen (2004). Among the dependent items, for example, the following were pertinent: 1) tends to be overly needy, requires excessive reassurance; 2) tends to be ingratiating; 3) fears rejection or abandonment; 4) goes to great lengths to avoid being alone; 5) tends to be unassertive; 6) tends to feel inadequate, inferior, or a failure; and 7) is indecisive when faced with choices. The relevant avoidant items were 1) fears embarrassment or humiliation, 2) tends to feel ashamed, and 3) is anxious. She also felt "misunderstood, mistreated, or victimized," a less frequently endorsed avoidant item but a very common paranoid trait.
>
> This catalog of dependent and avoidant traits does not tell the whole story. She called her daughter-in-law so often with questions, requests, and worries about the scheduling of visits that finally the daughter changed her phone number, and no further calls were permitted. She called me frequently also, often just begging to talk for a few minutes about nothing in particular. I found this behavior irritating and distracting and set firm limits about when and under what circumstances it was reasonable to phone me directly. In reaction, she became forgetful or sulky, expressing aggression passively—another quality mentioned by Shedler and Westen as being typical of dependent persons. Initially idealizing in her attitude toward me, she quickly became pouty and paranoid when I found it necessary to set limits. I was now seen as mistreating her.
>
> Her psychotherapy had been largely supportive and behavioral. I encouraged her to practice traveling unaccompanied by her companion, first for short distances, then for longer ones. Next I helped her to find students whom she could tutor in one of the foreign languages she knew. These efforts were intended to help make her less dependent on her mother, so that the latter's death would be less devastating. For a few months she was able to do these things, but then she gave up.

This patient's tendency to give up, no matter what the task, bespeaks a low level of *persistence*, another trait with important prognostic implications. Cloninger et al. (1999) identified persistence as a manifestation of temperament. They also discussed the importance of *self-directedness*, which is high in mature, resourceful people and low in immature people who are prone to discouragement (and depression). Because dependency is often associated with high motivation to remain in therapy—primarily to retain an attachment to the therapist—dependent persons often start out as "good patients" who are willing to come regularly to the sessions and to cooperate at least superficially with the various rules and demands of therapy. But in extreme cases, such as the one depicted in the previous vignette, therapy is stalemated, and the therapist's task is no less arduous and no more likely to succeed than with the less agreeable narcissistic types described in the earlier part of this chapter.

Personality-disordered patients at the "edge of treatability" thus include not only the egotistical and hostile types and those with one glaringly negative trait, but also those at the extremes of any DSM personality disorder—even those of the anxious cluster, where solid attachment to the therapist is the rule rather than the exception.

REFERENCES

American Psychiatric Association: Diagnostic and Statistical Manual of Mental Disorders, 4th Edition, Text Revision. Washington, DC, American Psychiatric Association, 2000

Carey B: Payback time: why revenge tastes so sweet. New York Times, July 27, 2004, p F-6

Chasseguet-Smirgel J: The Ego Ideal: A Psychoanalytic Essay on the Malady of the Ideal. Translated by Barrows P. New York, WW Norton, 1985

Cloninger CR: A unified biosocial theory of personality and its role in the development of anxiety states. Psychiatr Dev 4:167–226, 1986

Cloninger CR, Svraki D, Bayon C, et al: Measurement of psychopathology as variants of personality, in Personality and Psychopathology. Edited by Cloninger CR. Washington DC, American Psychiatric Press, 1999, pp 33–65

Costa PT Jr, Widiger TA: Introduction, in Personality Disorders and the Five-Factor Model of Personality, 2nd Edition. Edited by Costa PT Jr, Widiger TA. Washington, DC, American Psychological Association, 2002, pp 3–14

Esquirol E: Maladies mentales, Vol 2. Paris, Baillière, 1838

Fairlie H: The Seven Deadly Sins Today. London, University of Notre Dame Press, 1995

Freud A: The Writings of Anna Freud, Vol 4: 1945–1956: Indications for Child Analysis and Other Papers. New York, International Universities Press, 1968

Harmon-Jones E: Contributions from research on anger and cognitive dissonance to understanding the motivational functions of asymmetrical frontal brain activity. Biol Psychiatry 67:51–76, 2004

Harmon-Jones E, Sigelman J: State anger and prefrontal brain activity: evidence that insult-related relative left-prefrontal activation is associated with experienced anger and aggression. J Pers Soc Psychol 80:797–803, 2001

Harmon-Jones E, Vaughn-Scott K, Mohr S, et al: The effect of manipulated sympathy and anger on left and right frontal cortical activity. Emotion 4:95–101, 2004

Harpur TJ, Hart SD, Hare RD: Personality of the psychopath, in Personality Disorders and the Five-Factor Model of Personality, 2nd Edition. Edited by Costa PT Jr, Widiger TA. Washington, DC, American Psychological Association, 2002, pp 299–324

Kernberg PF: Narcissistic personality disorder in childhood. Psychiatr Clin North Am 12:671–694, 1989

Klein M: Envy and gratitude, in The Writings of Melanie Klein, Vol 3. London, Hogarth Press, 1957, pp 176–235

Lambert G: Natalie Wood: A Life. New York, Knopf, 2004

LaMotta J: Raging Bull: My Story. Englewood Cliffs, NJ, DaCapo, 1970

Millon T, Davis R: Personality Disorders in Modern Life. New York, Wiley, 2000

Ronningstam E: Identifying and Understanding the Narcissistic Personality. New York, Oxford University Press, 2005

Schimmel S: The Seven Deadly Sins: Jewish, Christian, and Classical Reflections on Human Psychology. New York, Oxford University Press, 1997

Schoeck H: Envy: A Theory of Social Behavior. New York, Harcourt Brace World, 1970

Shedler J, Westen D: Refining personality disorder diagnosis: integrating science and practice. Am J Psychiatry 161:1350–1365, 2004

Steiner R: On narcissism: the Kleinian approach. Psychiatr Clin North Am 12:741–770, 1989

Stone MH: The Borderline Syndromes. New York, McGraw-Hill, 1980

Stone MH: The Fate of Borderline Patients. New York, Guilford, 1990

Stone MH: Abnormalities of Personality: Within and Beyond the Realm of Treatment. New York, WW Norton, 1993

Streeck-Fischer A: Misshandelt—Missbraucht: Probleme der Diagnostik und Psychotherapie traumatisierter Jugendlicher, in Adoleszenz und Trauma. Edited by Streeck-Fischer A. Göttingen, Germany, Vandenhoeck & Ruprecht, 1998a, pp 174–196

Streeck-Fischer A: Über die Mimikryentwicklung am Beispiel eines jugendlichen Skinheads mit frühen Erfahrungen von Vernachlässigung und Misshandlung, in Adoleszenz und Trauma. Edited by Streeck-Fischer A. Göttingen, Germany, Vandenhoeck & Ruprecht, 1998b, pp 161–173

Temple-Raston D: A Death in Texas: A Story of Race, Murder, and a Small Town's Struggle for Redemption. New York, Henry Holt, 2002

9

UNTREATABLE PERSONALITY DISORDERS

In earlier chapters the term *treatability* was used to signify a combination of qualities—the capacity to submit to the rules and time demands of psychotherapy, as well as adequate motivation, reflectiveness, and ability to develop a working alliance with the therapist—that intertwined to conduce, some months or years later, to significant improvement in personality. Measures of such improvement include enhanced ability to get along with others, to form successful intimate relationships, to work, and perhaps also to develop constructive ways of handling leisure time. Freud summed up these outcomes in two words: when a reporter asked him what life was all about, he answered, "Liebe und Arbeit" (love and work).

Long-term follow-up of antisocial persons (Black 1999; Robins et al. 1991) has shown that some persons with severe personality disorders get better after many years without having received or benefited from individual or group psychotherapy. Sometimes the curative factor was the "tincture of time" (for example, among those who gave up most of their antisocial ways when they passed age 40 years). In other situations, institutionalization in a special rehabilitative center led to improvement; in still others, involvement in religion and envelopment in certain religious groups made the difference. Thus, some persons who started out with strong antisocial features were salvageable, even though they appeared initially to be untreatable.

This chapter concerns personality-disordered persons who are untreatable by any of the conventional psychotherapeutic means currently available. Two subgroups at this extreme end of the scale of treatability will be given special attention: the salvageable and the unsalvageable.

UNTREATABLE, BUT ULTIMATELY SALVAGEABLE PATIENTS

The fate of untreatable patients who turn out to be salvageable is revealed only through follow-up. When psychotherapy was initially attempted with these patients, the efforts failed, and the patients were regarded at the time as untreatable. The following examples, which come from the long-term follow-up study of patients treated originally at the New York State Psychiatric Institute (the P.I.-500 study [Stone 1990]), illustrate this point.

One-fourth ($n=137$) of the 550 patients who were included in the P.I.-500 study were younger than age 18 years when admitted to the hospital during the period 1963–1976. These patients were treated on the Adolescent Service, as it was then known. Seventeen (15 males and two females) met the criteria for antisocial personality disorder according to DSM-III (American Psychiatric Association 1980), the diagnostic system in use at that time.

> **One of these young men** was admitted because he was unmanageable at home, truant at school, and getting into trouble with the law because of petty thefts and shoplifting. He came to the hospital at the insistence of his mother. His troubles began 2 years earlier, shortly after his parents, a couple in solid middle-class circumstances, divorced. He was 15 years old at the time. He was noted to be rather surly and uncooperative on the unit, and he showed a defiant attitude toward the treating staff, including his therapist. He spoke very little about his problems or about his life in general and seemed just to be marking time until he could be discharged. Unbeknownst to him, the custom in that era was for patients to remain on the unit for about a year. Lengthy stays were especially common for adolescents, who often came from destructive home environments and who attended the special school within the hospital. Unbeknownst to the treating staff, his main symptom was alcoholism, but he said not a word about it to any staff member, and we were not astute enough in that era to ask him about his drinking habits. After 3 months on the unit, he eloped from the hospital.
>
> When I located him 20 years later, he reported that he had never sought

psychotherapy of any kind during the ensuing years but had instead traveled all over the country, often fleeing from a state where he was wanted for driving under the influence of alcohol. He lived by his wits, sustaining himself by means of temporary odd jobs and occasional thefts. Every so often he would be arrested and have to spend a few days in jail. In his early 30s, he met a woman who had a checkered past not unlike his own, but she by then was an ardent advocate and member of Alcoholics Anonymous (AA). She had also converted to Buddhism and regularly attended Buddhist religious functions. Through her influence he was persuaded to give these organizations a try. At first he went to these meetings just to please her. But in time, he found that both AA and Buddhism were appealing and helpful. He became abstinent, found a job in a hardware store, and by the time I met with him (4 years later, when he was 37 years old), he had become manager of the store and was engaged to marry the woman who had helped change his life.

Another patient who had an equally brief stay on the Adolescent Service was a 16-year-old girl who had run away from home. She was remanded to our hospital on what was euphemistically known as a PINS (person in need of supervision) petition. She had been truant at school and had become heavily addicted to heroin. For a brief time she had traded sex for drugs, but then she formed a relationship with her dealer as a way of reducing the number of sexual partners and ensuring a more steady supply of drugs. She had taken to the streets not because of the lure of drugs, but rather because of the need to escape from a father who had been abusing her mother physically for as long as she could recall and herself sexually since she was about 14 and a half years old. Before running away, she had made a number of suicide gestures by cutting her wrists. While she was on the unit, she was polite and well-behaved but restless and without any noticeable desire to unburden herself about her life or to cooperate with any of the therapeutic measures brought to bear on her situation. She received a diagnosis of "borderline with antisocial features."

After spending 4 months on the unit, during which she made a few friends among the other adolescent patients but made no real connections with the staff, she ran away—back into the arms of the drug dealer. Nothing further was heard from her until I located her 18 years later. Some months after she eloped from the hospital, she and her dealer friend had fallen on hard times and were living on the street. One morning she awakened with a start and said: "All of our friends are dying!" She was thinking about other heroin addicts who had recently died of overdoses. She and her friend decided then and there to quit heroin. Unaware that there were methadone clinics where they could be brought down gently, both simply stopped and experienced severe withdrawal effects. Afterward, they felt their best chance of escaping the lure of heroin was to choose an obscure rural place where illicit drugs were not readily available. They moved to a different section of the country and found jobs at a farm. They then married. By the time I found them, they had worked their way up to buying a farm of their own. The former patient had become successful in making and marketing a type of stuffed animal that became popular in their area. They bought a separate house nearby for her aging mother (the father having died in the meantime). Both were actively involved in parents' organizations of the school where their three children were enrolled.

The two previous examples concern patients who inspired pessimism in the hospital staff. Despite the intensity of the therapy offered to adolescent patients (three 45-minute and two 15-minute sessions per week), the two patients seemingly remained impervious to psychotherapy and any other interventions that were brought to bear on their conditions while at the hospital. The following example from my clinical work concerns a patient who proved to be untreatable in psychotherapy for a long time, at least while he was an outpatient, but who was ultimately salvageable:

A man in his late 20s had been living with his parents and a brother. He had graduated from college but afterward had worked only sporadically, at sinecure jobs arranged through friends of his father. He was moody and ir-ritable, had no real friends, and was unable to sustain any relationships with women. After the death of his father when the patient was about 25 years old, his behavior deteriorated. This change was not so much the result of any sadness over the loss of a parent as of the fact that he felt he could now get away with behaviors his father would not have tolerated. He began, for example, to make obscene phone calls, some to women he picked out of the phone book and others to female acquaintances. When several of the latter group complained to his mother, she insisted he go into treatment.

A psychoanalyst saw him three times a week and at one point referred him to a psychopharmacologist. The latter suspected there was an underly-ing bipolar condition and recommended a mood stabilizer. The patient, however, refused to take any medication. Matters grew worse at home. The father had maintained an expensive stamp collection. The family noticed that a number of the more valuable items were missing, as were some pieces of jewelry and antiques. It was discovered that the patient had been pawning these items and using (and losing) the money in gambling. Desperate to stanch the hemorrhage of pilfering from within the home, the mother placed locks on all the doors and locked any rooms in which valuable items were left temporarily unattended. These measures were only partly success-ful, because the patient had already secreted many expensive objects within his own room.

At this point the mother sought my advice about what to do. She had in the meantime learned that her son had told neither psychiatrist about the stealing. His dishonesty had in effect nullified their efforts. Hospitalization had also been recommended, but he turned that down, and he could not have been easily committed, because he was not suicidal or homicidal, as is required for involuntary commitment in New York. I persuaded the mother and other relatives in the family to take drastic steps. They were to pack his essential possessions in two suitcases while he was at work, change the locks to the house, and leave the suitcases outside with a note (along with some cash) suggesting that he stay at a hotel. The family paid the hotel bill in advance for a 2-week stay. My recommendation was based on my contention that there was no valid reason why a whole family should be brought to heel and ruined by the wrongdoing of one of its members. All of these steps were taken. The patient was permitted to stay an additional 2 weeks in the hotel, but by this time the desperation had shifted to himself. Unable to work productively and to sustain himself, he was now at least willing to enter a rehabilitation center. The family felt immense relief and was able for the first time in several years to lead a normal life.

I heard no more about the patient until I contacted the family 7 years later. Fortunately, the family's resources were ample enough to allow the patient to remain at the center for almost 4 years. His behavior was now exemplary. The director of the center had taken him under his wing and had helped him, through the center's vocational therapy program, to develop work skills and to stay at one task for an appropriate length of time. He became able to work half-time at a fairly complex job and to live in a residence for recovering patients. The family now welcomed him back at home at regular intervals. Mood-stabilizing medication was added to his regimen, and he took the prescribed doses faithfully. He had made no thefts or obscene calls since entering the rehabilitation center.

The patients in the three previous vignettes all had in common an adequacy of good character underneath the layers (much thicker in the last case) of impulsive and antisocial behaviors. Once those outer layers were stripped away—through AA for one patient and prolonged rehabilitation and a medication program for another—their decency of character and the ability to show appropriate concern for others finally surfaced, and these better qualities permitted the patients to pursue lives that were socially acceptable and far more gratifying than the lives they had been leading while under the influence of drugs or, for the last patient, of a chronic bipolar illness that had turned his life upside down during his 20s. These patients, who were untreatable by conventional psychotherapies, yet ultimately salvageable, showed antisocial features but were not psychopaths. This distinction is important, as highlighted recently by Herpertz and Habermeyer (2004), who wrote that the concept of psychopathy, as embodied in the work of Robert Hare, has proven a more reliable index of poor prognosis than is either the concept of antisocial personality (DSM-IV-TR) or dyssocial personality (ICD-10).

In some antisocial persons an unpredictable improvement occurs after many years of failed attempts at treatment during which they were written off as both untreatable and unsalvageable. In some cases, a fortuitous turn of events brought about a favorable change—a transformation, really—that led to their becoming as "pro-social" as they had been antisocial. I encountered several such persons at a treatment center in Sweden devoted to the rehabilitation of drug addicts who also had long records of criminal behavior. Many of the counselors were recovered addicts who had managed not only to conquer their drug habit and their criminal tendencies but also to ascend through the stages of 12-step programs to become major factors in the rehabilitation of other persons struggling with the same problems. The following example concerns a man who participated in a workshop I gave on antisocial personality. This treatment counselor, whom I shall call Sven, spoke to the audience about the downward spiral his life had taken until dramatic changes occurred when he was 47 years old:

> **Sven was a tall, 54-year-old man** with an athletic build, graying hair and beard, heavy jewelry, and large muscular arms adorned with multicolored tattoos. One could picture him as a rough "biker" on a Harley-Davidson motorcycle, which indeed had been his chief means of transportation when he was living free. He had been the only child of parents who were both addicted to amphetamines. His father was also alcoholic. Because of his parents' preoccupation with their drug habits, Sven was often neglected during his early years, although he was not mistreated physically.
>
> By the time he was 7 years old Sven showed a serious conduct disorder, a condition that would currently be considered incipient attention-deficit/hyperactivity disorder (ADHD). Wild and unruly in the classroom, he was placed in a special school at age 8 years. He got along reasonably well with one of the teachers, but a year later, a substitute, whom the pupils disliked, took over the class. Sven and some of the other pupils grabbed the new teacher, suspended her outside the window of a third-floor room, and let her fall to the ground. The teacher survived, but this act led to Sven's being transferred to a reformatory. Over the ensuing years, he spent a total of 27 years—one-half of his life—in correctional institutions, hospitals, and prisons. Many of his arrests and detentions over the years were for thefts connected with obtaining the funds to feed his amphetamine addiction. He was also arrested for assaults and fights in bars.
>
> He had been remanded to various treatment centers, either for alcoholism or drug abuse, but he found all the programs useless. Eight years earlier he had made another of his many attempts to go "clean" but was unsuccessful. He found himself unable to give up drinking, and he also began to inject drugs. He was put back in prison, where he came to the realization that "I have to do it myself." He said that he couldn't rely on therapy, because "people with criminal records like I've had tend to be lazy. Therapy doesn't reach us." At this time, he was once again put in an AA program, where he "clicked" with a particular sponsor. Since that time, Sven had not used drugs or alcohol. He was now a sponsor for other men who had been as out of control as he had been and who were trying to achieve abstinence and to acquire regular work skills. In discussing one of the 12 steps—in which one tries to make amends and seek forgiveness for past misdeeds—he said that he tried to locate the teacher he and the other pupils had once so grievously injured.

She had died in the intervening years. With genuine remorse, he expressed the hope that there might be a heaven where she could hear of the regret he now felt for the terrible thing he had done to her.

After hearing Sven's story, I commented that I didn't think he had done it all alone but rather that, in his late 40s, he had matured to the point where he was motivated to make something of his life. As long as he remained un-motivated, no therapist could influence him in a positive way. But once mo-tivated—either because of the maturity that age can confer or because of the special "chemistry" he had with his sponsor—he became reachable as a patient. Probably the effects of age and the influence of the sponsor con-verged in a synergy that fostered his pro-social growth. I speculated that the absence of parental brutality may have been another, hidden positive factor. His upbringing had been far from ideal, yet it had not been as dehumaniz-ing as growing up with constant verbal humiliation and senseless punish-ment. Ironically, he had self-medicated (and then had gone overboard) with a stimulant drug that, under other circumstances, might have been pre-scribed in more measured doses for his ADHD, had the condition been properly diagnosed and treated when he was in elementary school.

APPROACHING UNTREATABLE AND UNSALVAGEABLE PATIENTS

The previous chapters in this book have been organized according to the relative degree of amenability to psychotherapy within the broad domain of personality disorders, from the most treatable to the least. This chapter focuses on the far end of the spectrum—persons who are impossible to treat. The realm of the impossible is composed of two main groups. The first group consists of patients with personality disorders who are untreat-able and who, even after many years, do not get better by any means—not by conventional or unconventional rehabilitative measures; not by religion, special groups of various sorts, or military training; and not by finding an ideal sexual partner or by mellowing with age. The other main group is made up of persons who never cross paths with psychiatry or with mental health care practitioners of any sort and thus never submit to "patienthood" in the first place. Mental health professionals merely hear about patients in this group through the news media, read about them in biographies and his-tory books, or encounter them through sad personal experience.

The spectrum of treatability in the realm of personality disorders is de-picted in diagrammatic form in Figure 9–1. The spectrum has been divided into three main compartments.

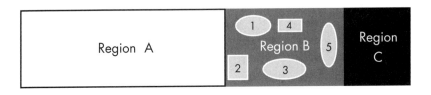

FIGURE 9-1. The spectrum of treatability for personality disorders: treatable (A), untreatable (C), and the "gray zone" (B).

Region A includes the bulk of patients with personality disorders—those whose negative attributes are counterbalanced sufficiently with positive qualities (for example, motivational, characterological, and psychological traits), such as those outlined in Table 1–1 in Chapter 1. Competent, experienced therapists from the various recognized schools of psychotherapy can do a creditable job of treating these patients and can look forward, with adequate time and patience, to significant improvement.

Region B includes patients for whom the resolution of personality disorder is more problematic and uncertain. This region is colored gray in the diagram, as it represents the "gray area" of treatability. For didactic purposes, I demarcated five small areas within this region. The precise dimensions of these areas are unknown and might vary from one locale or culture to another. Area 1 represents patients who could be treated successfully by one therapist but who may have failed to improve with one or with several others, for reasons that are not readily defined. Cultural compatibility of patient and therapist may be an important factor in successful treatment, but a counterintuitive factor, such as the therapist's "youthful enthusiasm" might also have an effect. Area 2 includes personality-disordered patients who respond well to a particular approach or treatment method but not to others. Here, the personality of the therapist emerges as less important than the method. Area 3 is occupied by patients who require an older, highly experienced therapist and who would fail to improve with less experienced therapists. Here, the successful therapist may be schooled in a particular approach or may be versed in several different techniques. In Area 4, one finds patients who fail with all standard methods, only to respond almost magically to a highly unconventional form of therapy that no clinician would have known to recommend. Area 5 includes personality-disordered patients who, after disappointing experiences with half a dozen therapists or more, finally "click" with a particular therapist and begin to make substantial improvement. As one former patient was quoted as saying (Carey 2004), "I've been through a whole lot and I can say that what ultimately is going to move someone toward healing and resolution, the most important factor, is the chemistry between client and therapist." To which Carey added, "Like the tango, psychotherapy takes two, and chemistry is hard to predict or measure."

A particularly compelling example of a patient in this intermediate gray region is a man who could be assigned to Area 4 in the diagram:

> **The patient had been admitted** to the New York State Psychiatric Institute in his early 20s. His personality was markedly avoidant, and he had developed a crippling agoraphobia. The analytically oriented therapy he had received for 3 years before his hospitalization had proven unsuccessful, but the year he spent in the hospital did not improve his condition either. Seventeen years of additional therapy followed, and toward the end of this period he was essentially housebound and living on disability payments. Finally, as he was nearing age 40 years, a friend mentioned a marathon therapy group conducted by a therapist in another state and urged the patient to sign up for one of the 3-day-long "sessions." He attended the marathon therapy session, and afterward, as I mentioned elsewhere (Stone 1990, p. 276), he was a changed man. No longer afraid of the outside, he teamed up with another man, with whom he went into the real estate business, and opened a small resort hotel that they eventually bought. By the time I visited with him, 26 years after he left the hospital, he was a contented and successful entrepreneur. Given the correlation between the marathon session and the abrupt turning point in his life, I don't see how one can argue with the claim that this highly controversial, not to say gimmicky, form of treatment was the decisive factor in this man's recovery.

Region C represents patients with untreatable personality disorders.

THE NARCISSISTIC SPECTRUM

Another way of approaching the realm of untreatable personality disorders, including the unsalvageable persons within this realm, is to consider a spectrum pertaining to the severe forms of narcissistic personality. Persons who are predatory in their relations with others are, by definition, exploitative, often to the point of being distinctly harmful, and are thus supremely egocentric and indifferent to the feelings and fate of others. Persons of this predatory disposition represent a subtype of severe narcissistic personality. To be antisocial is, among other things, to put one's own needs way ahead of the needs of others, if indeed one has any genuine concern for others at all.

It is important to remember that certain persons who meet the DSM-IV-TR criteria for antisocial personality disorder (American Psychiatric Association 2000) were nudged into antisocial patterns by harsh circumstances and that their antisocial patterns became a kind of patina superim-

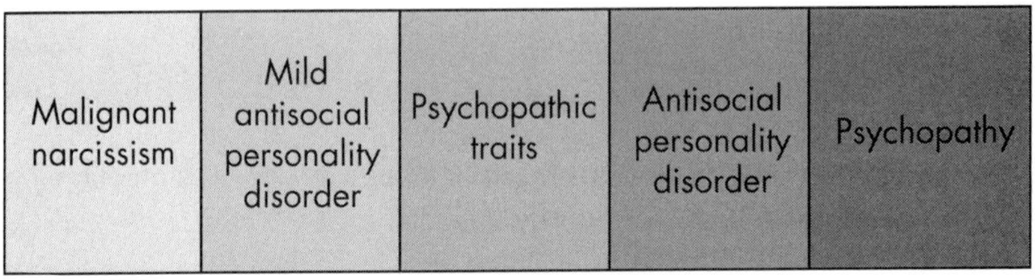

Malignant narcissism	Mild antisocial personality disorder	Psychopathic traits	Antisocial personality disorder	Psychopathy

FIGURE 9–2.   The narcissistic spectrum.

posed on an otherwise decent character structure. This evolution occurred in two of the patients described in the section on untreatable but salvageable patients earlier in this chapter. Another example concerns an adolescent in the P.I.-500 study (Stone 1990):

> **An adolescent's** mother died when he was 11 years old. His father married again, and the new wife behaved like the caricature of the wicked stepmother toward the son. He ran away from home at age 13 years, lived on the streets, took heroin, and stole to afford his habit. At age 18 years, he lay near death in an emergency room, having taken an overdose. After being rescued, he vowed to stop drugs altogether and went on, after some months in Narcotics Anonymous (NA), to become an NA counselor, lecturing to young people about the evils of drug abuse. He later made this work his career, married, and raised two children. For him, fortunately, antisocial personality was an ill-fitting coat he was eventually able to shake off, allowing his underlying decency of character to reemerge.

The compartments of the narcissistic spectrum outlined in Figure 9–2 are ordered in their degree of severity or, more specifically, in order of their departure from the ideals of normal, pro-social personality. An example of a malignant narcissist was given in Chapter 5 in the case vignette describing the businessman who hit his wife (pp. 130–131).

The distinctions and the similarities between DSM-IV-TR antisocial personality disorder and the concept of psychopathy are displayed in Table 9–1, which lists the various traits, attributes, and behaviors that pertain to these diagnostic regions. The first two columns to the right of the descriptors show the two main factors that can be derived from the 20-item Psychopathy Checklist—Revised (PCL-R) of Robert Hare and his colleagues (Hare et al. 1990; Harpur et al. 1989). Three original PCL-R items (criminal versatility, many short-term marital relationships, promiscuity) were found not to load onto these factors. The PCL-R items are scored 0, 1, or 2, allowing for a maximum score of 40. In the United States and Canada, a score of 30 or higher is used to establish the diagnosis of psychopathy;

TABLE 9–1. Items, traits, and attributes included in two models of psychopathy and in the criteria for DSM-IV-TR antisocial personality disorder

Item, trait, attribute	Psychopathy Checklist—Revised (PCL-R)[a]		Psychopathy model of Cooke and Michie[b]			DSM-IV-TR
	Factor 1: Interpersonal and affective	Factor 2: Social deviance	Personality	Affect	Behavior	Antisocial personality disorder
Aggressivity						+
Callousness	+			+		
Conning/manipulativeness	+		+			
Criminal versatility						
Early behavioral problems		+				
Failure to accept responsibility	+			+		
Failure to conform to social norms						+
Glibness/superficial charm	+		+			
Grandiosity	+		+			
Impulsivity		+			+	+
Irresponsible behavior		+			+	+
Juvenile delinquency		+				
Lack of guilt				+		
Lack of realistic goals		+			+	
Lack of remorse	+					+

TABLE 9–1.   Items, traits, and attributes included in two models of psychopathy and in the criteria for DSM-IV-TR antisocial personality disorder *(continued)*

Item, trait, attribute	Psychopathy Checklist—Revised (PCL–R)[a]		Psychopathy model of Cooke and Michie[b]			DSM-IV-TR
	Factor 1: Interpersonal and affective	Factor 2: Social deviance	Personality	Affect	Behavior	Antisocial personality disorder
Many short-term marital relationships						
Need for stimulation		+			+	
Parasitic lifestyle		+			+	
Pathological lying (deceitfulness)	+		+			+
Poor behavioral controls		+				
Promiscuity						
Reckless disregard for the safety of others						+
Revocation of conditional release		+				
Shallow affect	+			+		

Note.   The three italicized items were included in the original PCL-R but did not load onto factor 1 or factor 2.
[a]Hare et al. 1990; Harpur et al. 1989.
[b]Cooke and Michie 2001.

a score of 25 or higher is used in many parts of Europe. Scores in an intermediate range are said to accord with the presence of "psychopathic traits."

From the standpoint of prognosis, a person manifesting just some of the social deviance factor items (e.g., impulsivity, lack of realistic long-term goals, poor behavioral controls, irresponsible behavior) and the least offensive of the interpersonal and affective factor items (e.g., glibness, shallow affect) could end up with a score at or near the cutoff of 30 for psychopathic personality and yet not be unsalvageable. Some of the former P.I.-500 patients described earlier behaved in this way (and the emphasis here is on behavior) during their early years, engaging in drunk driving, drug abuse, petty theft, and a vagabond life. Untreatability and unsalvageability, in contrast, are much more closely associated with narcissistic personality factors per se, such as the interpersonal and affective factor items of callousness, lack of remorse, conning, and pathological lying.

The PCL-R was the outgrowth of experience primarily with forensic patients and incarcerated prisoners, hence the items "criminal versatility," which signifies arrest for many different types of crime, such as assault, vandalism, fraud, kidnapping, burglary, and "failure of conditional release," which has relevance only to those already incarcerated and then paroled. The PCL-R serves well as a criminological tool, and its predictive ability has been validated (Hart and Hare 1997; Hemphill et al. 1998a, 1998b). The recidivism rate, for example, of incarcerated offenders who were later paroled was significantly higher among those with PCL-R scores of 30 or higher, compared with those whose scores were in the 20s; rates were lower still for those with scores less than 20.

One drawback of the PCL-R is that it may not accurately reflect the severity of psychopathy in persons who do not have a criminal history. Some patients, especially those from wealthier families, show many of the *personality* (as opposed to the *behavioral*) traits of psychopathy but manage to elude arrest (thanks to family influence) or to avoid the temptation to steal (thanks to family money) and thus would have only modest PCL-R scores and would not be identified as psychopaths. Yet clinically and forensically, therapists would experience them as unquestionably psychopathic in personality.

Cooke and Michie (2001) sought to address this problem by first analyzing data from persons with clinically diagnosed psychopathy and then creating what they felt was a more accurate and widely applicable model. They argued that a partition of psychopathy consisting of three factors—personality, affect, and behavior—is superior. The items that made up those three factors are shown in Table 9–1. They also dispensed with the purely criminological items. Using their modification, one can identify as psychopathic those persons who show little besides the intensely narcissistic personality attributes of conning, glibness, grandiosity, and pathological lying, with perhaps with one or two affect-related items, such as callousness and lack of guilt. The items denoting lack of empathy in the criteria of Hare and colleagues signify primarily a lack of compassion. The lack of compassion is emphasized by Baron-Cohen (2003) in his comments on empathy and is distinct from the mere ability to "read others' minds" (that is, merely to *identify correctly* the feelings of others, without then feeling compassion for what the other person is experiencing), which many psychopaths can manage all too well.

Because the prognosis for treatability, let alone salvageability, is essentially nil in the presence of full-fledged psychopathy, the model of Cooke and Michie is particularly useful in the evaluation of offenders or highly narcissistic persons with no previous arrest record who were raised in more affluent circumstances. The phenomenon is hardly unknown to Hare and his co-workers: Hare, for example, devoted a chapter to "white-collar psychopaths" in his monograph on psychopathy (Hare 1993, pp. 102–123).

DSM-IV-TR antisocial personality disorder differs in some important ways from psychopathy. The overlap of the DSM antisocial personality disorder criteria with the narcissistic personality items of the psychopathy scales is confined to the traits of pathological lying and lack of remorse. As a consequence, the DSM-IV-TR diagnosis of antisocial personality disorder is more oriented to behaviors (aggressivity, impulsivity, etc.), as noted in Table 9–1, and is less useful in identifying the *core* of psychopathy—the extreme self-centeredness, exploitativeness, indifference to the feelings of others, and readiness to inflict hurt (whether psychological or physical) by way of advancing one's own desires and ambitions. The more favorable prognosis of some antisocial persons (who meet the criteria for antisocial personality disorder), compared with psychopaths, is a function of the definitions used. Symptoms, including symptomatic behaviors such as drunkenness, shoplifting, and engaging in brawls, are often easier to remediate or are more likely to diminish with time than are personality traits, which are, by definition, entrenched and enduring. This distinction accounts for the better outcomes in the antisocial (but not psychopathic) adolescent runaways described earlier.

Many psychopaths commit antisocial acts repeatedly and may thus be viewed as having a subtype of antisocial personality disorder. Prisons are full of persons with antisocial personality disorder, but only about one-fourth of them meet the criteria for psychopathic personality. Among violent offenders, the same is true—not all violent persons are psychopathic, and not all psychopathic persons are violent. However, the most untreatable and unsalvageable of all the personality disorders are those in persons who are at once psychopathic, habitually violent, and sadistic. The following examples concern persons who show the essence of psychopathy but whose fortunate social circumstances allowed them to escape arrest for their entire lives or to face arrest only after many years of predatory and unscrupulous behavior:

A 26-year-old man was referred for psychotherapy mostly because he seemed directionless to his family. He had held no steady job, flitted from one girlfriend to the next, and sometimes had sex with two or three women during the same period. He had ambitions that seemed grandiose and farfetched, given his lack of training in any area. He was one of five children born to parents with inherited wealth. His father served on the board of directors of the large corporation founded by the grandfather; he held this post as a courtesy, had no business skills, and did no work.

After the death of the patient's mother, when he was in his teens, the father's alcoholism grew worse, and he became emotionally remote from his children. Left to his own devices, the patient began to live on the "wild side," associating with a group of young persons who, like himself, lived off their trust funds. He went through a sizeable inheritance within just a year, flying back and forth to Europe to attend various parties. He crashed the sports car he received as a high school graduation gift 3 days after graduation, but he was able to keep this news from his father by purchasing an identical model. Along with some of his drinking buddies, the patient had gotten into a fight at a nightclub where someone was seriously injured. The police considered the patient a suspect, but they were persuaded by the patient's father's influence not to pursue the matter, and it was never determined if the patient had any role in the assault.

When I began working with this man, his most striking features were his impeccable attire, his charm and handsomeness, and his shallowness. He spoke at times of wanting to be a movie producer or an entrepreneur like his grandfather, but these thoughts appeared to be pipe dreams rather than true ambitions. He had no knowledge of filmmaking or of the business world, and he had no funds to invest anyway, having gone through his money with his jet-setting. My most immediate goal in therapy was to have him start working in a position where his pleasing facade could be turned to advantage. To this end, a family member offered him a job in his real estate company. Within a short time, the patient began to regale me with news about the "terrific deals" he had made selling buildings worth tens of millions of dollars and about how he was becoming a "factor" in the commercial real estate world. I had occasion to meet with two of his relatives who were partners in that firm. They assured me that the patient had sold nothing at all and that on the days when he showed up at the office, he did little but rest his feet on the desk while he read sports magazines.

Regarding this man's diagnosis, it will be noted that he showed all the traits of Cooke and Michie's psychopathy personality factor. He did not show callousness or lack of remorse and would thus have fit in a less severe category on the PCL-R ("some psychopathic traits") than he would in Cooke and Michie's schema. Here was someone who could be considered psychopathic but who was not violent or even identifiable as an offender. Had he been born into a less prosperous family similar in other ways to his own family, his life trajectory might have been much worse. He left treatment after 2 years, seemingly untouched by the process. I saw him as untreatable but salvageable. At follow-up some 18 years later, he had married and was the father of two children. He had settled down, was living mostly on a new inheritance, and was never in trouble with the law.

Whereas the person in the preceding example was essentially prodigal and passive rather than predatory, the next example concerns the more usual situation involving psychopathy, in which *predatoriness* is prominent and the person is neither treatable nor salvageable:

A woman in her mid-40s was in the midst of a custody battle over her young daughter. The father, from whom she had recently divorced, had been her fifth husband. She also had a son by her second husband. Born in humble circumstances to alcoholic parents, she parlayed her attractiveness and sexuality into a much higher social status. Although she claimed to have been pregnant only the two times, those who knew her well were aware that she had had at least eight abortions by her mid-20s.

She lured her first husband by promises that considerable wealth was soon coming her way through an inheritance, on the strength of which she persuaded him to lend her a large sum to be paid back within "a few months." After the wedding, the truth came out that she was no heiress and had no money at all except what her husband had lent her. Now that they were husband and wife, the debt was meaningless, but this situation soured her spouse, and the marriage soon ended. She then met a man who was keen on marrying a woman with a good education. She lied about having graduated from a prestigious university, when in fact she had never attended college. This marriage also ran aground because of her deceitfulness, although she had her son by this husband.

Before she was 30 years old, she married again. She bilked the third husband out of considerable money and ran off with another man after draining a joint checking account of a large sum. The fourth marriage was no more successful. Her husband began to tire of her drinking and lost patience over the stories that came his way of her infidelities. Aware that the winds were shifting against her, she sought to cement the marriage by claiming to be pregnant. This ploy backfired when her husband informed her he had had a vasectomy years earlier. If she claimed to be pregnant, he told her, she was either cheating or lying. Trust having been destroyed, this marriage ended abruptly also.

At age 35 years, she married again; this time her husband was a wealthy manufacturer. He sued for divorce 3 years after the birth of their daughter, when he caught her embezzling funds from his business. He moved to a different part of the country and gave her generous support, because she was the custodial parent. But he learned from friends that she would leave the child alone during the evenings while she went to bars to pick up men. Sometimes the girl would wander the neighborhood streets in the morning because her mother was still away. The neighbors would take her in and give her breakfast. On other occasions, her mother would take the girl with her to the bars she frequented and later expose her to sexual scenes with the various men she picked up during the evening. The father now sued for, and won, custody. But periodic weeklong visits with the mother were still permitted, and during these visits, the mother's behavior was as neglectful and inappropriate as before.

When the girl was about 5 years old, her mother began taking her with her when she went shoplifting. The mother shoplifted enormous quantities of toys, clothes, shoes, and small electronic devices and also taught her daughter to pilfer the more expensive items, calculating that the daughter was far too young to face arrest if she were caught. The mother was arrested several times but was often successful in seducing the policeman, the prosecuting attorney, her own attorney, and occasionally even the judge. She developed a cocaine habit and was arrested for possession of narcotics, but she extricated herself from possible incarceration by using the same techniques, which also served her well when she was arrested for driving while intoxicated.

Her ex-husband now sued for full custody and supervised visitation by the mother, on the seemingly irrefutable grounds that she was an unfit parent. A long journey through the labyrinth of the local court was required before he could persuade a less corruptible judge to clamp down on her predatory activities. Shortly before he gained full custody, she committed a fraudulent act whose artfulness showed that she was still a force to reckon with. Her now-teenage son had been with her on one of his rare visits. She knew that warrants for her arrest had been filed for several vehicular offenses. She had her son impersonate her by dressing up like her so that she could avoid arrest. After her daughter began living full-time with her father, the mother sent the girl large packages of toys and other items that she had obtained by shoplifting. The packages were forwarded to the court, and this evidence finally led to her conviction, when she was 45 years old, of crimes that cost her time in prison. Perhaps because her beauty was no longer as radiant as when she was younger, her attempts to seduce her way out of incarceration no longer met with success. When I evaluated her as an expert witness in connection with the custody trial, I found her PCL-R score to be 32, in the range where a diagnosis of psychopathic personality per se, as well as a diagnosis of any of the four Cluster B personality disorders, can be made.

This vignette concerns Fred Tokars (McDonald 1998), a man who showed all the personality factor traits included in either the PCL-R or Cooke and Michie's scale. Tokars hired a hit man to shoot his wife to death in 1992, when he learned that she had discovered that he was both cheating on her and cheating the government through his money-laundering activities. He had obtained a law degree from a mediocre school and then a doctorate from a diploma mill in a western state, after which he began calling himself "Dr. Tokars." He married Sara Ambrusko, the daughter of a surgeon. They had two children. Tokars became totally controlling, refusing his wife credit cards or a checking account. He also paid for everything in cash in order to sidestep the Internal Revenue Service. He abused his wife physically and forced her to take out a large insurance policy with himself as beneficiary. Addicted to alcohol and cocaine, Tokars began to defend drug dealers and criminals, which proved a very lucrative practice. As the marriage deteriorated, he took out still larger insurance policies, approaching a value of $2 million, "in case anything happened to my wife." When Sara sued for divorce, she also tried to expose his criminal activities. The hit man Tokars hired shot her to death in front of their two sons, but Tokars was unaware that his wife had already sent many incriminating documents to the authorities. This evidence played a crucial role in Tokars' conviction and sentencing to life in prison. To his psychopathy, Tokars added the elements of violence and sadism. He manifested one more than the minimum of four items needed to establish a DSM-IV-TR diagnosis of *sadistic personality disorder*: 1) uses cruelty or violence to establish dominance, 2) humiliates in the presence of others, 3) uses harsh discipline on a spouse or child, 4) intimidates, and 5) restricts others' autonomy.

Richard Minns (Finstad 1991) had become a health-spa tycoon with a chain of clubs and gyms in Texas by the time he was in his late 40s. Minns was also a compulsive bodybuilder who waged an all-out war against the passage of time, hoping to remain eternally youthful and powerful. Married with four children, he fell in love with a beauty queen and medical student, Barbra Piotrowski, with whom he carried on a torrid affair, lying to her about his age and pretending to be single. Among the more prominent of his personality traits, as documented in his biography, were sensation seeking, risk taking, hypomania (hypersexuality, intense "energy," and little need for sleep), litigiousness, contentiousness, extraversion, pathological jealousy, possessiveness, and marked stinginess. He was entrepreneurial, hard-driving, and intense, emotionally volatile and explosively angry, as well as dishonest, unethical, vindictive, arrogant, egotistical, paranoid, and manipulative. He threatened to blackmail various businessmen by revealing that they had mistresses. A charismatic man, he was "the flame next to whom others liked to dance." As to his braggadocio, he would have himself photographed in a bikini, holding up a gigantic fish he falsely claimed to have caught. After Barbra became aware that Minns was married, he tried to persuade her to kill his wife with an insulin injection. As the affair continued, Minns became increasingly jealous and controlling toward Barbra. The relationship deteriorated as she became intolerant of the extreme limitations he imposed on her autonomy. Once, when she was reluctant to change a dress as he had demanded, he punched her in the nose and then said, "I didn't do it! Something came over me!" Finally, when she mustered the courage to leave him, he hired hit men to kill her. In October 1980, when Minns was 51 years old, twice Barbra's age, they shot at her but succeeded only in rendering her paraplegic. Minns then fled to Europe, where he has remained for the past quarter-century, never having been brought to justice. In a civil trial, however, Minns was fined in absentia $60,000,000 in punitive damages, none of which Barbra has ever collected. Minns is of course as much "in absentia" from us as he is from his victim.

THE EXTREME OF THE NARCISSISTIC SPECTRUM

At the outer edge of the narcissistic spectrum are personality configurations where an extreme sense of entitlement and the psychopathic personality traits overlap. Often enough, sadistic personality is added to the mix, particularly the prototypic trait of enjoyment of the suffering that one inflicts on others. For mental health professionals (apart from those in forensic work), persons of this sort inhabit the dark side of the moon: their presence is suspected, but they are not actually seen. Examples from the news media are legion; they not only point up the more unflattering side of human nature but also carve out a territory where the concepts of *untreatable* and *unsalvageable* converge.

The untreatable component is a reflection of psychopaths' steadfast refusal to accept that anything could be wrong with their personality. A counterpart of this denial is contempt for psychiatry, which in the psychopath's view is simply an anodyne contrived for the weak and foolish (Hare 1993). Consistent with this attitude is the low (or often nonexistent) motivation for treatment noted in psychopaths housed in centers that emphasize the therapeutic community approach (Lösel 1998). From a psychodynamic point of view, the majority of violent and sadistic psychopaths were once on the receiving end of parental cruelty that fostered a craving for revenge (Stone 2001). From a neuropsychological point of view, cases of special interest are those where no such early history exists. Such instances must have a basis in genetic predisposition or unfavorable factors in the intrauterine environment that contributed to brain alterations affecting impulse control and the capacity for compassion and empathy; they may also result from brain damage affecting key areas in the frontal lobes that mediate empathy.

At least a "modest genetic predisposition" for psychopathy has been proposed by Raine (1993, p. 77). Raine and his co-workers (1996, 2000) also drew attention to the interaction of brain abnormalities, such as reduced prefrontal gray matter, and unstable family environment in antisocial persons. Porter (1996), in contrast, made a good argument for the development of what he called secondary psychopathy, where an extremely adverse family environment sets in motion an aberrant developmental pathway eventuating in psychopathic personality, even though genetic or constitutional factors may not have been prominent. Porter's concept may have special relevance to psychopaths who commit serial sexual homicide and other repetitive violent acts.

Regardless of the primary contributing factors to psychopathic personality in any given person, once the typical traits are firmly established, the trait of *entitlement* will be an accompaniment. A sense of entitlement is one of the descriptors of narcissistic personality disorder, but it has not been included specifically as a feature of psychopathy. This trait is so striking in severe cases, however, that Wilson and Seaman (1992) coined the phrase *Roman emperor syndrome* (p. 260) to describe this combination. These authors were drawing attention to the need of serial killers to subjugate and to exert total dominion over their victims, in the manner of Nero or Caligula.

This form of entitlement is hardly limited to the comparatively small group of serial killers. Many men who murder their wives through the agency of hired hit men or who stage the murder to appear as an accident are notorious for their belief that they are a law unto themselves, free to act with impunity to rid themselves of a marital relationship grown burdensome or to cash in on a hefty insurance policy taken out "in case anything happened to the wife."

In my study of 92 uxoricides (wife murderers) in the literature, 12 involved the husband's hiring of a hit man and 27 involved "staging"; the two types together accounted for 42% of the total. Those who hired a hit man included Fred Neulander (Francis 2002) and James Sullivan (Collins 2004); those who staged the murder included Howard Band (Band and Malear 2003), Kevin Anderson (Smith 2002), and Edward Post (McClellan 1993). Many of these men exhibited strong psychopathic personality (i.e., narcissistic) traits, including glibness, grandiosity, manipulativeness, deceitfulness, callousness, and lack of remorse, even though they functioned well in the community and showed few of the PCL-R social deviance attributes. Edward Post, for example, drove a long distance from a meeting he had been attending, drowned his wife in a bathtub, and then drove back to the meeting in the middle of the night to appear to have a solid alibi, so that he would be able to collect money from her life insurance policy and be free to marry the woman with whom he had been having an affair.

SADISM

I suggested earlier (Stone 1993) that at the extreme negative end of the personality continuum are persons, such as serial killers (Stone 2001), who, in peacetime situations unrelated to state-sanctioned or wartime behaviors, take delight in the humiliation and prolonged and systematic torture of others. Viewed from a different perspective, such behavior represents the farthest remove from the social conventions (such as the Golden Rule) that hold society together and a full 180-degree turn away from the lessons most of us are taught from earliest childhood—to respect the humanity of other persons and to refrain from subjecting others to psychological or physical pain.

Sadism in general is overwhelmingly a male phenomenon. Evolutionary psychiatry provides some hints as to why female sadists are a rarity. Women know which babies are theirs because they give birth to them. Fatherhood is guesswork. Men, to ensure that the children they provide for are actually, genetically, their own, have tended over the millennia to control women's sexuality to minimize the risk that they have been "duped" into supporting another man's child. Jealousy, harsh controls on women, social customs such as long engagements, and other measures have developed in our species to avoid this misallocation of resources. Sadism may be understood, in part, as an exaggeration of the male mechanisms for controlling women. Obviously, sadistic behaviors are sometimes mobilized in the service of various non-sex-related functions, such as exacting revenge for suffering inflicted by others. For some persons, sadism becomes the antidote for feelings of inferiority, inasmuch as the helpless victim of cruelty is vividly aware of the "superiority" of the sadist. As a corollary, the more exquisite the torture and the longer its duration, the wider the gap between the superiority of the victimizer and the inferiority of the victim, hence the greater the reassurance to the sadist's enfeebled self-confidence.

Most sadistic persons retain some sense of shame about the wrongness of their behavior and, through denial or rationalization, insulate themselves against the discomfort of self-recognition. Among the ranks of serial killers, however, I can think of at least four in whom not even the tiniest scintilla of shame is discernible and who furthermore have written extensively about their sadistic "philosophy." The most succinct testimonial comes from Mike DeBardeleben, who wrote concerning sadism:

> The wish to inflict pain on others is not the essence of sadism. The central impulse is to have complete mastery over another person, to make him or her a helpless object of our will, to become the absolute ruler over her, to become her god, and to do with her as one pleases—are means to this end. And the most radical aim is to make her suffer. Since there is no greater power over another person than that of inflicting pain on her. To force her to undergo suffering without her being able to defend herself. The pleasure in the complete domination over another person is the very essence of the sadistic drive." (Hazelwood and Michaud 2001, p. 88).

More insightful on the topic of serial killing per se is Ian Brady (2001), who for many years has been incarcerated in Ashworth Forensic Hospital in England. Brady is the famous Moors Murderer, who, with his accomplice and paramour, Myra Hindley, lured and killed five children in the years 1963–1965. Brady would strangle his victims and tape-record their screams to be replayed later as a kind of aphrodisiac for Myra and himself. Professor Jeremy Coid, a distinguished forensic psychiatrist in London, interviewed Brady and considered him the most narcissistic person he had ever encountered among all the offenders he had evaluated (J. Coid, personal communication, 1999). Colin Wilson (Brady 2001, p. 5) believed Brady to have pioneered, in effect, a new type of serial killing that was motivated not so much by sex as such as by a quest to restore *self-esteem*. Arguably the most intellectual of the serial killers, Brady saw himself, like the Marquis de Sade, as "being above normal morality" (Brady 2001, p. 6).

His psychodynamics, to the extent they can be grasped through his writings and the impressions of his biographers (Williams 1968), are different from those of most other serial killers. Unlike DeBardeleben, for example, who was brutalized during his childhood by his alcoholic and violent mother (Michaud 1994), Brady suffered no abuse of any kind. His father died shortly before he was born, and Margaret Stewart, his mother, gave him into the care of the Sloan family in Glasgow, who provided him with a warm and friendly home. But he emerged as a loner and a leader, a young man with a schizoid but also dominant personality, who engaged in burglaries from the age of 9 years. A few years later he took to burying cats and rabbits in the ground with only their heads exposed and then running a lawn mower over them. Arrested again at age 16 years, he was placed on parole on the condition that he live with his mother, who had remarried Patrick Brady, whose last name he now assumed. Arrested again a year later, Ian was sent to prison for more than 2 years, an experience that hardened him and turned him into an "antisocial rebel" (Brady 2001, p. 9). A voracious reader of the works of Tolstoy and Dostoevsky in his preprison days, he now read *Mein Kampf* and other Nazi literature. In 1961 he became enamored of a typist, Myra Hindley; she became totally infatuated with him and ultimately became his subservient "slave." His self-confidence now bolstered, Ian, with Myra's complicity, embarked on the series of child murders.

In the book Brady wrote during his incarceration (Brady 2001), he described serial killing as only someone who knows the subject from the inside can do. He made some remarkably insightful comments about his own personality and about the dynamics of other well-known serial killers, such as John Gacy. Gacy, the Chicago man who raped and killed many men during homosexual encounters, then buried them under his porch, had earlier been brutalized by his father. Brady mentioned that fear breeds hate and hate breeds violence and went on to say that "in an attempt to neutralize this fear and reinforce his masculinity, Gacy began by choosing homosexuals to beat up, torture and degrade, his acts simultaneously distancing and definitively proving to himself that he was superior to the breed" (p. 127). As for Richard Ramirez, the Los Angeles Night Stalker, Brady believed that his serial killing was motivated by a desire to dominate others, adding, "There is nothing in Ramirez' family history to indicate he had been mistreated by his father or that he harbored hatred for him" (p. 173). Brady seems not to have had access to a recent biography of Ramirez (Carlo 1996). Ramirez' policeman father, Julian, was extremely abusive physically toward Richard. In addition, Richard, who was hyperactive as a child, was knocked unconscious (and almost died) on several occasions before age 6 years and later developed temporal lobe epilepsy, aggressivity, and hypersexuality. In personality, Ramirez became a loner who was untrusting, stubborn, and completely amoral.

We do not know what peculiarities of cerebral circuitry predisposed Brady to develop as he did, in the absence of any severe environmental stressors, to become amoral, grandiose, devoid of compassion, domineering, sexually warped, and murderous—in effect, a "born" psychopath, in contrast to the environmentally "made" psychopaths such as Gacy and Ramirez. It seems clear that after the latter men embarked on their murderous careers, they were beyond treatment and beyond redemption. It is unlikely that Brady could have been salvaged no matter when he might have undergone psychotherapy. Besides being psychopathic and sadistic, Brady is schizoid, as is Ramirez and about one-half of the 127 serial killers ($n=63$, or 49.6%) whose biographies I have studied (Stone 2001). Schizoid personality disorder is uncommon in the general population, in which the prevalence is about 1% (Widiger and Rogers 1989), but it is 50 times more common among men who commit serial sexual homicide. The schizoid aloofness and detachment in these men appears to contribute both to their callous indifference to the suffering of their victims and to their untreatability.

Psychopathy and sadism were present to extreme degrees in a third serial killer who left autobiographical material, Leonard Lake (Harrington and Burger 1999; Lasseter 2000). Lake was born in San Francisco in 1945. His alcoholic father abandoned the family when Lake was 5 years old, just after the birth of his sister. Unable to support her three children, his mother left Leonard in the care of his maternal grandparents, who lived in comfortable circumstances and who treated him well. His mother took the younger two children with her to Seattle. Leonard was distraught over his mother's leaving and was never subsequently reunited with her. He was not known to have experienced traumata other than this abandonment.

By age 18 years he was having fantasies of enslaving women. His two brief marriages ended because his wives found him overbearing; the final straw for the second wife was her learning that Lake was eager to make "snuff" films (where a victim is photographed while actually being killed). His intense hatred of women came to the surface after his second wife divorced him in 1972. The divorce came a year after his discharge for psychiatric reasons from the Marines, where he had served from 1964 to 1971. While overseas with the Marines, he was consumed with jealousy about his wife, who had remained in the United States. Diagnosed with "hysterical neurosis," he was felt to be a danger to himself and others, and he underwent therapy at Camp Pendleton, with no appreciable benefit.

Afterward, Lake became a survivalist in remote sections of California and committed an extensive variety of crimes, including theft, murder (of his brother), robbery, auto offenses, sex offenses, fraud, illegal weapons possession, and kidnapping. He did form an attachment to a woman, Claralyn Balazs, but she eventually left him. Lake again felt devastated, but at the same time he felt free to do anything he wanted, because, as he later wrote, "[s]ociety is powerless against one who is not afraid to die." He carried a cyanide capsule with him at all times, to foil any attempt at capture.

He took under his wing Hong Kong–born Charles Ng, a fugitive from the Marines. Together they lured women to a hideaway, where they subjected them to violent sadistic sex and torture. They built a crematorium where they burned a dozen of their victims. Lake recorded his "philosophy" in a diary. One entry read, "The perfect woman is totally controlled, a woman who does exactly what she is told and nothing else. There are no sexual problems with a totally submissive woman" (Lasseter 2000, p. 150). Having kidnapped a woman, taken her baby away from her, and bound her, handcuffed, to a chair, Lake and Ng made a film of her psychological degradation and torture. At one point Lake told her, "You can cooperate with us. That means you will stay here as our prisoner. You will work for us, you will wash for us, you will f**k for us. Or you can say, 'No, I don't want to do that,' in which case we'll tie you to the bed, we'll rape you, and then we'll take you outside and shoot you. Your choice." (p. 217). Lake added, speaking on behalf also of his partner, Ng, "The fairness of what we're doing is, uh, not up for debate. We're not worried about whether we're fair or whether we're good. We're just worried about ourselves" (Harrington and Burger 1999, p. 61). Finally arrested in 1985 while he was using one of his many aliases, Lake committed suicide with the cyanide capsule.

In contrast to DeBardeleben, Brady, and Lake, Atlanta-born Gerald Schaeffer (London 1997) was born into an intact and well-to-do family. His father was alcoholic and abusive toward his wife, beating her often and calling her a "whore," despite her fidelity. Gerald himself became tormented with violent sexual fantasies from adolescence on, as well as by sharply polarized attitudes toward sex. He was voyeuristic, yet if he noticed a neighbor girl sunbathing, he would say that she was a "slut" and that he "would put a stop to that." He struggled with the idea of strangling her and dumping the body in the Everglades. For a time he dated Sondra London, whom he alienated with his violent talk but who later became the editor of his autobiographical material. At age 19 years he became a deputy policeman, and he used his uniform to lure women into his car on the pretext of their having committed a traffic offense. Additional paraphilic behaviors, particularly bondage, manifested themselves. He terrorized the women he handcuffed, until they involuntarily defecated. This tactic became his "trademark." A psychopath of the glib charmer type, he boasted of killing more than 80 women. After he was captured, he began writing autobiographical stories filled with nauseatingly explicit details of a coprological and sadistic nature. While in prison, he was stabbed to death by another inmate in 1995.

SADISM ACCOMPANYING ANTISOCIAL OR PSYCHOPATHIC PERSONALITY

With the exception of DeBardeleben, the examples just discussed concerned men whose sadistic behaviors and psychopathic traits seemed to have been set in motion more by *genetic* than by adverse *environmental* influences. This group includes other serial killers, such as David Berkowitz ("Son of Sam") (Klausner 1981) and Joel Rifkin (Eftimiades 1993), who had been adopted at birth into families known to have been warm and nurturing. Both men were schizoid and showed deterioration of personality after the death of an adoptive parent to whom they had grown strongly attached—the mother in Berkowitz's case, the father in Rifkin's.

Examples of men and women whose personalities have developed along psychopathic and sadistic lines as a result of *extreme and gratuitous parental abuse* are, in all likelihood, much more numerous. It is difficult to disentangle "nature" from "nurture" where the nurture has been particularly appalling. Bad outcomes in a good environment suggest *bad nature* as the cause; bad outcomes in a bad environment could stem from either or both factors.

Lonnie Athens (1992), however, made a compelling case that serious deformation of personality can arise from prolonged exposure to parental viciousness. Athens created a special vocabulary and outlined four stages to describe how relatively benign and ordinary children can end up as irremediably violent criminals after being victimized repeatedly by parental violence that amounts to torture. The emphasis here is on *irremediable* personality disorders that have crossed a line in the direction of sadism and antisociality and can no longer be fixed. In the first of Athens' four stages, the future criminals are subjected to *brutalization*. The brutalization might take any of several forms, including 1) *violent subjugation*, in which the child is the victim of coarse and cruel treatment at the hands of a parent or other caretaker; 2) *personal horrification*, in which the subject becomes the involuntary witness of the violent subjugation of another person (usually a sibling or parent); and 3) *violent coaching*, in which a parent or some other older intimate instructs and encourages a child to adopt violent means of dealing with various stressful interpersonal situations, or else ridicules the child for *not* getting revenge in a violent way for insults or criticism. Having absorbed a hefty measure of brutalization, the young person begins to develop an attitude of *belligerency*. In this second stage, the young person begins to brood over the brutalizing experiences previously endured. The former victim begins to reassess his options and resolves not to take any further such punishment "lying down." A decision is made henceforth to resort to violence, as the only reasonable means of redressing old wrongs. This decision ushers in a stage of *violent performances*. In this third stage, the subject "awaits only the proper circumstances to test his newly developed resolve to attack people physically with the serious intention of inflicting grave injury upon them" (Athens 1992, p. 63). If the subject, who by now is an adolescent or a young adult, has managed to score a decisive victory over an enemy by means of violence, he may make the transition to the final stage of *virulency*. Once virulency is established, there is no going back. The person now takes too much pride in the successful defeat of "enemies" through violence, has too much conviction that the world is a dog-eat-dog place, and is too entrenched in a paranoid assumption of the malevolence of most other people, which can be dealt with only with a kill-or-be-killed attitude.

The life of Gary Gilmore, recounted in the biography by Norman Mailer (1979) and in the moving account by Gilmore's brother, the novelist Mikal Gilmore (1991), shows dramatically the passage from violent subjugation to virulency. Gary was one of four brothers raised by a violent and irrationally punitive alcoholic father. All of the boys were beaten mercilessly by their father for trivial offenses. Gary drew the most fire, because he was the most rebellious and least "tamable" of the four. In his case, a genetic factor can be invoked as well, as he seems to have been born with the lowest tendency to "harm avoidance" (Cloninger 1986) and the highest tendency to impulse dyscontrol, compared with his brothers. Because he did not become obedient under the impact of his father's blows, his father, mindlessly operating as a kind of positive-feedback machine, simply struck harder and more often. The result was that Gary became a vicious and tyrannical dominator of the women in his life, terrorizing them into submission, and embarked on a career of criminal violence that ended after a botched robbery, when he shot to death a young gas station attendant whose wife was expecting their first child.

Athens in his monograph was concentrating on the overwhelming effects on personality development of a brutalizing family environment. Many of his clinical examples are truly horrifying, and there is no need to look further for the cause of the virulency that follows. But I suspect that even in such cases, minor differences in genetic and constitutional givens interact with the violent upbringing. We know that many brothers (boys being more prone to aggressivity than girls) of violent criminals become good and moral citizens. Temperament factors relating to harm avoidance and novelty-seeking make a difference, as do physical size and athletic prowess. Birth order may also be important, and there may be subtle factors, such as a child's being treating with less or greater affection because he happens to resemble either a despised or a much-cherished uncle or grandfather. But much evidence supports Athens' point that in many antisocial and psychopathic criminals of a markedly sadistic bent, parental violence was the *major* and *decisive* pathogenetic factor.

A DIFFICULTY IN EVALUATING THE EFFECTS OF TREATMENT

One of the problems confronting those who do therapeutic work with violence-prone persons, including certain juvenile delinquents and persons who harbor violent fantasies not yet acted out, is the difficulty of measuring a negative outcome. It is impossible to know whether a person who had the kind of history outlined by Athens but who was treated with psychotherapy early in the course of a disorder and did *not* commit murder "surely" would have done so if no treatment had been provided. The same goes for young persons who have a genetic or constitutional predisposition to psychopathic traits or to violent behavior but who are raised in stable families where they are not subject to violence. In the preceding chapter I mentioned the work of adolescent psychiatrist Annette Streeck-Fischer (1998a, 1998b) with young "skinheads" from the former East Germany. A proportion of her patients, had they been left untreated, might have gone on to firebomb the homes of immigrants or to kill the targets of their bigotry, but this number is not measurable.

Among the serial killers whose biographies I have reviewed, 38 (29%) had been treated or evaluated in psychiatric hospitals, often before their first murder. Four of them had spent stays of 5 years at California's Atascadero forensic hospital, including Arthur Allen and Ed Kemper. Allen, identified after his death from natural causes as the Zodiac Killer of the San Francisco Bay Area, had been remanded to Atascadero for pedophilic acts. He was not known at the time to have been a serial killer, and he resumed that career after his release. Kemper had been admitted after he shot his grandparents to death when he was 15 years old. His serial killing, which began with the murder of his mother, occurred only later. Gary Taylor, who had been hospitalized in Michigan after a series of assaults on women beginning in his adolescence, was allowed to leave Ypsilanti State Hospital if he promised to abstain from alcohol. A psychopath adept at conning the authorities, Taylor not only resumed drinking when he was released but moved on to serial sexual homicide, building a secret room in his house where he tortured his victims before killing them. Gary Heidnik, the Philadelphia man who chained a number of women to his cellar wall and raped and later dismembered them, had been hospitalized numerous times for suicide gestures. Later given a diagnosis of schizoid psychopathy, he had been severely traumatized by his alcoholic father, who used to suspend him outside the window when he was 4 or 5 years old and threaten to drop him if he didn't stop crying.

The men in this group either were treated at an appropriately early age, but only briefly and with no follow-through, or else were treated long after their propensity to violence had become well established. The majority of serial killers had never been treated at all or even identified as being in need of "help" until they were arrested. No one seemed to have noticed, for example, that Jeffrey Dahmer had, during his adolescence, been beheading dogs and cats and impaling their heads on sticks in his backyard. We have no way of speculating how salvageable he might have been, if someone had paid attention to this most serious of premonitory signs of future violence—animal torture—when it was first happening.

ANTISOCIAL PERSONALITY DISORDER, PSYCHOPATHY, AND FRACTURED FAMILIES

David Lykken (1995) drew attention to fatherlessness as an important factor in the development of antisocial personality. He wrote, "Most of our current harvest of antisocial youth were reared in homes without any resident biological father, most often by a poorly educated, poorly socialized mother subsisting on welfare" (p. 202). He pointed out that two-thirds to three-quarters of school truants, adjudicated delinquents, and prison inmates were reared in families in which the biological father was absent for long periods or never present from the start (p. 203). In addressing the topic of psychopathy, he underlined the evolutionary perspective, according to which primary psychopathy is a reflection of low genetic endowment in ordinary fearfulness (akin to Cloninger's concept of low levels of harm avoidance) or an innately weak *brain inhibitory system*. He ascribed secondary psychopathy to an overactive *brain activating system*, where excess impulse strength leads to a risky lifestyle (p. 226). The latter system strikes me as a different type of *innate* predisposition, with possible advantages in relation to adventurousness and pioneering, whereas I have confined the concept of secondary psychopathy to situations of extremely adverse family environments. Under ideal circumstances, the biological father serves as an external "brain inhibitory system," curbing—by means of the respect and fear he generates—the tendencies of his children, especially of his sons, to impulsive, socially unacceptable behavior. In time the rules he sets down become internalized, and his function as a "policeman" becomes less necessary.

It has been my observation in studying persons who commit violent acts, particularly repetitive acts of assault, rape, or murder, that the families of the offenders not only are often fatherless or permeated by an atmosphere of abusiveness, but in many instances are so fractured and structurally chaotic as to render their very charting next to impossible in any neat fashion. Instead of a simple genogram, one ends up with a cat's cradle of relationships that may include siblings born of incest, who are at once uncles or aunts as well as brothers or sisters; children born of a man with whom their mother was having an affair, rather than of the husband they assume is their biological father; and parents who have divorced and remarried several times and who entrust the rearing of their children to an ever-shifting array of stepparents, foster parents, or strangers. The net effect is to destroy any semblance of stability and to deprive the children of a consistently caring parent.

As illustrations of this situation, I have chosen a few examples from among approximately 500 biographies of murderers that I have studied. Figure 9–3 depicts the web of relationships of two psychopathic Vietnam veterans, John Wayne Hearn and Robert Black (Green 1992). Black, who had married Sondra Eimann, then divorced her 7 years later, only to remarry her the next year, had tired of her, much preferring his paternal cousin, Teresa, with whom he had been carrying on a clandestine affair. He became acquainted with John Wayne Hearn, who was an aficionado of *Soldier of Fortune* magazine, which features ads that can be construed as offering the services of hit men for hire. The son of Joe Pickett, who had died in World War II, John Wayne Hearn had been raised by his mother's second of four husbands, John Hearn, whose last name he took for his own.

He himself had been married four times, but he was obsessed with Debbie Sims Bannister, who was also on her fourth marriage. She saw in Hearn the means of getting rid of her husband and also the husband of her sister Marlene, to which end she affected being in love with Hearn, promising to marry him once her husband was out of the way. Robert Black was eager for similar reasons to avail himself of Hearn's services to unburden himself of Sondra, in the hope of freeing himself to be with Teresa. The plan did not work out as felicitously as anticipated. After Hearn killed the three "targets," Debbie had no more interest in him, and all three were caught and given severe sentences. My point here is to show that the murderer Hearn had grown up in a chaotic home with a succession of stepfathers and had later subjected his children to a succession of stepmothers, while in the meantime falling in love with an equally unstable woman, herself on her fourth marriage. I see this choice on Hearn's part as an example of *assortative mating*, in which persons with certain disorders gravitate toward mates with the same disorders. And I see the chaotic structure of his family as a factor that heightened the risk for the development of antisocial or psychopathic personality of a sort that becomes highly resistant to any psychotherapeutic measures. People with this kind of disorder rarely see themselves as ill and rarely seek treatment.

The next example concerns the Sexton family (Figure 9–4), the central figure of which is Ed Sexton, who murdered one of his sons-in-law (Cauffiel 1997). I will describe his story in more detail in the next section. Here I note that the genogram does not permit a simple linear presentation, by virtue of Sexton's having sired a male child by his own daughter, making the boy the half-brother of his aunts and uncles.

Similarly, the family structure of Karla Faye Tucker shows a pattern of fragmentation and instability. The genogram is depicted in Figure 9–5. Tucker and a male accomplice killed two people in Houston in 1983. Her mother, Carolyn, had two daughters by her first husband, Larry, whom Karla Faye assumed was also her father. She was actually the daughter of another man, with whom her mother had "cheated" while still with Larry Tucker. Carolyn and her mother, Zelda, were both sensation-seeking, "wild" women who were attracted to lawless men. Both were prostitutes, as was Karla Faye. Her mother taught her how to roll marijuana joints when she was 8 years old and supplied her with "johns" when she was in her teens. Karla Faye was expelled from school for getting into fights when she was 12 years old. By age 15 years she had already had a hysterectomy. She grew up essentially without parental control. Her stepfather, Larry, got custody of her when she was 10 years old, but by then she was already living with similarly wild, drug-abusing acquaintances in the streets of Houston.

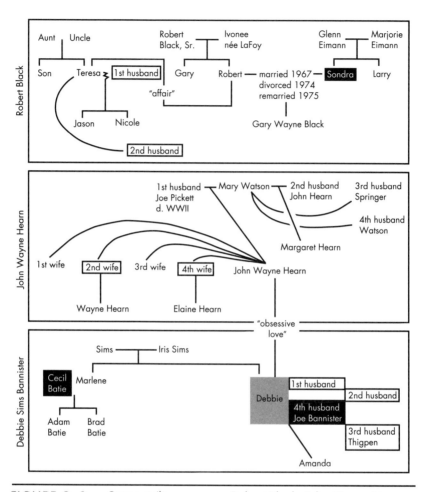

FIGURE 9–3. Crazy-quilt genogram: Robert Black, John Wayne Hearn, and Debbie Sims Bannister.

Note. Debbie persuades John Wayne to kill Joe, Cecil, and Sondra.

After she was arrested for the murders, Karla Faye spent 15 years on death row before her execution in 1998. While she was in prison, she became a born-again Christian and showed genuine remorse for the crime. Her story inspired a touching biography by Beverly Lowry (1992). The story is a tragic one of a woman whose antisocial personality came partly from the "wild" genes of her mother and grandmother but to a greater extent from the disordered life of drug abuse, fatherlessness, prostitution, and total lack of supervision induced by her chaotic family. She did not show sadistic, psychopathic, or narcissistic personality configurations, and she

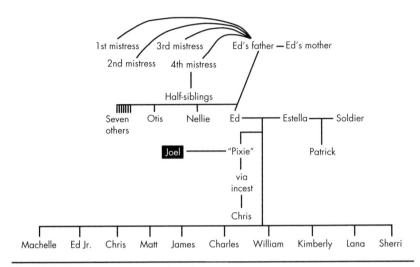

FIGURE 9-4. The Sexton family.

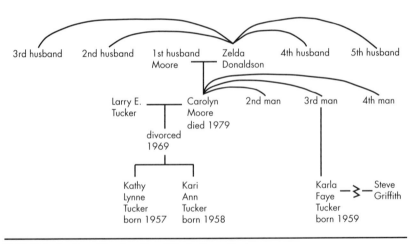

FIGURE 9-5. The family of Karla Faye Tucker.

seemed salvageable. But she grew up and lived her life far away from the conventional world, as though the concepts of therapy and medical help belonged to a planet she did not inhabit. Although Karla Faye was corrupted by her mother's antisocial "teaching," Carolyn loved her daughter in her own way. She did not brutalize Karla Faye and thus does not emerge as a "parent from Hell" like those described in the next section.

PARENTS FROM HELL

Parents with severe and essentially untreatable personality disorders can be divided into two broad groups: 1) those who commit depraved acts against or who murder their own children or their children's mates and 2) those whose depraved treatment of their children so warps the children's developing personalities as to predispose them to commit depraved or murderous acts as they enter adulthood. In the meantime, the offending parents in this second group continue with their lives, remaining very much in the background, never being arrested for any crime and never being compelled by any authorities to undergo psychiatric examination or treatment.

PARENTS WHO MURDER THEIR OWN CHILDREN OR THEIR CHILDREN'S SPOUSES

The psychological center of the Sexton family, depicted in Figure 9–4, was Ed Sexton. This West Virginia man, described in the book by Cauffiel (1997), had 11 children by his wife, Estella-May, whom he married just after being released from prison. A twelfth child, Patrick, was Estella-May's by a different father. Ed had incestuous relations with all five of his daughters. He abused Machelle physically as well, telling her "you get the belt till you're 16, then my fist." She was once beaten so badly she had to be hospitalized. He would humiliate his sons by making them stand naked in front of the whole family while Ed whipped them. All the children were warned that Ed would kill them if they talked to outsiders. He would at times lock them in a closet and spray roach spray in through the keyhole. One of the boys became severely ill and lost consciousness. He would tie them up for long periods, such that they ended up lying in their own waste.

His daughter Pixie became pregnant by her father. He then made her marry Joel, to make it appear as though the child was not born of incest. After she gave birth to Chris, Ed killed Joel, and Pixie killed Chris. When he was younger, Ed would kill cats and dogs, torture neighborhood children, and set fires. He encouraged his own children to have sex with one another and usually remained naked while at home, ready to have sex with whomever he pleased. The news of his sadism and depravity finally came out, and he was arrested for the murder of his son-in-law.

The torture and subsequent murder of other people's children, as in the case of Ian Brady, constitute a level of depravity that can be exceeded, I suspect, only by the torture and murder of one's own children. In this regard the example of Theresa Knorr (Clarkson 1995; Lohr 2004) is without parallel in the forensic literature. The younger of two sisters in a middle-class

California family, she was pathologically jealous of her sister although favored by their mother. Her first marriage was to Clifford Sanders. Increasingly jealous and possessive of him after the birth of their son, Howard, and daughter, Sheila, she murdered Clifford 2 years after they married, but she was exonerated in court because it was believed that she had killed in self-defense. Her second marriage, with Robert Knorr, by whom she had four children in rapid succession (Suesan, William, Robert, and Terry), lasted 4 years. Three brief marriages followed, the last to a man she married after knowing him for 3 days and divorced after 3 months. All the men rejected her because of her possessiveness.

Alone with six children in 1976, she began to put on weight and to drink heavily. She grew pathologically jealous of her own daughters' attractiveness and treated them with uncommon cruelty. Suesan ran away from home, but when she was found and hospitalized psychiatrically no one believed her stories of abuse. Theresa claimed the girl was lying, and Suesan was returned to her mother. Once back home, she was beaten repeatedly by her mother and also by her brothers, whom Theresa forced to join in the beatings. She was chained to her bed to make sure she didn't run away again. In 1982, when Suesan was 16 years old, Theresa began imagining the girl was a "witch" who was causing her mother to gain weight. Enraged, she shot and wounded her daughter with a .22 pistol. Later, she forced her 15-year-old son, Robert, to cut into his sister's back and retrieve the bullet. A few days later, Theresa bound Suesan's limbs, taped her mouth, packed all her belongings, and had her two brothers drive with their mother and sister to a remote spot. Theresa doused the girl with gasoline and burned her to death.

The following year Theresa forced Sheila, now age 20 years, into prostitution to supplement the family income. The beatings stopped for a time, thanks to the income Sheila was bringing in. But Theresa thought her daughter might be pregnant, at which point she beat her severely, bound her, and locked her in an overheated closet, tied to a pipe and deprived of food or water. Three days later, when the closet was opened, Sheila was dead. Again the boys were pressed into service to drive their sister's body to the same remote area, where it was dumped. The body was soon discovered but not identified. It remained for Terry, 8 years later, to reveal to the authorities about the two murders her mother had committed. Theresa was then arrested, convicted of two torture slayings, and sentenced to two consecutive life terms. Never in all this time had Theresa sought psychiatric help, instead giving vent to her murderous envy and hatred of her own daughters.

The phenomenon of the victim-turned-victimizer (van der Kolk 1996) is noticeable in the lives of certain parents who commit filicide. Judias Buenoano, for example, had been in an orphanage after the death of her mother, when she was 2 years old. She later returned to live with her father and stepmother, both of whom were extremely abusive and subjected her to beatings, starvation, and burning with cigarettes (Anderson and McGehee 1991). Years later, she poisoned her first son with arsenic and then drowned him in a faked accident, hoping to cash in on his insurance policy. Also for insurance money, she poisoned two husbands, tried to bomb the car of a fiancé, and burned two houses.

Although not reacting to childhood abuse, surgeon John Dale Cavaness (O'Brien 1989) brutalized his wife, four sons, secretaries, mistresses, and even his patients. He killed his first son, Mark, in 1977 for insurance money, and 7 years later killed a second son, Sean, for the same reason.

Another parent of similar narcissistic and sadistic characteristics, Dr. Debora Green (Rule 1997) was not abused in her early years, but she developed an abrasive, narcissistic personality with schizoid and psychopathic traits. A former high school valedictorian, fond only of her cats, she called her husband obscene names in front of their three children, was given to outbursts of rage that were exacerbated by her alcoholism, and tried to turn the two older children against their father. When her husband finally spoke of divorce and began an affair with another woman, Debora tried to poison him with ricin, which led to his being hospitalized 11 times before it became clear that she was trying to kill him. She then threatened suicide, at which point her husband committed her to the Menninger Clinic. She signed out after 4 days and warned her husband, "You'll get those kids over our dead bodies." She spread accelerant over their house and set fire to it, killing two of the three children. As for other facets of her personality, she also met the criteria for borderline personality disorder. During the few days she spent at the Menninger Clinic, she had fantasies of becoming a psychiatric resident, seemingly unaware that she lacked even the characteristics of a workable psychiatric patient, let alone those of a psychiatrist.

PARENTS WHOSE VIOLENCE PREDISPOSES THEIR CHILDREN TO VIOLENCE

Shengold (2000) used the term *soul murder* to refer to the brutalization of one's children. Prisons and forensic hospitals for mentally ill offenders include numerous persons whose parents subjected them to repeated and severe abuse and humiliation, contributing to the murderous careers of their offspring. Among the patients under my care at a forensic hospital was a man who, under the influence of "angel dust" (phencyclidine), attempted a multiple murder of three workmen. In his early history, the man had been beaten with an electrical cord by his mother for trivial offenses. His father on repeated occasions would get his son in a choke hold, rendering him unconscious, and would then sodomize him. By the time I met him, when he was 30 years old, he had become a silent volcano—outwardly polite but capable, if primed with alcohol or drugs, of explosive rages and murder. His PCL-R score was 30, and he met the criteria for both antisocial personality disorder and psychopathy. When he was first hospitalized, the story he told about his purchase of a pistol and the attempted murders was filled with deliberate distortions. After 8 years in the hospital, he recited the same story word for word. Efforts at treatment had made no impression at all.

The name Charles Manson (Bugliosi 1974) is familiar to all, although the details of his early life may not be. Manson was born in Kentucky in 1934 to a 16-year-old single mother, Kathleen Maddox, a prostitute who was in trouble with the law for auto theft and armed robbery and who disappeared for long stretches of time, leaving Manson in the hands of an uncle in West Virginia. Manson never knew his father. At one point the mother bartered her son for a bottle of beer to a "foster" couple. Charles was in and out of reformatories. His hatred for society was intensified after he was sodomized in prison. Paroled at age 19 years, he married briefly and had a son. By age 25 years, he had been arrested for a variety of crimes, including rape, drug use, pimping, theft, and fraud. Imprisoned again for rape, he was released in 1967, the year he went to San Francisco and used his charisma to become the leader of a group of hippies. The murders of Sharon Tate and others in August 1969 made Manson a nationally known figure. He is serving out a life sentence in Corcoran Prison in California. We know nothing about Manson's biological father, but Manson may have been burdened with risk genes for impulsivity and novelty-seeking from his mother.

If Manson's mother committed mainly *sins of omission*, the mother of Mary Bell, the girl who murdered two young boys in northwest England, was given to *sins of commission* of a most repugnant sort (Sereny 1998). The mother, Betty, was a neglectful prostitute, who forced her daughter from age 5 years to have sex with various men she brought home. Mary never knew who her father was; her mother may not have known either. Betty tried to kill Mary many times during her first year. Beginning when Mary was 6 or 7 years old, Betty would force her to perform fellatio on her clients and warned her of dire consequences if she ever told anyone. Both the men and Betty would force objects into Mary's rectum and would whip her. When Mary was 8 years old, her mother tried to drown her by pushing her head underwater. On other occasions, Betty throttled her daughter till she was unconscious. This modus operandi was adopted by Mary herself, who, when she was 11 years old, strangled birds and cats and then two boys (each of whom was 2 years old), for which she was sent first to a reformatory and, later, to prison. Considered a "vicious psychopath" at first, Mary became the object of nationwide obloquy. As time went on, she proved capable of being rehabilitated, morally and spiritually. She now lives under a different name and has married and has a child of her own. Whereas Manson became a sadistic psychopath, beyond treatment and beyond redemption, the sadistic psychopath in Mary's family was her mother, Betty, who was never brought to justice.

Parents from Hell, whose brutalizing, rejecting, and humiliating behaviors exert lasting effects on the personalities of their offspring, are hardly limited to the domain of violent criminals. It is of more than passing interest that many of the heads of state responsible for atrocities during the wars of the twentieth century had fathers whose brutality was later magnified a millionfold as their sons reached adulthood and acquired power. Hitler, according to his illegitimate half-brother, Alois Jr., was beaten "unmercifully with a hippopotamus whip" by their father and on one occasion was choked until he lost consciousness (Flood 1989, p. 7). Hitler had a loving mother, and one wonders what would have become of him if his father had been gentle and nurturing. Instead of seeking revenge on a massive scale, Hitler might have remained what he started out to be—an artist of modest talent, who would have left no mark on the world.

Stalin grew up with a violent hatred of his father, who "used to beat him when drunk, allegedly prompting the child to defend himself with a knife" (DeJonge 1986, p. 25). His mother, Ekaterina, used to thrash her son as well, with the result that Stalin loved no one and grew up with a hatred of all authority except his own. Mao Ze-dong's father was a prosperous farmer, and although he was "hot-tempered, miserly and excessively strict, frequently beating Mao and his brothers" (Short 1999, p. 28), he was not sadistic like the fathers of Hitler and Stalin. Mao, who was more rebellious than his brothers, nevertheless learned to hate his father, and their interaction appears to have fed Mao's vengefulness and contempt for traditional authority. Of Saddam Hussein's biological father, Hussein al-Majid, almost nothing is known, not even when or where he died. He may have been the father of Saddam's only full sibling, Siham, 2 years younger than Saddam. After fathering these children, the father apparently abandoned the family (Coughlin 2002, p. 6). The mother, Subha Tulfah, then married Hassan al-Ibrahim. Saddam was rejected, possibly abused sexually, and beaten regularly by his stepfather. Hassan used an asphalt-covered stick for the beatings and made Saddam dance in the dirt to avoid being hit. Whereas Hitler, Stalin, and Mao for the most part *ordered* the murders of others, Saddam's personal brutality is legendary. The categories of DSM do not do justice to the enormity of the acts committed by these men, for whom terms such as *sadistic, narcissistic, antisocial,* and *psychopathic* are shallow euphemisms. Psychotherapy would touch neither the fathers nor the sons.

PARENTAL DESTRUCTIVENESS IN THE FORM OF "PSYCHIC MURDER"

The phrase "soul murder," used by Shengold (2000), derived from an article written a century earlier by the Swedish playwright August Strindberg, who commented that although actual murder seemed to be decreasing, soul (or psychic) murder—the taking away of a person's reason for living—was on the increase. As Shengold explained, "the capacity to destroy a soul hinges entirely on having another human being in one's power" (which is inherent in the relationship between a parent and a young child), and he added that "in individuals, psychic murder is founded on the relations between hostile, cruel, indifferent, psychotic, or psychopathic parents and the child prisoners in their charge" (p. 19).

Many varieties of this phenomenon have already been described, with a focus on families where parental destructiveness contributed significantly, in many instances definitively, to violent criminality in their offspring. Numerous other examples exist where the outcome in the child was a deformation of personality that led to chronic depression, lack of fulfillment, or suicide. Such outcomes stem mostly from the *negative* narcissism of the parents. The catalog of attitudes Shengold listed—hostile, cruel, etc.—are variants of parental narcissism, with a negative twist in relation to the children. One could add parental hatred, envy, and contempt to this catalog. But *positive* narcissism may have dreadful outcomes also. Children can be literally "spoiled rotten" by parents, especially those in positions of great power, who grant undue license and who set no limits. In either case, there are severe narcissistic deformations of personality in the parents, who do not see themselves as needing help, do not seek psychotherapy, and remain quite outside the realm of patienthood, let alone of treatability. I chose the following examples from biographies of persons who were high in the social order (which led to their becoming subjects of biographies). Because the hostility of a spouse can sometimes exert equally shattering effects on the personality of a fragile partner, I include an example of that situation also.

According to her biographer, Craig Unger (1988), Rebekah Harkness, heiress and founder of the ballet company bearing her name, pursued her own interests throughout her adult life, to the detriment of her first child,

Edith. Born to the first of her mother's four husbands, Edith remained a stranger to the affection of her mother, whose indifference had led her to snap, "What do you want?" when Edith, age 7 years, entered her mother's room shortly after the death of her father (p. 387). In 1982 when Rebekah was dying of cancer, she was taking, and abusing, many kinds of drugs. With two of these drugs (amitriptyline and diazepam) plus alcohol, Edith committed suicide shortly after her mother's death. Edith had been seriously depressed much of her life and had become alcoholic after her marriage and worse so after the birth of her son. She felt she had no experience of having had a mother and no template for being a mother to her own child.

The life of Brenda Diana Duff Frazier (Diliberto 1987) illustrates the effects of gross manipulativeness by a self-centered parent of the "Hollywood mother" type, intent on *living through* her daughter to become the belle of the ball that she could never be in her own life. As beautiful as her mother was homely, Brenda Frazier was a wealthy debutante at age 18 years, already so famous in 1938 that her picture appeared on the cover of *Life* magazine and letters were delivered to her with just the address "Brenda Frazier, New York." Neglected by her mother (apart from her mother's ambitions for her) and raised entirely by nannies, Brenda grew up seemingly with no "backbone." A series of unhappy marriages ensued; she became alcoholic, developed bulimia, made self-mutilative gestures and suicide attempts, and ended her days as a recluse.

Both Edith Harkness and Brenda Frazier were in psychoanalytically oriented psychotherapy for many years and showed the combination of borderline personality, major affective disorder, and alcoholism that is associated with a greatly heightened risk for suicide (Stone 1990) and self-destructive behavior in general.

In the poignantly written account of his family by Geoffrey Douglas (1992), the author tells the story of his privileged but ill-fated parents. His father was a Wall Street broker, the son of an heiress. His mother was a fashion model from a Social Register family. But his father was intensely bigoted, a "weak, coddled, misguided, and cruel" man (p. 190) who was arrogant, controlling, and humiliating. His mother was fragile person who "believed [only] in her waist size, her smile, and her debutante's tool kit. When they were gone, she was a dance without music" (p. 190). She was admitted on a number of occasions to Silver Hill Hospital in Connecticut for depression and agoraphobia. The admitting psychiatrist once met with Mr. Douglas and had this to say about him: "As far as I'm concerned, he is the cause of Mrs. Douglas' illness.... He's about as intolerant a person as I have ever run into.... Desperately prejudiced, very rigid, and narrow-minded. Speaks of how Mrs. Douglas 'came home and started handing me this horse crap' that we are teaching here at Silver Hill.... To me the situation looks practically hopeless.... I don't see what we are going to do" (p. 173). The author's father lied and cheated on his mother and beat her. Another Silver Hill psychiatrist described Mr. Douglas as an "aggressive, ruthless man who hides behind a facade of assumed pleasantness, social grace, and charm. And further, he is an egotist" (p. 210). Thirteen years into their marriage, Mrs. Douglas committed suicide, a victim of "soul murder," this time by a husband rather than by a parent.

It is said that power corrupts, and absolute power corrupts absolutely. Examples abound, but that of Romania's Ceausescu family is particularly striking. Accumulating vast wealth while they ruled Romania, Nicolae and Elena Ceausescu feasted while the Romanian people suffered. In their boundless narcissism, they did not neglect their son, Nicu; instead, they spoiled him rotten. General Pacepa (1987), former head of Romanian Intelligence, wrote about Nicu's arrogance and contempt. At a dinner in honor of a party leader, a waiter came in with a platter full of oysters. Nicu asked, "Is there any seasoning on them?" The waiter replied, "They are just fresh and raw, Comrade Nicu," whereupon Nicu shouted, "They need seasoning, you idiot." Nicu then "climbed up onto the table and started urinating on them, careful to 'season' every oyster" and then forced the guests to eat them. When the dinner was mercifully at an end, Nicu raped one of the waitresses (p. 39). The only thing capable of humanizing narcissistic tyrants is failure, but failure came too late in the lives of the Ceausescus. When the Communist regime collapsed in 1989, Nicolae and Elena were executed. Their dissolute son, now without powerful parents to protect him, escaped to Vienna, where he died of alcoholism and cirrhosis in 1996, unrepentant and with his narcissistic personality untreated.

As the preceding vignettes and others in previous chapters (such as the story of the temporarily mute incest victim mentioned in Chapter 1), show, the sacredness and relative impenetrability of the family allow some parents with marked narcissistic and psychopathic personalities to commit criminal acts against their children and yet remain, throughout their lives, untreated by any therapist and unpunished by the courts.

REFERENCES

American Psychiatric Association: Diagnostic and Statistical Manual of Mental Disorders, 3rd Edition. Washington, DC, American Psychiatric Association, 1980

American Psychiatric Association: Diagnostic and Statistical Manual of Mental Disorders, 4th Edition, Text Revision. Washington, DC, American Psychiatric Association, 2000

Anderson C, McGehee S: Bodies of Evidence: The True Story of Judias Buenoano: Florida's Serial Murderess. New York, Lyle Stuart/Carol Publishing, 1991

Athens LH: The Creation of Dangerous, Violent Criminals. Chicago, IL, University of Chicago Press, 1992

Band C, Malear J: Shattered Bonds: A True Story of Suspicious Death, Family Betrayal, and a Daughter's Courage. Far Hills, NJ, New Horizon Press, 2003

Baron-Cohen S: The Essential Difference. New York, Basic Books, 2003

Black DW: Bad Boys, Bad Men: Confronting Antisocial Personality Disorder. New York, Oxford University Press, 1999

Brady I: The Gates of Janus: Serial Killing and Its Analysis. Los Angeles, CA, Feral House, 2001

Bugliosi V: Helter Skelter: The True Story of the Manson Murders. New York, WW Norton, 1974

Carey B: For psychotherapy's claims, some skeptics demand proof. The New York Times, August 10, 2004, p F1

Carlo P: The Night-Stalker: The Life and Crimes of Richard Ramirez. New York, Kensington, 1996

Cauffiel L: House of Secrets. New York, Kensington, 1997

Clarkson W: Whatever Mother Says: A True Story of Mother, Madness, and Murder. New York, St. Martin's Press, 1995

Cloninger CR: A unified biosocial theory of personality and its role in the development of anxiety states. Psychiatr Dev 3:167–226, 1986

Collins M: The Palm Beach Murder: The True Story of a Millionaire, Marriage, and Murder. New York, St. Martin's Press, 2004

Cooke DJ, Michie C: Refining the concept of psychopathy: toward a hierarchical model. Psychol Assess 13:171–188, 2001

Coughlin C: Saddam: King of Terror. New York, Ecco/HarperCollins, 2002

DeJonge A: Stalin, and the Shaping of the Soviet Union. New York, William Morrow, 1986

Diliberto G: Debutante: The Story of Brenda Frazier. New York, Knopf, 1987

Douglas G: Class: The Wreckage of an American Family. New York, Henry Holt, 1992

Eftimiades M: Garden of Graves: The Shocking True Story of Long Island Serial Killer Joel Rifkin. New York, St. Martin's Press, 1993

Finstad S: Sleeping With the Devil. New York, William Morrow, 1991

Flood CB: Hitler: The Path to Power. Boston, MA, Houghton Mifflin, 1989

Francis E: Broken Vows: The Shocking Murder of Rabbi Fred Neulander's Wife. New York, St. Martin's Press, 2002

Gilmore M: Family album. Granta 37 (autumn):11–52, 1991

Green B: The Soldier of Fortune Murders: A True Story of Obsessive Love and Murder-for-Hire. New York, Delacorte, 1992

Hare RD: Without Conscience: The Disturbing World of the Psychopaths Among Us. New York, Pocket Books, 1993

Hare RD, Harpur TJ, Hakstian AR, et al: The revised Psychopathy Checklist: reliability and factor structure. Psychol Assess 2:238–241, 1990

Harpur TJ, Hare RD, Hakstian AR: Two-factor conceptualization of psychopathy: construct validity and assessment implications. Psychol Assess 1:6–17, 1989

Harrington J, Burger R: Justice Denied. New York, Plenum, 1999

Hart SD, Hare RD: Psychopathy: assessment and association with criminal conduct, in Handbook of Antisocial Behavior. Edited by Stoff DM, Maser J, Brieling J. New York, Wiley, 1997, pp 22–35

Hazelwood R, Michaud SG: Dark Dreams: Sexual Violence, Homicide, and the Criminal Mind. New York, St. Martin's Press, 2001

Hemphill JF, Hare RD, Wong S: Psychopathy and recidivism: a review. Legal and Criminological Psychology 3:139–170, 1998a

Hemphill JF, Templeman R, Wong S, et al: Psychopathy and crime: recidivism and criminal careers, in Psychopathy: Theory, Research, and Implications for Society. Edited by Cooke DJ, Forth AE, Hare RD. Boston, MA, Kluwer, 1998b, pp 375–399

Herpertz SC, Habermeyer E: "Psychopathy" als Subtyp der antisozialen Persönlichkeit. Persönlichkeitsstörungen: Theorie und Therapie 8:73–83, 2004

Klausner LD: Son of Sam. New York, McGraw-Hill, 1981

Lasseter D: Die for Me: The Terrifying True Story of the Charles Ng and Leonard Lake Torture Murders. New York, Kensington, 2000

Lohr D: The case of Theresa Cross Knorr. Available at: http://www.crimelibrary.com/notorious_murders/family/theresa_cross/index.html. Accessed May 29, 2004.

London S (ed): Killer Fiction. Venice, CA, Feral House, 1997

Lösel F: Treatment and management of psychopaths, in Psychopathy: Theory, Research, and Implications for Society. Edited by Cooke DJ, Forth AE, Hare RD. Boston, MA, Kluwer, 1998, pp 303–354

Lowry B: Crossed Over: A Murder. A Memoir. New York, Knopf, 1992

Lykken DT: The Antisocial Personalities. Hillsdale, NJ, Erlbaum, 1995

Mailer N: The Executioner's Song. Boston, MA, Little, Brown, 1979

McClellan B: Evidence of Murder. New York, Penguin, 1993

McDonald RR: Secrets Never Lie. New York, Avon, 1998

Michaud SG: Lethal Shadow: The Chilling True Crime Story of a Sadistic Sex Slayer. New York, Onyx, 1994

O'Brien D: Murder in Little Egypt. New York, William Morrow, 1989

Pacepa IM: Red Horizons: The True Story of Nicolae and Elena Ceausescus' Crimes, Lifestyle, and Corruption. Washington, DC, Regnery Gateway, 1987

Porter S: Without conscience or without active conscience: the etiology of psychopathy revisited. Aggress Violent Behav 1:179–189, 1996

Raine A: The Psychopathology of Crime: Criminal Behavior as a Clinical Disorder. New York, Academic Press, 1993

Raine A, Brennan P, Mednick B, et al: High rates of violence, crime, academic problems, and behavioral problems in males with both early neuromotor deficits and unstable family environments. Arch Gen Psychiatry 53:544–549, 1996

Raine A, Lencz T, Bihrle S, et al: Reduced prefrontal gray matter volume and reduced autonomic activity in antisocial personality disorder. Arch Gen Psychiatry 57:119–127, 2000

Robins LN, Tipp J, Przybeck T: Antisocial personality, in Psychiatric Disorders in America. Edited by Robins LN, Regier DA. New York, Macmillan, 1991, pp 258–290

Rule A: Bitter Harvest: A Woman's Fury, A Mother's Sacrifice. New York, Simon & Schuster, 1997

Sereny G: Cries Unheard. New York, Metropolitan Books/Henry Holt, 1998

Shengold L: Soul Murder. New Haven, CT, Yale University Press, 2000

Short P: Mao: A Life. New York, Henry Holt, 1999

Smith C: Death of a Doctor: Two Doctors, Obsessive Love, and Murder. New York, St. Martin's Press, 2002

Stone MH: The Fate of Borderlines. New York, Guilford, 1990

Stone MH: Abnormalities of Personality: Within and Beyond the Realm of Treatment. New York, WW Norton, 1993

Stone MH: Serial sexual homicide: biological, psychological, and sociological aspects. J Personal Disord 15:1–18, 2001

Streeck-Fischer A: Misshandelt—Missbraucht: Probleme der Diagnostik und Psychotherapie traumatisierter Jugendlicher, in Adoleszenz und Trauma. Edited by Streeck-Fischer A. Göttingen, Germany, Vandenhoeck & Ruprecht, 1998a, pp 174–196

Streeck-Fischer A: Über die Mimikryentwicklung am Beispiel eines jugendlichen Skinheads mit frühen Erfahrungen von Vernachlässigung und Misshandlung, in Adoleszenz und Trauma. Edited by Streeck-Fischer A. Göttingen, Germany, Vandenhoeck & Ruprecht, 1998b, pp 161–173

Unger C: Blue Blood: The Story of Rebekah Harkness and How One of the Richest Families in the World Descended Into Drugs, Madness, Suicide, and Violence. New York, William Morrow, 1988

van der Kolk B: The complexity of adaptation to trauma: self-regulation, stimulus discrimination, and characterological development, in Traumatic Stress: The Effects of Overwhelming Experience on Mind, Body, and Society. Edited by van der Kolk B, McFarlane AC, Weisaeth L. New York, Guilford, 1996, pp 182–213

Widiger TA, Rogers JH: Prevalence and comorbidity of personality disorders. Psychiatr Ann 19:132–136, 1989

Williams E: Beyond Belief: A Chronicle of Murder and Its Detection. New York, Random House, 1968

Wilson C, Seaman D: The Serial Killers: A Study in the Psychology of Violence. New York, Carol Publishing Group, 1992

AFTERWORD

O wad some Pow'r the giftie gie us
To see oursels as others see us!
It wad frae monie a blunder free us
An' foolish notion:
What airs in dress an' gait wad lea'e us,
An' ev'n Devotion!

Robert Burns, "To a Louse, on Seeing One on a
Lady's Bonnet at Church"

Nature saw fit to have our eyes point outward. This way we can spot the dangers and delights of the outside world in ways that enhance our survival. One drawback to this arrangement is that we are not so good at seeing ourselves. This idea was behind the poet's gentle mocking of the aristocratic lady in church, unaware of the bug that only others could see on her bonnet, spoiling her otherwise elegant image. In contemporary terms, her narcissism (her "airs") would be punctured if she were as aware of how she appeared as were those near her. There is an analogy here to our concept of *personality*, the self we project to the outside world, which ends up being more visible to others than to ourselves.

Everybody has a personality, and for most people, their personality is adaptive socially. Even in the privacy of our homes, we do not show many traits that offend those with whom we share our intimate lives. We may have one or two traits or eccentricities that we, or others, would wish to change, but that is about all. Extreme situations aside, a degree of subjectivity exists in the measure of the more unwelcome or maladaptive traits—some people find them annoying, but others find them not at all bothersome, or even charming.

Where there are enough unwelcome traits to trigger a personality dis-

Therapy not needed	Treatment likely to be beneficial	Treatment difficult	Outcome uncertain	Beyond treatable
Mild quirks	Some bothersome traits	Cluster A disorders	Borderline personality disorder, antisocial personality disorder	Psychopathy (high in callousness, remorselessness, and deceitfulness)
	Most Cluster C disorders	Narcissistic personality disorder, milder borderline personality disorder	Rigid obsessive-compulsive personality disorder	"Fanatical paranoids" and terrorists
	"Hysteric character"			Sadistic personality disorder
	"Depressive-masochistic"	Histrionic personality disorder	Hypomanic personality	
			"Malignant narcissism"	
			Highly arrogant narcissistic personality disorder	
			Highly suicide-prone borderline personality disorder	

FIGURE 1. Overview: personality disorders and their treatability.

order diagnosis, we have crossed over into a territory where we feel "something ought to be done." This situation is portrayed in Figure 1, which encompasses the total realm of personality. On the left is the domain (proportionally much larger than is indicated in the diagram) of normal or quasi-normal personality, where no more than a few quirks are present and psychotherapeutic intervention is not needed. This region shades gradually into a territory where there are enough bothersome traits to warrant treatment.

A surplus of the *inhibited* personality types is found in this territory, although, as I emphasized in earlier chapters, the likelihood of benefit and the ease with which benefit can be achieved are not as promising with very rigid obsessive-compulsive persons, slavishly dependent persons, and profoundly phobic and avoidant persons. The extremes of the otherwise more treatable types, that is, are more challenging to treat than are the milder narcissistic or even borderline personalities.

In the region I have labeled "difficult," one finds persons with the Cluster A disorders and some of the less severe Cluster B disorders.

The realm of the less treatable personality types includes borderline patients of the more self-destructive types, including those who are highly suicide prone. The latter may present with qualities of self-reflectiveness and motivation that make for good treatability, yet they may be susceptible to sudden and unpredictable downturns, even to suicide, much as an otherwise airworthy plane may encounter wind shear and plunge without warning to the ground. Outcome is also uncertain when dealing with patients Kernberg (1992) described as malignant narcissists. Persons who show antisocial behavior but whose underlying character structure is not predominantly of the sort Cooke et al. (2004) called the "arrogant and deceitful interpersonal style" may have uncertain, but ultimately favorable, outcomes, even though positive social change may occur more through the maturation that comes with time than through a prolonged course of therapy.

Finally, in the realm of the untreatable are found the paranoid fanatics, including political and religious fanatics (such as neo-Nazis, Ku Klux Klansmen, Islamists), the vast majority of whom do not view themselves as disturbed or disordered, do not seek treatment, and, in all but a few instances, would not be amenable to change if remanded or forced into treatment. An example of an exception might be the adolescent neo-Nazi "skinheads" described by Annette Streeck-Fischer (1998a, 1998b), some of whom have responded well to the psychotherapy devised for them.

When an antisocial person proves untreatable, an underlying psychopathic personality (of the arrogant, deceitful type) is likely to have preexisted and to have predisposed the person to the antisocial behavior. Cooke et al. (2004) made a similar point, referring to antisocial behavior as a consequence rather than an inherent symptom of psychopathic personality, especially as many psychopaths have no history of antisocial behavior per se (Cleckley 1941). Perhaps it is more accurate to say that many psychopaths may engage in offensive or illegal behaviors, yet manage to avoid confrontations with the law. The clever ones, for example, know which naive tourists, having been sold a fake Rolex, will not complain to the authorities.

In the meantime, we need to learn more about brain *differences* (which, beyond a certain point, can amount to *abnormalities*) that may in extreme cases make psychopathy an all but inevitable outcome. Are there, for example, persons with such risk for novelty-seeking, low empathy and compassion, low P300 reactivity to startling stimuli, and high impulsivity that they are as much at risk for psychopathy as certain persons appear to be for developing schizophrenia? Matthysse and Kidd (1976) introduced the idea of a "schizophrenia quotient," or "SQ," analogous to IQ, that quantified the degree of genetic risk for schizophrenia. Those with the highest SQ may be vulnerable to the psychosis, no matter how protective and nurturing the family. Might there be others with a comparably high "PQ" (psychopathy quotient) whom the most ideal family could not protect against the development of psychopathic personality?

Persons exhibiting habitual sadism likewise belong on the other side of the line between treatability and untreatability. Some are motivated by a combination of grandiosity, vengefulness, the need to control through humiliation, and the psychopath's lack of compassion (Baumeister et al. 1996). They do not seek treatment, and when therapists encounter them in forensic settings, they do not respond to treatment. Sadistic personality of this sort should not be confused with the sadistic behaviors manifested during times of armed conflict by men who out of malice or vengefulness torture soldiers and civilians of the opposing side. Among the more prominent Nazis, for example, Julius Streicher, "a bully and intimidator of the worst sort" (Zillmer et al. 1995, p. 148), was sadistic in personality before he joined the movement, whereas Adolf Eichmann, as Hannah Arendt (1965) made clear, was markedly ambitious, but not sadistic. Both men committed evil acts, but of the two, it was Streicher who was an evil person, day in and day out, throughout his life.

Another group of essentially untreatable persons who do not seek help and would not commit themselves to a course of therapy at the urging of others are the "parents (or spouses) from Hell," some examples of whom I sketched in Chapter 9. Narcissistic traits dominate their personality structure, along with a marked insensitivity to the feelings of others.

From an epidemiological standpoint, the size of the realm of the scarcely treatable or altogether untreatable personality disorders cannot be estimated. In this realm are patients and persons who do not identify themselves as patients and for whom successful outcomes would not be achieved by any therapist, no matter the school of training or orientation. The ranks of all mental health professionals—collectively adding up to a substantial army of potential therapists—would be considerably outnumbered by persons with very difficult or impossible-to-treat personality disorders. It becomes important to discern which such persons could benefit from available treatment methods and which are least likely or totally unlikely to benefit. The more we know about the prognosis of the different personality disorders and their combinations, the more accurately and successfully we can direct therapeutic efforts. Other variables unrelated to personality that affect prognosis—such as intelligence and age—need to be factored in. An older person who is reflective and open may, for example, show more positive changes in personality than someone much younger who is rigid and not at all psychologically minded.

The need for therapists to husband their resources is relevant not just to those in forensic work, where the extremes of "negative" personality are encountered with greater regularity, but also to those in the wider community of nonforensic therapists. At the same time, improvements in therapists' ability to work effectively with borderline, schizotypal, certain antisocial, and other "difficult" personality disorders have been made in the last generation. A book such as this one must be seen as a work in progress. The recommendations made here about the boundaries between the treatable, the scarcely treatable, and the untreatable may shift in a more favorable direction as further progress is made in the coming years. Even so, there will probably always be a residue of eternally untreatable persons— serial rapists and serial killers, inveterate swindlers, political tyrants, confirmed bigots, and the like—who will remain of interest *to* psychiatry but immune to the methods *of* psychiatry. It is useful for clinicians to recognize the limitations, as well as the powers, of these methods.

REFERENCES

Arendt H: Eichmann in Jerusalem: A Report on the Banality of Evil. New York, Penguin, 1965

Baumeister RF, Smart L, Boden JM: Relation of threatened egotism to violence and aggression. Psychol Rev 103:5–33, 1996

Cleckley H: The Mask of Sanity. St. Louis, MO, Mosby, 1941

Cooke DJ, Michie C, Hart SD, et al: Reconstructing psychopathy: clarifying the significance of antisocial and socially deviant behavior in the diagnosis of psychopathic personality disorder. J Personal Disord 18:337–357, 2004

Kernberg OF: Aggression in Personality Disorders and Perversions. New Haven, CT, Yale University Press, 1992

Matthysse SW, Kidd K: Estimating the genetic contribution to schizophrenia. Am J Psychiatry 133:185–191, 1976

Streeck-Fischer A: Misshandelt—Missbraucht: Probleme der Diagnostik und Psychotherapie traumatisierter Jugendlicher, in Adoleszenz und Trauma. Edited by Streeck-Fischer A. Göttingen, Germany, Vandenhoeck & Ruprecht, 1998a, pp 174–196

Streeck-Fischer A: Über die Mimikryentwicklung am Beispiel eines jugendlichen Skinheads mit frühen Erfahrungen von Vernachlässigung und Misshandlung, in Adoleszenz und Trauma. Edited by Streeck-Fischer A. Göttingen, Germany, Vandenhoeck & Ruprecht, 1998b, pp 161–173

Zillmer EA, Harrower M, Ritzer BA, et al: The Quest for the Nazi Personality: A Psychological Investigation of Nazi War Criminals. Hillsdale, NJ, Erlbaum, 1995

INDEX

*Page numbers printed in **boldface** type refer to tables or figures.*